ONE TREE, MANY BRANCHES

ONE TREE, MANY BRANCHES
The Practice of Integrative Child and Adolescent Psychotherapy

Edited by
Bozena Merrick and Di Gammage

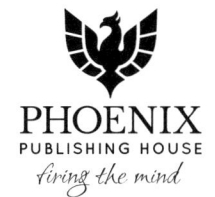

PHOENIX
PUBLISHING HOUSE
firing the mind

First published in 2024 by
Phoenix Publishing House Ltd
62 Bucknell Road
Bicester
Oxfordshire OX26 2DS

Copyright © 2024 to Bozena Merrick and Di Gammage for the edited collection, and to the individual authors for their contributions.

The rights of the contributors to be identified as the authors of this work have been asserted in accordance with §§ 77 and 78 of the Copyright Design and Patents Act 1988.

All rights reserved. No part of this publication may be reproduced, stored in a retrieval system, or transmitted, in any form or by any means, electronic, mechanical, photocopying, recording, or otherwise, without the prior written permission of the publisher.

British Library Cataloguing in Publication Data

A C.I.P. for this book is available from the British Library

ISBN-13: 978-1-80013-220-7

Typeset by Medlar Publishing Solutions Pvt Ltd, India

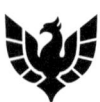

www.firingthemind.com

Contents

Acknowledgements ix
About the editors and contributors xi
Introduction: seeds sown xix
Bozena Merrick and Di Gammage

Part I
Therapeutic holding

1. Ecopsychotherapy with children and young people in mind: attachment to place, nature, and landscape 3
   Alix Hearn

2. Airy creatures: using somatic countertransference to ground autistic states in child psychotherapy 21
   Magda Raczynska

3. The absent other: reflections on the absence of male integrative child and adolescent psychotherapists 45
   Jamie Butterworth

Part II
Race and cultural identity

4. Meet them where they are: integrative psychotherapy with refugee children and young people   65
   Evania Inward

5. Unveiling racial trauma in the practice of the integrative child and adolescent psychotherapist   95
   Audrey Adeyemi

6. Understanding the trauma and implications of female genital mutilation (FGM) through child psychotherapy   117
   Irene Mburu

7. Working with children and young people in the Orthodox Jewish community   145
   Zisi Schleider

8. Go well: bearing witness to the grief of young clients in therapy   163
   Tasha Bailey

Part III
Neurodivergence and differently wired brains

9. Working therapeutically with uniquely wired children   185
   Sasha Morphitis

10. Is it too late? The contribution of the integrative child psychotherapist to those affected by fetal alcohol spectrum disorder   213
    Anna Tuttle

Part IV
Systemic issues and working within systems

11. An ongoing conversation … What (really) works in therapeutic residential care? 245
    Kelly Brackett

12. Working through play on the mentalizing capacity of controlling-caregiving children who suffered early relational trauma 279
    Nadja Rolli

Index 303

Acknowledgements

To all students, graduates, tutors, and staff at Terapia for co-creating an amazing organisation where profound learning now benefits the children, young people, and families we work with.

To the contributors who agreed to come on board this project and share their learning, insights, and clinical experiences.

To our editor, Kate Pearce, who believed in the book from the outset and has supported us throughout.

Special thanks to Alix Hearn for stepping forwards and offering her steady, skilled hand in the editing process.

Bozena and Di

About the editors and contributors

Editors

Di Gammage, MA, UKCP, trained as a drama therapist and play therapist in the 1980s and early 1990s respectively. In 2010, she completed her training in Buddhist psychotherapy at the Karuna Institute, Devon. Di was accepted onto the UKCP child psychotherapy register in 2013. Di has worked in charities, including the NSPCC Child Sexual Abuse Consultancy in Manchester with Anne Bannister, the NHS, and in the private sector as a psychotherapist and supervisor. She has taught at Terapia since 2006 on the play therapy residential, drama therapy, and working with children and young people who have experienced sexual abuse. Di is the author of *Playful Awakening: Releasing the Gift of Play in Your Life* (JKP, 2017). She currently practises in an independent foster care agency in the South West together with her private practice as a therapist, supervisor, and trainer. She completed a Masters in Creative Writing with Teesside University with a distinction and continues to explore the therapeutic power of creative writing with her clients. Di lives in Devon.

Bozena Merrick, MSc, UKCP, CPC, is the founder of Terapia, Training in Child and Adolescent Psychotherapy and Counselling. She is also the visionary behind Terapia Centre for Young People and Children and the Bothy restoration project. Bozena has over thirty-five years of experience in working with children, adolescents, adults, and groups as a psychotherapist, counsellor, clinical supervisor, trainer, lecturer, and group facilitator. She gained her MSc in clinical psychology abroad and has a background in psychiatric settings and social work. Bozena is the chair of the Child Psychotherapy Council (CPC) and has over twenty years' experience in child psychotherapy regulation through her work for the United Kingdom Council for Psychotherapy (UKCP).

Contributors

Audrey Adeyemi is a trainee Terapia integrative child and adolescent psychotherapist. She enjoys working with young people in the five- to twenty-four-year-old range. Working in a diverse city such as London, Audrey has worked with young people from different racial, ethnic, and cultural backgrounds who experience issues such as gender dysphoria, social anxiety, PTSD, bereavement, autism, and violence in the home. Her integrative psychotherapy training has provided a broad lens for understanding her clients' underlying difficulties. Audrey is mother to a teenage boy. Following attempts to help her son with the challenges he faced as an energetic, inquisitive, neurodiverse, primary-school-aged Black boy, she realised both the threshold for psychological and behavioural support and the financial commitment required were barriers for many children and their caregivers. This awareness inspired Audrey to embark on her own integrative psychotherapy training and to make psychotherapy accessible to less privileged children. As a fifty-year-old woman of West African heritage, Audrey has experienced both covert and overt forms of racism and has reconciled her own internalised racism. She writes this chapter galvanised by her personal and clinical insight and the research she has done into the psychological impact of racism in adolescent Black males and how racism can inform identity formation.

Tasha Bailey, MA, UKCP, is an integrative child and adolescent psychotherapist, specialising in trauma, anxiety, identity, and intersectionality with clients of all ages. She strives for therapy to be relevant, real, and inclusive, bringing humour, creativity, and compassion to meet the client where they are. Tasha has previously worked as a therapist in schools, pupil referral units, charities, and drama schools. She currently works in private practice with adults from marginalised communities who have experienced childhood trauma. Her work includes collaborating with brands such as Spotify and Nike to facilitate conversations around mental health and self-care in corporate or community spaces. In addition to being a graduate of Terapia, Tasha has worked there as Pastoral Support Tutor, giving emotional and reflective space throughout the Masters programme. Tasha is also a content creator and writer who hopes to influence positive change in the world of mental wellness and therapy, especially for younger generations entering adulthood. She does this on social media through her Instagram platform @RealTalk.Therapist, where she makes psychoeducation easily digestible. Tasha is the author of It's Real Talk: Lessons from Therapy on Healing & Self-Love (2023, Radar/Octopus).

Kelly Brackett, MA, UKCP, is an integrative child and adolescent psychotherapist working in therapeutic residential care (TRC) with children in the care of a local authority ("looked-after children"), the corporate parents. As a "child-in-care warrior", her purpose is to strengthen the voices of society's most vulnerable children. Kelly's professional journey includes numerous roles supporting adults, children, and families through adversity, trauma, and poverty within the domains of homelessness, alcohol and substance misuse, residential care for looked-after children, and supporting mothers to breastfeed and bond with their babies. Kelly qualified as a humanistic counsellor and worked with adults including asylum seekers and ex-offenders. However, she was deeply touched by her earlier relationships with the children in TRC and qualified as a child and adolescent psychotherapist, where she undertook research. This research was Kelly's cathartic attempt to "make sense" of the minefield of TRC and the "care system". She wanted to understand *how* TRC served the child. Kelly further studied in leadership and management and analytic network coaching. Kelly is a proud mother and values precious family time.

Jamie Butterworth is a trainee integrative child and adolescent psychotherapist, currently working in school services across London. He is an advocate for working systemically with families and schools when supporting children with complex emotional issues, as well as exploring the role of psychotherapy in assisting neurodiverse children and those who have experienced developmental trauma. Jamie's background is in music and the performing arts, achieving a bachelor's degree in popular music studies at Leeds University, where he became interested in the connection between creativity and mental health. It was during this time that Jamie decided to pursue a career as a psychotherapist later in life. Prior to training, Jamie gained experience as a volunteer mentor and non-directive play therapist with charities in North and East London. During this period, Jamie completed a certificate of higher education in counselling at Birkbeck College, followed by a foundation course in psychoanalysis at the Association of Group and Individual Psychotherapy (AGIP). Following a successful career in the live music industry and the birth of his first child, Jamie chose to become a stay-at-home parent. Jamie's experience as a male primary caregiver sparked his interest in gender stereotypes and led him to contemplate societal attitudes towards men's roles in children's lives.

Alix Hearn, MA, PgDip. Supvn., UKCP, CPC, is a Terapia-trained integrative child and adolescent psychotherapist and ecopsychotherapist with over ten years' experience of specialist work with children, young people, and families. She has worked within schools, specialist trauma teams, child and adolescent mental health services, and private practice. Alix specialises in the areas of developmental trauma, adoption and fostering, and rape and sexual abuse. She is particularly interested in and passionate about the fields of youth justice/youth offending and ecotherapy and how they can be brought together. Alix is a huge advocate for child therapy and is a tutor and trainer at various child and adult therapy training organisations across London. She is also a qualified clinical supervisor to both child and adult psychotherapists and counsellors. Alix is vice-chair of the Child Psychotherapy Council (CPC), which promotes best practice and professional standards within the field of child psychotherapy. Currently, she is drawn to rites of passage work and facilitation of grief ceremonies. Alix is working on a number of non-fiction books including writings on grief and ritual within nature.

Evania Inward has always worked with people and has a passion for liberty, equality, and justice for those who do not have as much as many in the West. Previously, as a care worker, she worked to provide dignity, humility, and independence for the elderly and people with physical, mental, and learning disabilities. As a race equality officer, she worked for many years with employers and public services through different projects to reduce discrimination and promote equality and diversity. In community development, working alongside a range of minority ethnic and refugee communities, she supported individuals from the community to become more empowered and to advocate for and represent their community's needs to authorities and funders. Evania is experienced in a range of roles within primary and secondary schools to develop services for children and families, working for the last few years as an integrative child and adolescent psychotherapeutic counsellor to children and adolescents of all ages, parents, and adults. She currently works as a complex case therapist with an inner-city specialist school and psychotherapy charity. She has a bachelors in psychology and human biology, a masters in social anthropology, a postgraduate diploma in integrative child and adolescent psychotherapeutic counselling, and is a trainee in integrative child and adolescent psychotherapy. Evania believes it is soul work and a privilege to be a therapist and that each and every client has something to teach us.

Irene Mburu is a trainee integrative child and adolescent psychotherapist at Terapia. During her professional career, Irene has worked with a diverse range of clients in secondary and primary schools and private practice, supporting them to work through social and relational issues, depression, anxiety, anger, trauma, low self-esteem, gender dysphoria, and other life challenges. Irene enjoys working relationally with children and young people and is committed to delivering client-centred holistic support. Her work is fundamentally child-led, and she draws on different theoretical models based on the needs of each client. She strives to foster a good working alliance that enables her to understand the client's internalised world, which informs the mode of intervention. Irene identifies as an ethnic minority and it is against this backdrop that she writes on the topic of female genital mutilation (FGM), which is a common practice within this group. The World Health Organization has classified FGM as child abuse. This transgenerational cultural practice is shrouded in mystery and shame. In her chapter, Irene highlights the long-term mental and psychological health implications brought upon the young person who undergoes FGM and brings into perspective the seriousness of this vice. She explores how the consequential trauma can be addressed through psychotherapy, and what the therapist needs to be aware of in the work with the victims.

Sasha Morphitis, MA, UKCP, completed her MA at Terapia prior to which she had worked as an actor/singer, a drama teacher, a special educational needs playworker, a learning support assistant, and an early years teacher. She discovered DIR (Developmental, Individual-Difference, Relationship-Based) Floortime first as a psychotherapist and a parent, and was guided to support her own children under the inspiring guidance of Sibylle Janert. After completing the Floortime training herself, it became part of her professional approach. Sasha identifies as neurodivergent and can relate to this demographic of client both from a personal and parental perspective. She became head of clinical services at Terapia for a time, helping to set up and run the new therapeutic services provided in Terapia's bespoke Bothy as well as local schools and services within Barnet. Since then she has worked for BytheBridge, a therapeutic foster agency, as a regional therapist supporting foster parents and developing and delivering a trauma-informed approach to parenting. She currently lives and works in North London in private practice, working predominantly with children and parents. She teaches the autism module at Terapia and more widely provides training in working therapeutically with neurodiversity.

Dr Magda Raczynska, PhD, MA, UKCP, CPC, is an integrative child and adolescent psychotherapist trained at Terapia. She works mostly with adolescents and young adults in her private practice, specialising in anxiety, developmental trauma, and attachment difficulties. She works psychodynamically with a strong relational focus, prioritising growth through playfulness and safety. She supervises students at Terapia, where she also teaches on transference and countertransference. In addition to her therapeutic credentials, Magda holds an MA in contemporary art theories from Goldsmiths College, London, and a PhD in sociology from the University of Warsaw. In her pre-clinical life, she was a co-founding editor of *Krytyka Polityczna* and an author of numerous essays and articles on the intersties of art and politics. For twelve years, she created and curated a programme for promoting Polish literature in the UK for the Polish Cultural Institute in London.

Nadja Julia Rolli, MA, UKCP, BACP, is an integrative child and adolescent psychotherapist. Formally a primary school teacher, she initially trained in Switzerland in psychomotor therapy, a somatic psychotherapeutic approach, integrating elements of play and art therapy into the clinical work. After relocating to London in 2006, she studied at Terapia, completing the MA in integrative child and adolescent psychotherapy. Nadja has worked for a number of years at primary and secondary school settings and is now working in private practice in West London. She is working intensively with children who have experienced abuse and neglect and who demonstrate ongoing problems related to attachment and trauma.

Zisi Schleider, MA, UKCP, is a Orthodox Jewish Terapia-trained child and adolescent integrative psychotherapist. Zisi works within the Orthodox Jewish community and in the wider community, both in private practice as well as within the public-school sector, and in a number of Jewish Orthodox schools. Zisi works individually with children as young as three years old, adolescents, and adults, and also in groups. She regularly gives presentations to different age groups, students, and staff in school settings. Zisi may work with parents to facilitate them to support their children, rather than directly with a child, benefitting not only the originally referred child but also other siblings in the family. Being a psychotherapist and belonging to the Orthodox Jewish world, Zisi brings a specific perspective to her work. In her chapter, she explores how other therapists can acquire skills and qualifications to work effectively with minority groups, such as the Orthodox Jewish community. Her work assists in bridging this gap and giving definition to the Orthodox Jewish Community, which can appear shrouded in secrecy.

Anna Tuttle, UKCP, is a clinical psychotherapist working with children, young people, families, and adult clients. Anna is the CEO of NESTT CIC (Nurture, Empowerment & Skill through Therapy & Training Community Interest Company) in Yorkshire, an organisation committed to providing systemic therapeutic interventions to families whose needs and circumstances may mean that therapy is less accessible. This may be due to financial constraints or traditional service thresholds of needs or complexity of intervention not being met. NESTT is also a counselling and psychotherapy training institute. Anna has developed the developmental, attachment-focused, relational and neurophysiological perspective (DARN) clinical model at NESTT to work systemically. Anna is particularly committed to developing models of working with the adults in a child's life so that the child is not left to carry out the therapeutic work on the family's behalf. Anna is also a lecturer in Counselling Psychology, Child Psychology, and Forensic Psychology. Before training as a psychotherapist, she worked within mental health and learning disabilities services for over twenty years, most recently leading inpatient and community learning-disability services for the NHS. Anna is particularly interested in working with individuals affected by pre- and post-birth developmental trauma. She is passionate about developing psychotherapeutic understanding and interventions for fetal alcohol spectrum disorder (FASD) and drug exposure in utero, due to the impact she sees in her client work, the lack of awareness in the psychotherapy community, and her own experiences as both an adoptee and adoptive parent. Anna has undertaken the conversion training in child psychotherapy at Terapia.

Introduction: seeds sown

Bozena Merrick and Di Gammage

The saplings

In developing this book, we revisited our early connections. On our first meeting, we discovered we had each worked as a residential social worker in the same London borough a quarter of a century ago. As we delved deeper, to our astonishment, we learnt that we had worked in the same children's home, one filling the residential social work (RSW) vacancy left by the other. We knew the same children, colleagues, and mid-1980s culture of "caring for" traumatised children and young people. We both shared the experience of working in an environment where there was no real understanding of, much less a psychological framework for, working with traumatised youngsters. The staff were often little more than teenagers themselves; there was no training, no clinical supervision, and, not surprisingly, a very high turnover of workers. Just as a young person might be beginning to build any semblance of trust with an adult, the adult would leave, never to be seen again. Survival was the goal—for everyone, staff and young people alike. Physical restraints prevailed, and the burliest amongst the RSWs were sought out and praised for their ability to instil control, often replicating the environments of domestic violence from which the children had been removed.

Our young people were antisocial, aggressive, disrespectful, violent. They were also vulnerable and in desperate need of safety and understanding. There was no culture of therapy and psychological inquiry, yet some of the RSWs knew intuitively that this was fundamental for healing the horrendous wounds these children carried. Some of those wounds were visible to both of us, a testimony to the trauma and abuse that lead to their admission to the home. We both tried to negotiate with the management for the possibility of offering a confidential space wherein the young person could disclose and be allowed to tell their story, and for us to create an opportunity to work with the trauma that led to them being cared for by us. We saw how institutional choice sacrificed the young person's chance to share and have their trauma witnessed.

Award-winning poet and advocate, Lemn Sissay, knows well the experience of a child in the care system, saying, "How society treats those children who have no one to look after them is a measure of how civilised it is" (2016). Seeds were sown in each of us, knowing our traumatised children and young people's emotional and psychological needs should be recognised and responded to appropriately in our civilised society.

The roots

Integrative child psychotherapy owes much to the psychoanalytical child psychotherapy developed at the Tavistock Institute in London. The Tavistock has been a leading teaching and research institute in psychoanalytical psychotherapy in the UK and beyond.

Historically, the advancement of child psychotherapy follows the establishment of adult psychotherapy as a valued intervention in the field of mental health. Created by Sigmund Freud in the late nineteenth century, adult psychotherapy found its place in Western societies as a valid treatment for psychological distress as well as for personal development. Freud and his colleagues worked on the premise that practically all psychological distress and mental illness in adulthood begins in early childhood. Children constitute a fifth of most societies' populations, and despite the growing body of evidence, including empirical findings in neuroscience to indicate the importance of early interventions, it is baffling how it took decades for child psychotherapy of all modalities to become an equally recognised psychological profession. Furthermore, if we are truly to address and serve our societies, we need to encompass research derived from pre- and perinatal sources (Maret, 2007).

Over the past quarter of a century, the demand for child and adolescent psychotherapists within our society has grown. In order to respond to this demand, child psychotherapy needs to develop to reflect society's myriad needs. Child psychotherapists must be prepared and trained to work with children from diverse social and cultural backgrounds of differing ages and developmental stages and abilities, who may present with a wide range of emotional, developmental, social, and behavioural issues. To meet this task, child psychotherapists need to be equipped with knowledge and skills gleaned from a spectrum of appropriate theoretical models.

Although the psychoanalytical modality in the field of child psychotherapy is well established and well researched, we consider that a single theoretical approach to therapeutic work with children is no longer relevant to the diversity and complexity of the issues child psychotherapists work with in today's modern practice. Integrative child psychotherapy embraces the new developments in the field, including new findings in related modalities.

Integrative child psychotherapy has been working its way into the mainstream of therapeutic interventions over the last twenty years with the development of new non-psychoanalytic child psychotherapy trainings in the UK. With the support of the Child Psychotherapy Council (CPC) and the United Kingdom Council for Psychotherapy (UKCP), the two main voluntary regulatory bodies for the integrative psychotherapy profession, it is now possible to put integrative child psychotherapy on the map of psychological interventions.

There are a number of practitioners and contemporary child psychotherapy training organisations that have contributed to the emergence of the integrative approach to child psychotherapy in the last twenty years. The Institute for Arts in Therapy and Education, the Northern Guild, and the Centre for Counselling and Psychotherapy Education all provide professional training in this field, alongside Terapia, one of the leading child and adolescent psychotherapy and counselling training organisations in the UK, with which the two editors of this book are involved. Bozena established Terapia as a charitable organisation two decades ago and Di has been a Terapia tutor since 2005. Terapia training has been accredited by the UKCP and is currently going through the accreditation process with the CPC.

At the foundation of the Terapia programme is an understanding of core therapeutic values, a theory of mind derived from psychodynamic psychotherapy, and an awareness of interpersonal relationship, power dynamics, and social humanistic psychotherapy principles. We view relationship as absolutely paramount to any healing process. The therapeutic space and appreciation of the ethical and complex dynamics of relationship are imperative to the healing process. The psychotherapist's self-knowledge and self-awareness are fundamental. It is crucial that, in receipt of such responsibility, the child psychotherapist can challenge their own assumptions and judgements gathered from their own social context and personal history, both of which impact on the therapeutic relationship.

The trunk

Recent studies estimate that one in eight children and young people are likely to be impacted by mental ill health in England, with this estimate rising to one in six during the COVID-19 pandemic:

> Mental health disorders experienced in childhood and adolescence not only impact the short and long-term health, wellbeing, socioeconomic trajectories and family life of children and young people, but also exert pressure and a financial toll on the health and social care systems and the State through its impact on mental health services, the cost of interventions and pressure on the State benefits system. (University of Bristol 2022)

The world of the child has been rapidly changing and will change for evermore. The lives of children in Western societies over the last few decades have altered unrecognisably with the development of the internet and social media and with changes to societal structures and norms. The world of children and young people has become more complex, demanding the ability to navigate their lives in different families' and social systems, often without parental holding or an extended family. Child psychotherapists need to track these changes, and the field of child psychotherapy needs to constantly diversify and update itself alongside the changing world of children and young people. Thus, child psychotherapists must be trained and continuously updated in the latest developments in neuroscience, child development, mental health, and new therapeutic interventions, and must be provided with an understanding of the challenges faced by children and young people today in order to be able to work with clients in an informed and relevant way.

The pith

This book celebrates the achievements of Terapia's trainees, tutors, and staff over the last two decades. All contributors to this book are graduates from Terapia's training, and the chapters are inspired by the teaching and the work provided at the centre.

Terapia is a strong voice for child psychotherapy as a distinct and specialist profession. We do not believe that the child is a small adult. Therapeutic work with children requires a different set of skills and knowledge to that required of adult psychotherapists; child psychotherapy is also different to adult psychotherapy in the way it needs to address emergent issues in the session. As noted above, adult psychotherapy addresses the presenting problem and its roots in the client's childhood and primary relationships, relying on the client's own narrative, agency, and ability to make change. The child psychotherapist needs to find ways of accessing the internal world of the client where talking therapy techniques are not applicable. The work relies on nonverbal communications in play and metaphor. It looks into arrestment of development or aspects of development and seeks ways of helping the child to meet their potential. This requires involvement with the system around the child, including parents, the wider family, and professionals. Crucially, it also requires the practitioner to manage the conflicting agenda of the issues mentioned above and to act on behalf of the child.

There is no one-size-fits-all approach in child psychotherapy, and practitioners are required to draw on a broad range of skills to support children, depending on the age and development of the individual.

The crown

> *All our wounding happens in relationship and all our healing happens in relationship.*
> —Franklyn Sills, Director of the Karuna Institute, Devon, and author of *Being and Becoming*

At the core of most integrative child psychotherapies lies the humanistic understanding that a therapeutic change takes place in the relationship between therapist and client. Although the theory of mind tends to be derived from psychodynamic psychotherapy, the awareness of interpersonal relationship, power dynamics, and social awareness adhere to core humanistic psychotherapy values. Integrative child psychotherapists view relationship as unequivocally primary to any healing process. Practitioners know how to hold the therapeutic space.

The important task of integrative child psychotherapists is to respond to the complexity of the child's world within the system around them. There have been extensive societal changes which cause children to question their place in the family, in peer groups, in culture, and in their own bodies. For a multitude of reasons, some financial, the established services designed to help children to achieve their own potential, such as Child and Adolescent Mental Health Services (CAMHS), Social Services, and educational establishments, are no longer able to respond in a timely or, in some cases, helpful manner. Integrative child psychotherapists work with various professional communities, often advocating for the child's emotional and psychological needs within multidisciplinary teams and agencies.

There is an urgent need to respond to wide cultural changes and, particularly since the killing of George Floyd, society's raised awareness of racism, diversity, and intersectionality. We are aware of migrating communities and that they bring with them uprooted and traumatised children. Integrative child psychotherapy must respond to this task not only with careful and informed interventions but by taking responsibility for the cultural and racial diversity of the profession itself.

The recent events related to the pandemic, war in Europe, and the climate emergency bring particular responsibility into the work with children and young people. Child psychotherapists need to be aware of children's anxieties around these events and how to respond to them in a sensitive, culturally informed, and resourced way. The child psychotherapist appreciates that their role can also demand that they help children make some sense of what has happened to them and find meaning in their lives and for their future. To address this, we draw on the theory and practice of existential and transpersonal psychotherapies.

Integrative child psychotherapists must actively engage with the systems around the child. Consideration of parents, siblings, extended family, professionals, peer groups, and social media groups are important in understanding the internal world of a child and a young person. These systems are constantly changing, and we need to be able to adopt and adapt to them in an informed and age-relevant manner or we will fundamentally fail to meet the child where they are. To enable the child psychotherapist to work effectively, ethically, and confidently with families and carers, and to promote partnership work with families and other related professionals, systemic family therapy needs to be an aspect of the integrative training.

Terapia's approach to integrative psychotherapy requires each trainee to develop their own model of integration within the agreed framework which, apart from the taught modules at Terapia, will embrace their previous trainings, life experiences, and personal philosophies. The experiential and theoretical modules of the programme, as well as the self-development aspects of the training, are designed to support the exploration of the psychotherapist's understanding of theories and how they correlate, and their individual style of relating, pace, and ways of integrating therapeutic tools into their clinical practice. The training strives to create and maintain a forum that can facilitate the trainee's individual discovery of their personal philosophy of psychotherapy.

The chapters in this book illustrate how, in order for child psychotherapy to be relevant to the client's world, one-to-one, behind-closed-doors therapy provision may no longer be applicable to the child's world, instead looking at opening up exciting and pioneering new approaches to meeting the multifarious needs of children and adolescents today.

The bark

At Terapia, we believe that the practice of child psychotherapy cannot exist without engagement with politics in the external world of the therapist (Samuels, 2015). Child psychotherapy requires practitioners to engage with the system around the child and many therapeutic interventions are constrained by the politics of those systems.

We take a view on private practice in working with children, particularly small children. A parent who accepts that their child will form a close attachment to another adult and that disclosure will take place in that relationship is probably already a "good enough" parent (Winnicott, 1953). Children who would most benefit from psychotherapeutic intervention are often in situations where it is impossible for parents to feel secure enough to bring a child to such a service. It is also often impossible to access private therapy for financial reasons. Terapia's graduates are encouraged to strive for a balance of working environments to provide their services to hard-to-reach and diverse communities and to develop links with external agencies and multidisciplinary teams. We see this as a significant aspect of a child psychotherapist's social responsibility. As a registered charity, Terapia endeavours to model this stance for our trainees through the way the training is run and through the many charitable activities we are engaged in.

This is understood and accepted within the organisation, as there is an understanding that many candidates for training in the therapy profession enter programmes as "wounded healers" (Barr, 2014). Trainees need to evidence their resilience and their readiness to engage with personal material and past traumas from their own childhood in order to be available to their clients' material without their own traumas being reactivated in the work; and when they are, to recognise them and take the necessary course of action, usually additional personal therapy, to further process their own traumatic material.

Our own childhood trauma is not a prerequisite for the psychotherapy profession; however, engagement with society, with its many challenges and injustices, is.

The taproot

The work of a child and adolescent psychotherapist is particularly challenging. Our practice exposes us to the suffering that is a consequence of the neglect and abuse experienced by clients who have little or no power to change or influence the circumstances of their lives. As practitioners, this can lead us to feel powerless. In addition, the children and young people themselves can cause others much distress, injury, and trauma. Trauma begets trauma. In this vicious cycle, wounded people wound others and themselves. Our work is to support a child to heal from the trauma they have experienced, thus limiting the possibility that they will perpetuate the same destructive cycles in the future.

As child psychotherapists, we are often expected to meet adults' expectations of behaviour management and anger management, or to provide a brief intervention so that the young person no longer "acts out" or "seeks attention". It can be challenging to manage the conflicting agenda of the adults around a child whilst trying to build a reliable therapeutic relationship by remaining alongside them, and validating, empathising, supporting, witnessing, reflecting, and exploring with them.

These extraordinary demands require extraordinary resilience. It is, therefore, essential for us as child and adolescent psychotherapists to resource ourselves in our work to prevent burnout, and to sustain our capacity to be reflective and to respond using our constantly replenished reservoir of creative interventions and thoughtful responses.

Resources, according to Peter Levine (2005) and Franklyn Sills (2008), are those qualities, factors, practices, and relationships that can be drawn upon in times of need. For the child psychotherapist, these would include their own clinical supervisor, psychotherapist, colleagues, training, and ongoing Continuing Professional Development (CPD). They may also include the psychotherapist's professional, political, and personal values, beliefs, and practices, such as regular exercise, meditation, recreational hobbies, creativity, regular rest periods, good nutrition, and social activities.

During the psychotherapy training at Terapia, trainees are introduced to the practice of resourcing through creative methods, such as story-making and projective techniques, so that they might discover, reconnect to, reclaim, and grow their own resources. A resource is only supportive if the psychotherapist is aware of it and is able to access it at times of need. Otherwise, it may as well not exist.

Recognising and practising resourcing benefits not only the psychotherapist and, therefore, the child; it is also a significant area of work for the psychotherapist to explore directly with the young person in questions such as: Who or what might support you in managing this situation? Who was there for you at that time? What might enable you to face this challenge in your life with self-belief, courage, confidence? The child psychotherapist can explore each of these aspects in non-threatening and reflective ways with the child.

Many branches

We are delighted to bring you a book that we hope will contribute to the field of integrative child and adolescent psychotherapy. We are presenting to you some of the sterling work that has been developed at Terapia and carried out by our graduates in a variety of diverse placements and organisations. In order to best serve a child, it is necessary for the psychotherapist to pay attention to the child's wider system—influences—and to hold these in mind, to engage with them, and still maintain an unwavering focus on the child.

As a reflection of the way in which work with each child is unique, we have encouraged, and supported, the contributors to find their own voices through which to articulate their passion in this work. All case material is fictionalised, drawing on contributors' personal and professional experiences so that no one child or child's individual situation will be identifiable in these narratives.

In Chapter 1, Alix Hearn discusses how the ever-changing and dynamic field of ecopsychotherapy can meet the needs of vulnerable children and young people. The author reflects on how working therapeutically outdoors enables a re-rooting into relational knowing and connection with oneself, with others, and with our place in the world. She explores different ways of working in and with nature so that we can understand more about our clients' internal landscapes and sensory, embodied experience. Alix highlights the importance of eco-anxiety/eco-grief and how the potential of loss affects clients and therapists alike.

In Chapter 2, "Airy creatures", Magda Raczynska explores the meanders of embodied working with the unconscious and uncommunicated. Focusing on the case of fourteen-year-old Flora, the chapter shows how to use somatic countertransference, that is, the therapist's capacity to employ her body and its somatic signalling to work with withdrawn, detached, autistic clients.

In Chapter 3, "The absent other: reflections on the absence of male integrative child psychotherapists", Jamie Butterworth explores the meaning and impact of gender disparity in the field of child psychotherapy, and the sociocultural barriers, including negative assumptions, that underpin it. He explores the meaning of gender roles in the therapeutic alliance between a child client and a male therapist and how this influences clinical outcomes. How should contemporary integrative child psychotherapy address the mother-centric theories of child development and male students' experiences of infant observation? Do child and adolescent psychotherapy trainings present unique barriers for men?

Evania Inward, in Chapter 4, explores the complexities of working with refugee children and young people, highlighting the distinctive, multiple, and cumulative traumas they may carry. The author raises questions around power and politics when working with these vulnerable clients, offering the clients a thoughtful, compassionate, and hopeful "other" who can attend to both external, practical realities and internal psychological warfare. Evania highlights the need for a strengths-based approach, and reflects on the continued need for safety and building of trust with a child or young person who has experienced and/or witnessed horrific violence and transgenerational trauma.

In Chapter 5, Audrey Adeyemi addresses the impact of racial trauma experienced by children and young people from ethnic groups. In "Unveiling racial trauma", the author presents two cases studies and, drawing on the acculturation framework proposed by Berry (2006, 2007), she explores strategies such as integration, assimilation, separation, and marginalisation to illustrate creative approaches that help to reveal deep-seated suffering. Audrey discusses the challenges and benefits of being a brown-skinned psychotherapist working with children and young people in such communities. She highlights the clashes in expectations, ideologies, and perceptions of first-generation immigrants and their children's schools, and how the psychotherapist can act as an advocate, bridging the gap between the child and others.

In Chapter 6, Irene Mburu addresses the highly emotive and culturally sensitive subject of female genital mutilation (FGM) and how, as in this case, a child psychotherapist's own culture can pertain to the practice. Irene highlights the need for the therapist to have ongoing emotional support in order to best serve the child and to play a vital role in the safeguarding of other children at risk of this form of abuse.

In Chapter 7, "Working with children and young people in the Orthodox Jewish community", Zisi Schleider addresses the need for more non-Orthodox child psychotherapists to work with Orthodox Jewish communities and guides us through her unique experiences of working with this client group. She invites child psychotherapists to cross invisible borders and shows how to navigate through the intricate social and cultural norms of the child-client and the family. As integrative child psychotherapists committed to intersectionality and the multicultural values of our clinical practice, are we giving enough attention to this distinctive ethnic group? Societal stigmas impact both sides of therapy room. What do practitioners need to know about how the Jewish worldview is affected by anti-Semitism and what the client's possible responses to a secular therapist are?

In Chapter 8, Tasha Bailey contextualises what it means to bear witness when a child is holding and processing their grief. The author describes theoretical approaches to understanding grief for children and young people and the benefits of using play and metaphor as vessels for making the unbearable bearable. The chapter looks at this through case studies which demonstrate individual grief, collective grief related to social injustice, and grieving the end of the therapy.

In Chapter 9, "Working therapeutically with uniquely wired children", Sasha Morphitis demonstrates the requirement to develop one's own skill and practice as a child psychotherapist when working with a specific client group. The author illustrates how she has enhanced her capacity to serve children and young people with neurodiverse brains and their families, and their carer and support systems, by integrating the practice of Developmental, Individual-difference, Relationship-based (DIR), also known as Floortime (Greenspan & Weider, 2006), into her practice as an integrative child psychotherapist.

In Chapter 10, Anna Tuttle asks, "Is it too late?", in relation to fetal alcohol syndrome disorders (FASDs). The author shows how many children and young people seem resistant to conventional one-to-one psychotherapy that may indicate undiagnosed FASD. She identifies the need for a multiagency approach in working with this often-unrecognised client group, identifying primary, secondary, and tertiary implications and the crucial need to address this issue before further damage is caused. Anna proposes a holistic treatment programme within which the child psychotherapist can support others in the system to understand and address this widespread and far-reaching condition.

Kelly Brackett, in Chapter 11, acknowledges the failings in the residential care system and invites engagement in the ongoing conversation of what really works for some of society's most vulnerable children. Drawing on her extensive experience of working in this sector, the author applies her psychological thinking developed as a child psychotherapist and proposes a much-needed, and very much overdue, reflective, collective approach for our looked-after children and young people.

In Chapter 12, Nadja Rolli highlights the link between disorganised attachment behaviour and early relational trauma as a result of emotional neglect and the unavailability of the primary carer. She writes about the impact on the child's emotional and psychosocial development leading to controlling-punitive and controlling-caregiving behaviours. The author reflects upon how, through play and the therapist's capacity to mentalize and be a "marked mirror" of the child's expressions, the child learns to integrate inner experiences and create moments of repudiating and reaccepting the object, without the risk of being overwhelmed and dysregulated.

We hope you find the chapters informative, helpful, and as moving as we have, and may you use them within your own endeavour to enrich and improve the quality of the lives of our children and young people.

References

Barr, A. (2014). What is a wounded healer? Website: the green rooms. https://thegreenrooms.net/wounded-healer-counsellor-psychotherapist-research/ (Retrieved 15 January 2014).

Berry, J. W. (2006). Acculturative stress. In: P. T. P. Wong & L. C. J. Wong (Eds.), *Handbook of Multicultural Perspectives on Stress and Coping*. Boston, MA: Springer.

Berry, J. W. (2007). Acculturation and identity. In: D. Bhugra & K. Bhui (Eds.), *Textbook of Cultural Psychiatry* (pp. 169–178). Cambridge: Cambridge University Press. Available at: https://www.cambridge.org/core/books/abs/textbook-of-cultural-psychiatry/acculturation-and-identity/EC9F0ABA9650A3C75D0D9160750E54F3 (last accessed 22 December 2022).

Greenspan, S., & Wieder, S. (2006). *Engaging Autism: Using the Floortime Approach to Help Children Relate, Communicate and Think*. Boston, MA: Da Capo Press.

Levine, P. (2005). *Healing Trauma: A Pioneering Program for Restoring the Wisdom of your Body*. Boulder, CO: Sounds True.

Maret, S. (2007). *The Prenatal Person: Frank Lake's Maternal-Fetal Distress Syndrome*. Lanham, MD: University Press of America.

Samuels, A. (2015). *The Political Psyche*. London: Routledge.

Samuels, A (2019) *Politics on the Couch: Citizenship and the Internal Life*. London: Routledge.

Sills, F. (2008) *Being and Becoming: Psychodynamics, Buddhism, and the Origins of Selfhood*. Berkeley, CA: North Atlantic Books.

Sissay, L. (2016). Orphans, foundlings and fostering in literature: a child's view of belonging. *The Guardian*. 1 January 2016.

The University of Bristol (2022). A survey of the mental health of children and young people in care in England in 2020 and 2021. School for Policy Studies, University of Bristol.

Winnicott, D. W. (1953). Transitional objects and transitional phenomena. In: *Playing and Reality*. London: Routledge, 2005.

Part I

Therapeutic holding

CHAPTER 1

Ecopsychotherapy with children and young people in mind: attachment to place, nature, and landscape

Alix Hearn

> [T]hus the greening of the self helps us to reinhabit time and own our story as life on Earth. We were present in the primal flaring forth, and in the rains that streamed down on this still-molten planet, and in the primordial seas. In our mother's womb we remembered that journey, wearing vestigial gills and tail and fins for hands. Beneath the outer layer of our neocortex and what we learned in school, that story is in us—the story of a deep kinship with all life, bringing strengths that we never imagined.
>
> —(Macy, 2009, p. 245)

"What's this fucking thing?" Rakesh began to prod at the fungus with the end of his brand-new trainers. I felt a spark of hope whilst wishing he wouldn't prod at the fungus quite so fiercely, in case it became uprooted. "Hmm, what do you think"—we bent down to look at his discovery more closely. I asked Rakesh what he perhaps liked about it. "The colour," he replied, "it's sick." It was indeed—the scarlet elf cup aflame in the shady woodlands. "You're right, it is." Rakesh, a thirteen-year-old boy of mixed heritage, had recently been taken into care, having started a fire in his family home. He, too, had been uprooted. Rakesh then noticed a piece of bark next to the fungus—crusty yet crumbling, still holding itself together even though the rains had sunken the soil around us. He began to peel the skin, strip by strip. "It's, like, red"—he commented, sounding surprised by what he had found underneath. "Yes, just like the fungus," I replied. "What do you think about the colour red?" "Blood. Innit."

He continued to peel at the outer layer of bark, until the redness below was visible. Rakesh's movements reminded me of the phrase "tearing a strip off"—Rakesh recently disclosing that his stepfather beats him with a belt. I thought of Rakesh's skin being hurt, torn, stripped off him, his need for a "second skin" (Bick, 1968, p. 484) perhaps to keep himself together, to not acknowledge the hurt. Of what is visible and not yet seen. My mind went to Rakesh's mother who, too, had grown up in care, and the sense of repeated hurting and uprooting—where was safe to land, to be.

I began to notice other "more-than-human" beings to and with Rakesh—plantain, nettles, dock—all with their own unique healing properties and gifts; those with capacity to hurt as well as heal, not unlike humans. Seeking, finding, a way of playing hide-and-seek together through and with nature; safer relationally for a young person who has experienced relationships other than safe. A form of a developmentally reparative relationship (Clarkson, 2003) that can also be kept at bay and its intensity managed. After all, it is "*joy to be hidden but disaster not to be found*" (Winnicott, 1963, p.186, original emphasis).

I was struck by Rakesh's encounter with the scarlet elf cup—why had he noticed a fungus amongst all the many plants and other natural elements? I was aware of the possible transgenerational aspects to Rakesh's story—uprooting, dislocation and disconnection from land, from home, from family. Rakesh was now part of a different system of networks—the oft-named "team around the child". How could we all form our own mycelium network around this vulnerable young person who had to set something ablaze so his distress could be seen? How might being in and with nature help Rakesh to soften his own "hard" skin-bark, if, when, this became safe-enough to do so?

Re-rooting ourselves home

Ecopsychotherapy is the therapeutic practice of being in and with nature—that, as humans, we are part of something greater than ourselves, that we are not only part of human systems, but ecosystems too;

that our relationship to the earth and the world around us matters—to our sense of well-being and all our attachment relationships. Indeed, for our very survival and nourishment. American-Russian psychologist Urie Bronfenbrenner (1979) provided a useful map in his ecological systems theory to explore some of this terrain; how children and young people are part of interrelated and interconnected systems that impact upon one another and inform their development and growth. The term ecopsychotherapy is itself an expansive term, branching off into differing approaches and perspectives. There is no one way of being an ecopsychotherapist or practising working alongside and with nature. Many practitioners may call themselves ecotherapists, ecopsychologists, wild therapists, embodied-relational therapists, or nature-based therapists. It seems that the field itself refuses to be labelled and tamed. I am reminded of wild rambling brambles offering flowers and fruits, growing free and unfurled.

Ecopsychotherapy with children and young people can take many forms and draws upon varied and wide-ranging disciplines depending on the clinician's background and approach. It may include "walk and talk" therapy for adolescents and young adults; wilderness therapy (immersive experiences in nature involving eating, cooking, living together in the wild); adventure therapy, including outdoor experiences such as hiking, rafting, abseiling; and working either in groups or one-to-one on and with the land, focusing perhaps on working with nature as a co-therapist (Berger & McLeod, 2006, p. 87).

When working with children and young people in particular, there can be many systems at play. There might be caregivers, key workers, medical practitioners, psychiatrists, social workers, school staff. Our work can be complex and requires many hearts and minds working in conjunction, weaving and holding a supportive scaffold together, sometimes a safety net, for the child. Spider's webs are strong—can we model our own human systems of support on Grandmother Spider? For me, knowing that I am part of something more than human systems, which may be frail or fallible, helps to ground and resource me in my clinical practice. If I can stay rooted in my own knowing and foundation, then that will serve my clients.

Many of us know that the idea that we are interconnected and impacted by the physical environment around us is not new; that we may need to only reconnect to our early ancestral roots, wherever they may be, and ancestral knowing of land and other-than-human wisdom. Many communities and cultures continue these threads of embodied knowing and connection to land and/or animal medicine. Psychologist and ecopsychologist Craig Chalquist states:

> roughly nine to eleven thousand years ago, when Europeans began farming to compensate for dwindling game, the first fences went up to separate domesticated from wild, human from non-human, settled from nomadic and personal from terrestrial … It seems to divide everything: matter from spirit, feelings and thoughts, yours and ours, us, and them. (Chalquist, 2009, p. 69)

He goes on to ask: "Why is there no psychology of homecoming—of how to live in accord with the rhythms and needs of our home world?" (ibid., p. 69).

In my clinical practice, I often return to Stern's thinking on "psychic isolation" (1998, p. 126) as opposed to psychic communion. How unsettling and brutal it can be for our sense of self and our well-being to feel so alone, adrift, untethered. How much of our current distress is part of our wider disconnection to the land and our environment around us, of our forgetting about, and our yearning for, something that we have already known within us? Systemic psychotherapist Roger Duncan writes of the "toxic legacy that we are still struggling to understand" (Duncan, 2018, p. 15) and yet hopefully asserts that "despite alienation from nature and urbanization of populations, humans are still drawn to and emotionally moved by the aesthetics of the natural world" (ibid., p. 15)

Ecopsychotherapy with children and young people therefore seems even more pertinent, especially in our current climate. Many children and young people struggle with being in the therapy room, particularly those who may have experienced early developmental trauma. No matter how cosy, it can be too intimate, too frightening, too "clinical", too exposing to be tolerated. If part of our work as therapists is to help our clients reconnect to their body, to their sense of embodied self, to help them feel or make sense of what is happening inside them, then being in nature is vital in resourcing both our practices and offerings for our clients. We are in the realm of Stern's "vitality affects" (1998, p. 53)—it's not just the experience but the quality of that experience which we recall and hold onto.

Being in nature could be sentimentalised but in reality, it is alive and kicking—there might be battering wind or rain, there might be jagged and jarring obstacles in the way, there might be insects which tickle or bite, the sun may be too hot. I can hear a red kite's cries or smell a passing honeysuckle. I may scratch myself on a holly bush or be bitten by a wasp. Being in nature and landscape is therefore an alive, dynamic relational process (Jordan, 2015). Daniel Siegel refers to the "neurobiology of we" (Siegel, 2010, p. 60); perhaps ecopsychotherapy enables the building of a neurobiology of us.

Similarly, when working outside, there is a heightened awareness and aliveness of our client's body and our own body in space and time. Many practitioners have commented on the potential losses of working on digital platforms through, and since, the pandemic. We cannot see our clients' bodies and they cannot see ours. We need to smell our clients; they need to smell us too. I can see how my clients might walk around a muddy patch, or run down a slope, or climb a tree. They can also witness how my body responds and reacts. Being outside, therefore, can enable an increased sensitivity to our nervous system and sensory attunement to our bodies. This can be particularly helpful if a client experiences disassociation or hyper-aroused states. Outdoor psychotherapist Hayley Marshall states:

> I think that in outdoor therapy, therapists have golden opportunities to explore a somatic immersion in the dynamic experience of their clients, consequently finding out more about the lived physical reality of their past and present worlds. (Marshall, 2016, p. 155)

Arguably, there is both safety and an increased window of tolerance (Siegel, 1999) for client and therapist when working in nature. Being outdoors may also take us out of our own comfort zone. There is potentially more safety in the consulting room for the therapist, but not necessarily for the client. As a child psychotherapist, I must consistently attend to the power dynamics and power imbalances that may be at play when working with vulnerable children and young people. With this in mind, I find working outdoors and with nature to be a gentle way of addressing some of these power dynamics. We are not working in "my" room but in a shared liminal space that I do not have control over. Ronen Berger, a child psychologist and ecotherapist working in Israel, outlines in his therapeutic model of nature therapy (Berger, 2009) how dynamics of hierarchy and authority may be worked with differently when nature is our co-therapist.

Confidentiality, too, needs careful thinking through when working outdoors in nature. Contracting and transparent discussions with clients are an important part of the process here, particularly around any intrusions or someone overhearing—perhaps easier to attend to directly with adolescents and young adults than younger children. But it is worth remembering that working outdoors specifically, regardless of whether we are in a more private, contained space or a more public one, requires an enlivened response to situations or other people/beings that may share the therapeutic space. Our work therefore elicits a perhaps more fluid response to the metaphorical temperature changes, when and however they occur, in landscape. Of course, this is all to be worked with and to bring into the sessions, just as we would inside the therapy room. Martin Jordan highlights some of these practice issues when moving outdoors, suggesting that the importance of the therapeutic frame and the therapeutic presence are key here.

> An important thing to realise is that the therapist holds an internal psychological frame around the work with the client, in so doing trusting their own confidence and competence to be able to hold a much more dynamic and fluid process which unfolds in an outdoor context. (Jordan, 2015, p. 93)

Essentially, there has to be a kind of surrender when working outdoors and in contrasting and unpredictable natural environments. As a clinical supervisor and trainer of child psychotherapists, I may invite students and supervisees to check in with what weather system they are feeling like today: perhaps a cold, breathing wind echoing across a deep valley; a tentative sun emerging after a rain shower. When working outdoors in nature, we are embedded in that weather system, in that landscape—everything is in the "here and now", felt experience.

David Abram, in his book *The Spell of the Sensuous* (1996), writes about the necessity of this sensory, sensuous experience, as a way of making contact with our body through contact with the earth:

> by acknowledging such links between the inner, psychological world and the perceptual terrain that surrounds us, we begin to turn inside-out, loosening our psyche from its confinement within a strictly human sphere, freeing sentience to return to the sensible world that contains us. (Abram, 1996, p. 262)

Winnicott wrote about the connection between mind and body, or psyche and soma; through the processes of being held, physically, emotionally, and psychically, we become embodied, we have a sense of Winnicott's "indwelling" (1960, p. 45). I wonder about the links between being embodied and emplacement, which Craig Chalquist (2009) describes—having a sense of place, of being here, in this world, right now; how nature can facilitate these key, necessary paths towards safety in one's own body, one's place in the world, and being in relationship with others.

Nature as co-therapist

Inherent in the wider aspect of ecopsychotherapy is how nature heals, that nature can be our co-therapist, another layer of container (Bion, 1962a, 1962b, 1970) for the meeting of human therapeutic relationships. Sometimes other sentient beings can be safer for our scared and dysregulated clients. Many children and young people who have experienced trauma are activated by the most micro of expressions or movements on the human face or body—a too visceral reminder of what came before—without this even being in their cognitive awareness. We might want to anthropomorphise nature, but these are projections, and ecotherapy can attend to some of these and untangle them, through the safety of nature as our co-container.

Brady was a six-year-old boy who struggled to stay inside a usual therapy room. He had witnessed severe domestic violence and had stopped speaking—instead making sounds and throat gurgles. Following a neurodevelopmental assessment, he had been diagnosed with attention deficit hyperactivity disorder (ADHD) and subsequently prescribed Ritalin. His school was very concerned about his behaviour, and he was on the brink of being excluded. He would often run out of class, or hide under tables, refusing to get out. Outdoor therapy was deemed to be his last chance before exclusion. Brady and I met in a safe and contained outdoor space with many trees and a meadow nearby. When I first met Brady, I could feel my heart beating out of my chest, his distress immediately palpable and transmitted, his nervous system on red alert. I wondered how best I could contain him and keep him safe but not constrict him—always a difficult balance therapeutically anyway, but particularly when working outdoors. Would he run off as he did so often at school? I decided that we had to start with safety, that perhaps we needed to make lots of safe homes outdoors in nature. I wondered about Brady's places of sanctuary within himself and outside of himself, his own sense of an internal container.

Nature would provide another level of container as we spent endless sessions making nests, making caves, making graves, Brady burying himself in the ground and enjoying throwing soil around and at me. I took the soil and made mud pies, sitting alongside him, offering these to him later as our "dinner". I wondered whether Brady would be able to "take in" the "good" food I was trying to offer him. Sometimes he would let me help him build his many variations of home; other times he would turn his back on me, or occasionally make intonations whilst making hand gestures. There were many beautiful birds around where we met, including some corvids. After many sessions of nests, and caves and graves, Brady began to notice the birds and their calling to each other. He started to copy their sounds, and enjoyed listening to their sounds back. Perhaps they were communicating back to him, perhaps not. It didn't really seem to matter. Brady was making a connection to something other than himself. I began to join in (my desire to come into relationship with Brady and offer him an attuned presence). Brady would shush me, putting his finger on his lips, sometimes putting his hands near my face. I took a metaphorical step back—my role was to allow nature to be the main facilitator for a while, and I would still be there, to midwife, as and when necessary (Berger & McLeod, 2006).

The work with Brady required patience, time, and care—all-too-often missing in our therapeutic practices when we feel the demands to "make better" and do it quickly. But he needed that time, we needed that time, together. Brady began to track the birds, not just their sounds, but their appearances and disappearances—we started to pretend to be birds, and then he allowed me to make noises too and verbalise more of his experiences. Over time, Brady started to say small words—pointing more, waving me over to look at something. He found a swing in the woods, and he allowed me to push him on the swing—his delight visceral and moving to witness. He became calmer in school and started to approach teachers for a cuddle when feeling overwhelmed, nestling into their bodies for comfort. Brady was beginning to allow himself to seek out others as points of safety rather than of threat.

Working therapeutically as a nature-based practitioner or ecotherapeutically doesn't necessarily have to occur outside. After all, we *are* nature. I find that nature finds its way into those in-between spaces of client and therapist as the client arrives or as we say goodbye for another week; perhaps noticing the weather outside or saying what they might do next in that transition space. I notice I feel different when I can see a tree, or a plant, or a bird outside of my therapy room window. I wonder whether my clients can sense that difference in me too. Bringing natural elements (twigs, rocks, shells) into the therapy room can also facilitate ways of being ecologically minded and can enable ways of engaging with both inner and outer worlds in parallel. Nature can appear in our clients' dreams, in images, in multiple symbolic forms. Can we allow our clients' "ecological self" (Barrows, 1995) and our own to emerge within the therapeutic process?

Nature as mirror/metaphor (the art of soulwork)

Nature is perhaps the most powerful mirror there is—trees, plants, and rocks just … are. One can have projections towards natural environments, of course, but the gaze which is received back is clear, without prejudice or judgement. If we are open to receiving it, nature has much wisdom to share with us.

Within ecopsychotherapy sessions, I might ask a client to see what path they want to follow, or what they notice around them—do they find themselves stuck in bramble bushes or feel lost at deciding which path to take through the woodlands. How might these be mirrors for their own lived experience? Is this familiar? Is this a pattern they notice? Is this something they may have encountered before? We can ask ourselves questions as to why we are drawn to certain landscapes or places, or how unconsciously and without intention we always end up in the tangled branches rather than a clear, poppy-filled meadow.

Just as we might draw upon objects or images to represent symbolic aspects of a client's process within the therapy room, so too can nature provide profound and unexpected insights and imaginings. Working in and with nature in this way has ancient and sacred roots—medicine walks and vision quests (also known as vision fasts) were held within Native American communities. Many traditional cultures would look to the use of ritual and ceremony as part of these sacred journeys. In contemporary practices are invitations to observe and pay attention to mirrors within the natural environment—they may initially be mundane, or not look quite as we would imagine or hope. Following these sacred journeys, the guides, as elders leading the participants through these experiences, mirror back through imagery and metaphor what they have heard from the participants' retelling of their walks and fasts. Certain plants or animals may appear and reappear on these walks—what do they have to show us, if we can be receptive and open? For me, psychotherapy is soul work. And yet, at times, I have felt a disconnection from this within the four walls of overwhelmed and tested human systems. Being outdoors and working alongside nature, as well as having my own personal experiences of being guided by nature, enables a remembering of something more-than-human.

As Bill Plotkin (2003) writes:

> the individual human soul is one element of the fabric of nature. You are not in any way separate from nature. The wild world reflects your essence back to you just like a still lake reflects your image. Is that reflection in you or in the lake? Neither. Both you and the lake are in the world, and the lake reflects that fact back to you. In the same way, your soul, your essence, is in the world, and nature mirrors that fact back to you. (Plotkin, 2003, p. 216)

Nell was a nineteen-year-old young woman who decided to seek some support following a period of intense anxiety attacks. She was articulate and imaginative, a brilliant artist who found herself becoming paralysed by panic. I suggested to Nell we go on a medicine walk and that I would be alongside her, offering the invitation to be witness and to pay attention to where she was being drawn to within the landscape and to what may emerge as we walked along the common together. Nell had expressed to me she didn't like mud, though she really didn't know why. She hoped to avoid it on our walk and find higher ground where she felt safer. It was deep autumn and it was quite wet on the ground, so there were many shining leaves under our feet. We soon found ourselves heading into a patch of mud—I hesitated. Perhaps I had made a mistake, as I knew that Nell wanted to avoid the mud rather than move towards it. How interesting that we had found the very thing that Nell had wanted to steer away from. Nell began to cross the muddy patch, determined to get through it. She froze as she felt her boots enter the earth. She was stuck. Or so it seemed. I encouraged her, asking her to stay connected to me and her breath, and she made it across. We sat down nearby on a blanket to talk about what had happened and to process her experience of being "stuck in the mud".

Nell said she had felt panicky and breathless in her chest, trapped. I invited her to think about what she had said to me earlier about not liking mud, and not knowing why, and her recent panic attacks. I wondered with her about this feeling of stuckness, of being trapped, and asked her whether this felt familiar or when, perhaps, was the last time she had felt this? Nell suddenly began to sob, recalling a car accident when she was fifteen years old in which her best friend had been left with life-changing injuries. Nell had remembered that feeling of panic in her chest as she had been trapped in the car and unable to help her friend. Nell had assumed she was "over it", as she had tried to not think about the horror of the accident and what had happened, throwing herself into her studies afterwards and achieving high grades. The mud had been a mirror for Nell's experience on that day and had, in that moment, offered an opportunity to connect to something deeply painful—hopefully beginning a process of recovery and healing for Nell.

I am reminded that Bill Plotkin says, "the mirror of nature is not always pleasant or comforting" (2003, p. 237). The work of psychotherapy involves confronting these painful and difficult aspects of our lives, and ecopsychotherapy, through nature as our guide and witness, enables us to be in contact with parts of ourselves or parts of our lives we have disconnected or split off from.

Tending to our grief

I find myself returning again and again to the themes of connection and disconnection. For me, this feels like a constant theme in my clinical work too—how to stay connected to oneself, how to become connected to others, without losing contact with oneself. How to come back into contact after disconnection. This relational dance between self and other, or self with other (Stern, 1998), is a fundamental developmental task.

If I, we, can connect to Mother Earth in all her forms and re-formings, if we can allow ourselves to really feel this depth of holding and containment, if we allow ourselves to remember the interconnectedness and interdependence of all, then we also must keep on attending to our relationship with the natural world, including our grief at its destruction and loss.

Lizzie had been only six years old when her mother had suddenly died. Lizzie was bright and lively, eight years old now, and she loved being outside. There had been some concerns that she had never really talked about her mother's death, that she "seemed ok" in her presentation, had taken on caregiving roles towards her younger sister and father. We were fortunate to have access to a self-contained garden at school, and so we spent time outside together. There was a small pond in the garden, and Lizzie and I would gather together around it, wondering what new beings might emerge from the murky green. One time a tiny, speckled frog appeared. Lizzie calling out in delight to me at finding this new playmate. I thought of the importance of shared attention and shared intention—how it is through the intersubjective playful space of relationships we learn about ourselves, and the world around us (Stern, 1998). I thought of Lizzie's loss, of no longer being able to call out to her mother to share these reciprocal moments of togetherness.

Lizzie began to build a temple of stones, a home in case the frog wanted to return, carefully choosing each stone until her stone-people castle was complete. Internally, I noticed how, unconsciously perhaps, she had created a cairn—a marking place for a burial site, for those who have been lost. I thought of her mother's sudden death, of Lizzie's intolerable pain, of perhaps having to seem okay. I was reminded how grief is not a linear process, but rather a puddle-jump—how we might remember, then forget, then remember again. How we can feel sad, and then return to life and play. I began to feel deeply sad, a possible countertransference response, and gently reflected this back to Lizzie— I wondered whether Lizzie could bear her own sense of sadness that was perhaps emerging. Lizzie nodded and asked whether "she" was ok. I wondered about the "she". "My mummy," she whispered, as she began to link some daisies together through their stems.

We spent the rest of the session collecting flowers together, Lizzie commenting that she used to do this with her mum, threading the daisies together and making necklaces and bracelets. Separate, yet connected. I was left with a sense of Stern's "evoked companion" (Stern, 1998, p. 121), of Lizzie's "going on being" (Winnicott, 1956, p. 303), and that of her mother within and around her. I was grateful for the frog and their medicine—in creating a home for the frog to return, Lizzie had also made a home for some of her grief to be held. How, through simple ritual and ceremony in nature, again and again, we can return to feeling, allowing for what emerges from our own deep inner ponds (Berger & McLeod, 2006).

Therein lies the rub. In letting ourselves feel in and towards our natural environments, we also encounter grief. If something matters, then it matters when it's no longer there. What are we if we are no longer part of the natural world? Many young people in the therapy room have brought their relationship to the natural world—this may be to their love of animals, or a fear of their pet dying. Sometimes it can be easier to relate to the more-than-human world than the human one. Many young people have looked me straight in the eye and spoken of fear for their future— why does no one care? Why does no one care about what's happening? There is anger, yes, and it is justified. Why are we not all angry?

I have no answer, or not one in any way that would be sufficient or that might really be able to hold their depth of frustration, rage, and grief. And if no one does care, or only some people care, then why should young people care about others and the world around them? Why are we shocked on hearing about county lines, and more stabbings, and young people hurting each other and/or themselves when we all co-exist in a world of not-feeling and not-caring? It is no wonder, then, that distress is manifested in the most disturbing and provoking of ways—how can our children and young people do anything other than this? Many children and young people I worked with in deprived boroughs of London have never seen a sheep or a cow, or seen the sea—how can they care about something that is so abstract or even non-existent in their minds?

If we connect to the thoughts and feelings around eco-anxiety, the fear of climate change and destruction—in effect, eco-grief—then this may be useful figural ground to the ever-increasing numbers of children and young people seeking help for their mental health. This may not be in any of our conscious awareness, but it's there. It may also provide a useful scaffold for widening our lens, keeping our curious minds open and attentive, to what is, what could be, what might be. As child psychotherapists, staying curious, bearing the "not knowing" is our Bionian legacy. Psychotherapist, researcher, and lecturer on climate psychology and eco-anxiety Caroline Hickman, in her 2020 paper, suggests we reframe eco-anxiety within an attachment lens, that it's because we care that we become distressed or disturbed by what is happening around us to our natural environments, and could be termed "eco-empathy, eco-compassion, eco-care and eco-awakening" (Hickman, 2020, p. 422).

Anita Barrows (1995) highlights the importance of the child's "ecological self", a key part of their development, of their becoming. And if this is the case,

> if we see the child as inextricably connected not only to her family, but to all living things and to the earth itself, then our conception of her as an individual, and of the family and social systems in which she finds herself, must expand … How would an expanded vision alter our efforts to affect the child's environment, to look beyond her object relationships for the sources of depression, agitation, apathy, violence or chronic illness. (Barrows, 1995, p. 108)

I am left wondering how it serves us to think we are not connected to place, nature, and landscape. Would this mean we have to systemically and politically address things we do not want to attend to, nor consider? Better for the pathology to be located in an individual child or family, surely? Because, perhaps, we then don't need to feel our own individual and generational displacement and disconnection, our own lost yearnings and rememberings of what has been severed.

Hickman (2020) invites us to consider that

> eco-anxiety in children and young people should be seen as an emotionally congruent healthy response to the climate and biodiversity crisis, and adults can help by understanding and validating all their feelings through "internal activism", helping to build their emotional resilience and understanding how many children feel; in partnership with "external activism", taking action in the world; both feeling sad and recycling, feeling angry and lobbying politicians, feeling guilty and planting bee friendly plants, feeling grief and supporting school climate strikers. We can both take action in the outer world and also give attention to inner relational landscapes, our inner emotional climate crisis. (p. 422)

So, what next?

I am heartened at times when it seems as if we are moving away from a behavioural-medical model, and yet the slow pace of emergence can be a painful one at times. I feel a resonance with Nick Totton's call for therapy itself to be rewilded (2011), a return to therapy as "wild" work, rather than a standardised set of worksheets to be taken through. Child psychotherapy, after all, is intended to be a relational process, not a "doing to", but a "being with". And yet, there are days when it feels far from that, as therapy has become increasingly manualised and digitalised with a brevity of "treatment" as its core.

The thought of risk assessments/outdoor first aid/not being a qualified mountain leader/being outdoors and holding a containing safe space with a vulnerable child or young person may prove overwhelming for those who have followed a more traditional training route. These are valid, common fears, and yet I encourage my fellow practitioners to perhaps reconnect themselves to their own natural landscapes, both within and around them. The practice of ecopsychotherapy can be expansive as well as foster more intimate moments of reciprocity between client, therapist, and nature.

In my end, is my beginning—working within nature is about belonging and kinship. To feel a sense of belonging and part of something is one of our basic human needs. That, perhaps, as many others feel, part of our "sickness" at an individual, societal, and cultural level is our lack of kinship with the world around us, the environment that we belong to, just by being here, alive, in this moment.

I would like to finish this chapter with some invitational enquiries:

What is your own relationship to nature, place, and landscape?
What is your own earliest memory of being outside?
What nourishment does nature resource you with?
And how can these reflections infuse your work with those who need this sense of connection the most?

Stay wild, folks.

References

Abram, D. (1996). *The Spell of the Sensuous: Perception and Language in a More-than-Human World.* New York: Vintage.
Barrows, A. (1995). The ecopsychology of child development. In: T. Roszak, M. Gomes & A. Kanner (Eds.), *Ecopsychology: Restoring the Earth, Healing the Mind* (pp. 101–110). London: Sierra Club.
Berger, R. (2009). Nature Therapy—developing a framework for practice. A Ph.D. University of Abertay, Dundee: School of Health and Social Sciences.
Berger, R., & McLeod, J. (2006). Incorporating nature into therapy: a framework for practice. *Journal of Systemic Therapies*, 25(2): 80–94.
Bick, E. (1968). The experience of the skin in early object relations. *International Journal of Psychoanalysis*, 49(2): 484–486.
Bion, W. R. (1962a). Learning from experience. In: *Seven Servants.* New York: Aronson, 1977.
Bion, W. R. (1962b). A theory of thinking. In: *Second Thoughts.* New York: Aronson, 1967.
Bion, W. R. (1970). Attention and interpretation. In: *Seven Servants.* New York: Aronson, 1977.
Bronfenbrenner, U. (1979). *The Ecology of Human Development.* Cambridge, MA: Harvard University Press.

Chalquist, C. (2009). Ecotherapy research and a psychology of homecoming. In: L. Buzzell & C. Chalquist (Eds.), *Ecotherapy: Healing with Nature in Mind* (pp. 69–82). Berkeley, CA: Counterpoint.

Clarkson, P. (2003). *The Therapeutic Relationship* (2nd ed.). London: Whurr.

Duncan, R. (2018). *Nature in Mind: Systemic Thinking and Imagination in Ecopsychology and Mental Health.* London: Routledge.

Hickman, C. (2020). We need to (find a way to) talk about … Eco-anxiety. *Journal of Social Work Practice, 34*(4): 411–424. https://doi.org/10.1080/02650533.2020.1844166

Jordan, M. (2015). *Nature and Therapy: Understanding Counselling and Psychotherapy in Outdoor Spaces.* London: Routledge.

Macy, J. (2009). The greening of the self. In: L. Buzzell & C. Chalquist (Eds.), *Ecotherapy: Healing with Nature in Mind* (pp. 238–245). Berkeley, CA: Counterpoint.

Marshall, H. (2016). A vital protocol—embodied-relational depth in nature-based psychotherapy. In: M. Jordan & J. Hinds (Eds.), *Ecotherapy: Theory, Research & Practice* (pp. 148–161). London: Palgrave.

Plotkin, B. (2003). *Soulcraft: Crossing into the Mysteries of Nature and Psyche.* Novato, CA: New World Library.

Siegel, D. J. (1999). *The Developing Mind: How Relationships and the Brain Interact to Shape Who We Are.* New York: Guilford.

Siegel, D. J. (2010). *The Mindful Therapist: A Clinician's Guide to Mindsight and Neural Integration.* London: W. W. Norton.

Stern, D. (1998). *The Interpersonal World of the Infant: A View from Psychoanalysis and Developmental Psychology.* New York: Basic Books.

Totton, N. (2011). *Wild Therapy: Undomesticating Inner and Outer Worlds.* Ross-on-Wye, UK: PCCS Books.

Winnicott, D. W. (1956). Primary maternal preoccupation. In: *The Maturational Processes and the Facilitating Environment.* London: Hogarth, 1965.

Winnicott, D. W. (1960). The theory of the parent–infant relationship. In: *The Maturational Processes and the Facilitating Environment.* London: Hogarth, 1965.

Winnicott, D. W. (1963). Communicating and not communicating leading to a study of certain opposites. In: *The Maturational Processes and the Facilitating Environment.* London: Hogarth 1965.

CHAPTER 2

Airy creatures: using somatic countertransference to ground autistic states in child psychotherapy[1]

Magda Raczynska

How do you know what the client may be feeling if they cannot tell you about it because they cannot feel it themselves or are unable to communicate it?

This chapter presents a case study from my clinical work with fourteen-year-old Flora. Although autism spectrum disorder (ASD) was never mentioned, she presented close to how Fordham saw autistic states as defence mechanisms that enable someone to cut off the external environment to either defend the inner world from impingements or to protect it from imploding (Fordham, 1987; Case, 2005). My focus here, however, is not on her state as such, detached from her feelings, but rather on how I worked with that disconnection by relying on my somatic countertransference. I define the latter as the therapist's capacity to use their body and its somatic signalling to pick up and track the client's as yet unsymbolised affective experience, chew it over in reverie

---

[1] For the purpose of this publication, all characters and events have been fictionalised, including the code name, which I always see as a starter for getting the feel of the client by accessing my projections of what she evokes in me, perhaps in parallel to how her parents named her to reflect theirs.

(Bion, 1962) until something of that unconscious emotional communication induced in the therapist's body becomes clearer, and then use it to inform clinical thinking and possible interventions. Showing how this works, I draw on my earlier theoretical research (Raczynska, 2019) and its conceptual framework.

Bring up the bodies

Considering that effective therapeutic process demands that the client feels understood by the therapist, including their unconscious material transmitted by impact, the therapist's capacity to use her body is essential. Since we are putting our bodies, not only our minds, in the room with our clients, we want to use the visceral information they provide, together with our imagination and capacity to unpack what is going on. It is valid for all kinds of psychotherapeutic encounters. Nonetheless, considering that working with young people often involves non-verbal means of communication related to play and creativity, it seems particularly fitting to know how embodied energies work in this field. Yet available literature on somatic countertransference in child psychotherapy is nearly non-existent.

There is a growing recognition of interpersonal brain-to-brain communication (Schore, 2001, 2009)—the acceptance that clients discharge their repressed arousal by somatically pinging it to their therapists (Carleton, 2009), much as infants project their states onto their carers (Bion, 1962; Casement, 1985; Thomson-Salo, 2018). Yet major neuroscience-inspired and body-oriented therapeutic approaches (Siegel, 1999; Payne, Levine, & Crane-Godreau, 2015; Ogden & Fisher, 2015; Fisher, 2017) seem to ignore the concept of countertransference, at least in the published materials (Ogden, 2020). On the other hand, until quite recently, most of the mainstream psychodynamically oriented literature on countertransference, including a smaller body of work on this phenomenon in child psychotherapy, has reduced it to mind-related impact: words, images, feelings, and associations evoked in the therapist by the client (Wolstein, 1988; Tsiantis, Sandler, Anastosopoulos, & Martindale, 1996; Vulcan, 2009). Clearly, something is missing. We facilitate the body–mind integration for our clients, yet we stay split as their therapists.

We put our bodies in the room with them but then seem to ignore the visceral information they provide. We teach our clients to observe their sensations but then blank out our own physical processing. What seems to be lacking, therefore, is a reflection on the use of the therapist's body in empathic communication with the client's affective experience.

Filling this gap began nearly three decades ago (Samuels, 1985; Field, 1988; Orbach, 1995) and has gained strength in the past few years, drawing interest even among psychoanalysts (Brothers & Sletvord, 2022). Nonetheless, the available literature on somatic countertransference, although growing, is still focused on working with adults.

We have always engaged our bodies as child psychotherapists. We know how to do it—we just lack the published reflection on it. We play hide-and-seek, doll's houses, "it", doctors, and marbles. We build slides and retreats to hide from sharks, ghosts, and monsters. We get dirty in clay, splashed in paint, and fed imaginary food. We witness sand-tray dramas and puppet shows. We also stay with selectively mute, compliant, or highly defended children for months, tracking what may be going on for them based on what we see and feel, our loneliness in this task mirroring and containing theirs. This chapter tells the story of one of those withdrawn children, aiming to expand the study of somatic countertransference into working with young people.

Case study: frozen child

Flora's older sister, Alice, who worked as an assistant curator in one of London's independent galleries, brought her to sessions. Every week, she dropped Flora outside the building and waited for her in the car. Alice sought therapy for Flora, worried about her little sister's increasing isolation, exacerbated by lockdowns and online schooling, which had recently evolved into emerging school avoidance.

Their French mother was an award-winning translator of literature working with major publishing houses and for years struggled with recurring depression manifesting in bouts of agoraphobia, missing her family as well as the Mediterranean weather and jovial sociability. Their father was a British professor of law and finance at Oxford. Shy and quirky as a child, he was sent to boarding school to toughen up and continued the line of multigenerational academic achievement and emotional unavailability. The parents hoped therapy would support Flora in developing the social and communication skills they valued highly and thought she was lacking.

I held my breath when I first saw Flora, and that congested sensation in my chest reminded me of how Alice described her little sister as frozen during our initial phone conversation. The code name Flora came just then, carrying the juicy, blooming energy of early springtime flowers, as if I needed to hold on to it to feel again. She looked tall for her age, yet was so delicately built that it felt like I might blow her away with a sigh. With her pearly pale, makeup-free face surrounded by dark blonde, wavy hair, she looked uncannily graceful—less Disney's Sleeping Beauty, more a gothic Madonna. Her speech was strikingly rigid, however, like the wood these Madonnas were made of in the Middle Ages. She spoke rarely, her thin lips tight and eyes looking down, initially limiting her answers to my questions to "fine", "awkward", or "I don't know how to say it". Her voice was flat, wispy, and somewhat guttural, words coming out in fast, chopped, and muffled bursts, often additionally blocked by her hand, which she used to cover her mouth.

We worked in a small room devoid of typical child psychotherapy trinkets, the only one available at the time she could make. I brought my own capsule collection of postcards, story cubes, and sand-tray miniatures, fearing I was offering an impoverished experience. But Flora seemed content, and each week, for months, chose the same lilac pencil and a piece of A4 paper, my box untouched in the corner. She sat stiffly at the edge of her chair, not once brushing the chair's backrest or arms. I often thought of that air cushion surrounding her, ensuring distance to objects, material and human, and how this tiny, barely furnished room might actually add to that safety too.

Flora is an anglicised version of the Gaelic Fionnghuala. The name comes with a story of a young princess turned into a swan and banished to a remote, freezing exile for nine hundred years by her stepmother Aoife, jealous of Fionnghuala's warm, loving attachment to her father. In return, angry at his new wife's deed, King Lir turned Aoife into a terrifying demon of the air. The name also means "white" or "fair shoulder". Its significance will make sense later. For now, it is suffice to say that a shoulder happened to be involved in a pivotal moment for my understanding of Flora's therapeutic process: my shoulder that signalled Flora's pain; Flora's shoulder that she thought was ugly; and finally, a blemished shoulder of one of the creatures she drew—admittedly, not a swan like in Fionnghuala's story, but a winged horse.

I knew only a few bits about Flora's background. Her mother was in the middle of a big translation project and could not be distracted, so sent Alice to accompany Flora to the assessment instead and quietly deflected my further attempts at contact. Her father was out of reach entirely, spending working days in Oxford, where the family owned a small, comfortable flat. It was Alice who sorted out payments and parental consent and emailed occasional updates about the home situation. Parental absence felt keen, and I often wondered how lonely Flora must have been in their big house in North London, shared with her busy mother and bright and gregarious sister, too old for mutual interests except for Taylor Swift's music, which they all loved, seeing Dad only on weekends. I mirrored her desertion in how frustrated and resigned I frequently felt in my role as her therapist, as if I were an incompetent fixer or unimpressive entertainer, and wondered if some of it could be how she felt.

Alice briefly mentioned Mum's brief postnatal depression, as well as Gina Ford's method (1999), which her parents eagerly followed, their anxiety reassured by its promise of training the baby to disciplined sleep and feed by controlling the time and silencing frustration by leaving the baby to cry. Alice was born when they were young and aspiring. With their careers established, there was less tolerance for entropy, so the needs of their second baby had to be quickly contained. Little Flora was described as a healthy, shy, and rather unproblematic child who only threw occasional tantrums, especially around joining her family at restaurant dinners, private views, and other social outings. To somewhat placate her paternal grandparents, the family, unused to children's unruly behaviour, turned it into a joke, nicknaming her Spike after one of the main characters from her beloved TV series *My Little Pony*—a baby dragon who had fiery hiccups and belched out green flame.

Mapping the territory

My interest in somatic countertransference is grounded in the concept of "emotional revolution" (Schore, 2014, n.p.). Schore proposed this term for a paradigm shift across various disciplines towards acknowledging that affects determine all areas that constitute who we are. Following this new paradigm, it takes five steps to explain why feelings matter. One, feelings are not fluffy ideas that belong to an abstract realm of thoughts or images represented through language but are grounded in specific, describable bodily sensations. Two, feelings constitute a part of a broader system of reactions to, and indicators of, experience and thus determine a sense of self. Three, feelings are relational, meaning they are co-created, shared, and communicated between interacting individuals. Four, their transmission is embodied. It occurs on the unconscious level of body-to-body communication before it reaches consciousness and can become symbolised and verbalised. Five, and most importantly for this chapter, an ability to attune to this somatic relay is what makes for a sense of connection and healing.

Translating these five theoretical principles to clinical actions allows us to envisage how to use somatic countertransference to enhance affective communication with our clients. One, how do I recognise when my client embodies a feeling? Two, how do I make sense of the sensation the client evoked in me? Three, how do I realise its relational potential? Four, what is the nature of that relational space? And five, how can I use it to attune to the client?

Figure 2.1 summarises these steps. It is an outcome of my theoretical research in which I reviewed twenty articles discussing the adult therapist's somatic experience during therapeutic process, focusing on those that were frequently cross-referenced and freely available online or directly from the authors (Raczynska, 2019). I excluded the only two articles on that subject in child psychotherapy I could find at that time as not sufficient to make the sample, and only later grounded my core findings in the available literature on general countertransference in child work. The sample ultimately consisted of mostly qualitative, phenomenological research studies and practice-based publications: seventeen published in peer-reviewed journals (Samuels, 1985; Orbach, 1995, 2004; Shaw, 2004; Stone, 2006; Dosamantes-Beaudry, 2007; Forester, 2007; Egan & Carr, 2008; Vulcan, 2009; Booth, Trimble, & Egan, 2010; Athanasiadou & Halewood, 2011; Gubb, 2014; Lemma, 2014; Margarian, 2015; Martini, 2016; Hartung & Steinbrecher, 2018; Godsil, 2018), one as a book chapter (Orbach & Carroll, 2006), one in a post-conference publication (Schellinski, 2013), and, finally, an expanded blog post on a respected website (Orbach, 2012).

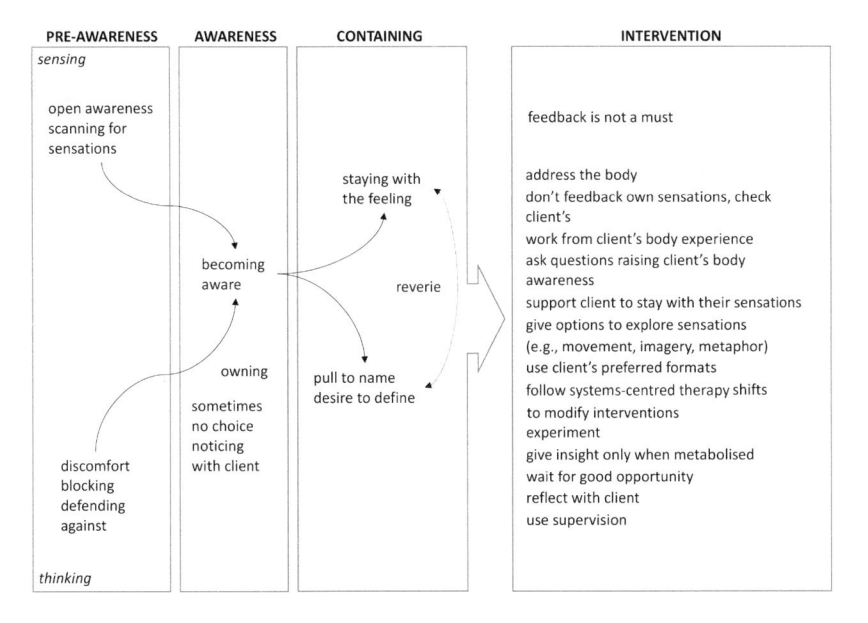

PRE-AWARENESS	AWARENESS	CONTAINING	INTERVENTION
sensing			
open awareness scanning for sensations		staying with the feeling	feedback is not a must
	becoming aware		address the body don't feedback own sensations, check client's work from client's body experience ask questions raising client's body awareness
		reverie	support client to stay with their sensations give options to explore sensations (e.g., movement, imagery, metaphor)
	owning	pull to name desire to define	use client's preferred formats follow systems-centred therapy shifts to modify interventions experiment
	sometimes no choice noticing with client		give insight only when metabolised wait for good opportunity reflect with client
discomfort blocking defending against			use supervision
thinking			

Figure 2.1 Stages of managing somatic countertransference (SCT) in adult therapy

The therapist begins working with somatic countertransference before it enters her awareness, that is, before she registers specific physical symptoms. Two different states of mind may alert the therapist to recognise such dynamics. She may notice physical discomfort and the urge to defend against it because of a lack of awareness (Schellinski, 2013), embarrassment, unresolved issues, poor experience, or insufficient training or supervision (Athanasiadou & Halewood, 2011). Consequently, somatic signalling puts the therapist into her mind and activates its defences. Alternatively, the therapist may be actively looking for the signals of embodied communication using "open awareness, scanning for sensations" (Forester, 2007, p. 127) when she feels grounded enough to stay in the body.

Obviously, it helps if the therapist has "the ability to reflect on somatic experience" (Forester, 2007). Nonetheless, both ways of becoming aware of embodied dynamics prove effective, even if the therapist feels she has no choice but to own her physical states (Athanasiadou & Halewood, 2011). Tuning in to the arising sensations does not have to mean "feeling in tune" with the client (Samuels, 1985, p. 53). Feeling harmoniously connected in countertransference is not required to gain access to the client's experience. It is the capacity to attune to somatic states, whatever they are, that is essential. Otherwise, the therapist cannot follow the client in their process, especially when the latter dissociates (Egan & Carr, 2008).

Once aware that something is physically "babbling" (Martini, 2016, p. 8), the therapist enters the stage of containing. There, she finds herself pulled in two different directions again: to stay with the observed sensation or to move on to understanding it. Forester (2007) shows that even somatically conscious therapists feel the desire to react and quickly nail, name, and define what they are sensing—to know the story. She argues, however, that recognising her defensive urge to flee from the feeling allows the therapist to stay curious instead of rushing to interpretation.

Ultimately, these two energies—to experience and to understand—can be harnessed in reverie, when the therapist engages in internally oscillating between feeling and thinking, between "symbol as image and symbol in the body" (Schellinski, 2013, n.p.). This way, she gradually becomes able to gauge the nature of the sometimes uncomfortable or overwhelming sensation she is experiencing against the backdrop of the client's affective material and story. The capacity to stay in the reverie seems to be an essential stage in exploiting somatic countertransference. It allows the therapist to hold and contain the client's raw and unbearable energy. Taking her time and internal space, the therapist digests the affective communication she is receiving (Forester, 2007; Gubb, 2014; Lemma, 2014; Martini, 2016), relying on her imagination to translate from the somatic to the symbolic (Schellinski, 2013).

Once ready, if only tentatively, the therapist can now choose how to return the client's somatic transmission she has absorbed and digested. The spectrum of possible interventions spreads from suppressing it to verbally interpreting embodied communication back to the client. These two extreme responses are rarely used in a clear-cut form. The former is seen as a defence against the intensity of somatic communication that is potentially harmful to the therapist, the client, and the process. In the realm of adult therapy, interpreting somatic countertransference, on the other hand, seems widely accepted. Nonetheless, it also comes with caveats and conditions, which are a significant part of the possible interventions listed in the last column of Figure 2.1.

Interestingly, feedback as such is not a universal requirement—unlike the awareness of and ability to survive the intensity of somatic communication by staying regulated. That is what sustains connectedness and enables the client to experience relating (Orbach & Carroll, 2006; Martini, 2016). Orbach (2004) recommends holding one's physical sensations in mind and waiting for a good opportunity to respond. Carroll adds that feedback can come in many forms, varying from interpretations to images to noticing body states, and argues that the therapist needs to adjust the form of feedback to the client's "preferred sense (vision, hearing, and proprioception) and a preferred mode of access" (Orbach & Carroll, 2006), integrating it, for example, through spontaneous movement, dream work, or talking. Stone (2006) adds that instead of feeding back sensations such as feeling suffocated, the therapist may use his experience as an inspiration to check with the client what is happening in the corresponding part of their body—the client's chest, in his case. The therapist may also check with her client whether her somatic intuitions are meaningful for them (Shaw, 2004; Martini, 2016) or offer interpretations in small chunks to verify that resonance (Lemma, 2014). Interpreting somatic countertransference too early can lead to adverse outcomes, including premature termination of the therapy (Shaw, 2004; Godsil, 2018).

Most clinicians tend to focus on selected aspects of managing somatic countertransference within a session or case, but sometimes a full sequence emerges (Dosamantes-Beaudry, 2007; Forester, 2007; Lemma, 2014; Martini, 2016; Godsil, 2018; Hartung & Steinbrecher, 2018). Far from being clean and direct, it involves messy miscommunications, half-expressed intuitions, and unobvious meanings. Schellinski (2013), for example, describes how she asks her client to elaborate on a particular part of their story that evoked her physical reaction. Then she observes her inner response to this new material and how it increases the strength of her physical symptom. She feeds back to the client her sensation, checks what is going on in their body, and then asks another clarifying question. Following that, she hears the client respond with an insight—able to connect to something previously inaccessible. Finally, she observes the disappearance of her somatic symptom.

Grounding therapeutic work in the body facilitates, Carroll says, the client's increased awareness "of sensory elements, impulses, breathing, feelings and defences" (Orbach & Carroll, 2006, p. 63). It allows the therapist to assist the client in the difficult task of staying with their sensations instead of evading them, and to investigate them safely through movement, imagery, or metaphor (Dosamantes-Beaudry, 2007). Orbach stresses that the therapist must keep her focus on the client's body and not rush into searching for symbolic meanings of physical needs (1995, 2004, 2012).

Consequently, the body of the therapist can serve several different purposes in this process. It can work as a "diagnostic tool" (Orbach & Carroll, 2006, p. 74), which Orbach describes as "if I'm feeling this, it's either a version of what you are feeling or it's what you need" (Orbach & Carroll, 2006). It can become the "auxiliary" body (Orbach, 2004, pp. 144–145) to contain the split-off aspects of the client's physical self. It can function as a transitional object (Dosamantes-Beaudry, 2007; cf. Winnicott, 1953) when the client uses the therapist as an extension of their self during more regressed stages of their therapeutic process. Finally, the therapist can use her body to regulate the client (Martini, 2016), similarly to how a mother takes a few deep breaths to ground herself when calming down her child from a tantrum. In my work with Flora, my body did it all.

Case study: solid ground

Flora's childhood love for ponies grew into a continued interest in researching and sketching winged horses. She drew many in our sessions, and it evolved from Winnicott's squiggle game (1968), which I once softly offered to shift a moment of wooden silence. My nervous system could tolerate it, but I felt it was too much for Flora. Her gaze became glazed, her breath indiscernible. As if in response, my forehead went heavy, and my mind played the familiar G–E♭–A♭–B♭ sound of a PC shutdown. Flora's body—via mine—was signalling that she was out of her already narrow window of tolerance.

Siegel (1999) describes this as an optimal level of excitation in the nervous system that allows one to stay connected with one's experience instead of crashing into hyper- or hypo-arousal. Although therapy needs to hover around these edges to gradually expand the client's tolerance and capacity to regulate, it must also stay within this window to be safe—there is no work done with the nervous system offline.

Flora was going hypo and needed some up-regulation—but it had to be very gentle so as not to extinguish her arousal completely. Her mother was emotionally unavailable when depressed or immersed in her work but also commanding around Flora's early routines of feeding, sleeping, and sociability. It suggested that baby Flora's capacity to learn how to regulate her arousal, through interacting with the other, who would attune to her emotional states and accordingly spark her *up* or calm her *down* (Stern, 1985, pp. 196–197), was compromised from both ends: not only neglected but occasionally hijacked too. As a result, Flora learnt to curb her awareness and expression of her own emotional needs to avoid the pain of unbearable, unrealistic longing for having them met—or failing to compete with Mum's. As a result, she could tolerate an extremely narrow range of affective experience, including that coming from others.

Drawing her favourite creatures allowed her to stay in her comfort zone. Each one took most of the session, leaving about ten to fifteen minutes to talk. She sketched in silence, meticulously, not taking her eyes off her work. She tolerated my "So, who is this one today?" and then patiently explained its mythical origins, features, and qualities. Those were the rare moments when words flowed, even though her speech and body remained stiff, and I often thought about how this buffer against the pressure of surviving the therapeutic hour was also a bridge to her own affective experience, communicated through her delicately outlined and intricately ornate flying creatures.

Wise children

Schowalter issued his widely cross-referenced call to reappraise countertransference in child psychotherapy in the same year—1985—as Samuels pioneered the inclusion of embodied countertransference in mainstream therapy. It was also the year when Zbigniew Religa performed the first successful heart transplant surgery in Poland, where I was born. I appreciate how these two parallel calls to incorporate children and the body into transferential thinking coincide temporally and how the act of transferring the heart as a physical organ from one body to another symbolises this correspondence. Consequently, I want to argue that all countertransference is embodied by nature, and suggest that every time the term "countertransference" is used in the therapeutic context, especially in child therapy (but not limited to it), it connotes an integrated psychosomatic experience. In what follows, therefore, I discuss the fundamental qualities of child psychotherapy that convey its inherently embodied nature. Then I consider how the management of somatic countertransference differs in work with young people from adult therapy, referring to Figure 2.1.

The nature of child psychotherapy exceeds language. Play and creativity go beyond the limit of ideas expressed through words; action outweighs reflection (Schowalter, 1985; Anastasopoulos & Tsiantis, 1996). Also, play demands physical proximity, which shortens the spatial and clinical distance between the client and the therapist, making their relational experience more immediate (Holder, 1996). Children's capacity to mentalize is developmentally limited (Luyten & Fonagy, 2015), especially if their carers have failed to model it (Fonagy & Allison, 2012). Therefore, young people tend to stick to their primary process: instinctual and unconscious, closer to dream work or psychotic dynamics (Ekstein & Wallerstein, 1956; Anastasopoulos & Tsiantis, 1996; Benveniste, 2005). Consequently, their natural and often healthy defence mechanisms can feel as forceful as those of adult psychotic clients, resulting from the intense use of splitting and projective identification (Benveniste, 2005; Anastasopoulos & Tsiantis, 1996). Finally, weaker containment of child aggression and sexuality increase the likelihood of the therapist's regression (Schowalter, 1985). This means that the energies the child unleashes can activate the practitioner's own unresolved early wounding, parenting dynamics, and sibling relations, especially if she has children who are close to her client's age or have similar problems (Schowalter, 1985; Anastasopoulos & Tsiantis, 1996).

As a result, the child psychotherapist is for the most part faced with "communication by impact" (Casement, 1985, p. 72; Boehmer, 2010); that is, embodied transmission of affects, similar in its nature to how an infant conveys her experience to her mother (Bion, 1962; Stern, 1985). This is consistent with Stone's (2006) suggestion that borderline, narcissistic, or psychotic clients rely on somatic countertransference to communicate their experience. Consequently, the feelings children evoke in their therapists tend to be more extreme than those aroused by adult clients (Abbate, 1964; Schowalter, 1985; Anastasopoulos & Tsiantis, 1996).

Nonetheless, for the sake of the healing process, the therapist, like the mother, has to find ways of surviving such intensity.

At the same time, however, it is harder for the child therapist to metabolise her client's material when she is on all fours escaping a roaring lion or hiding from ghosts under a dark blanket. Often, there is no time to reflect with a child who cannot sit still (Anastasopoulos & Tsiantis, 1996) nor space enough to verify therapeutic processing with one whose expression is thwarted by anxiety. As a result, the child psychotherapist rarely has a chance to properly immerse herself in the reverie, the critical stage in employing embodied awareness.

Two other aspects of work with children modify the management of somatic countertransference in comparison to adult therapy. These are the presence of the child's primary objects—parents, siblings, or grandparents—and the sensitivity around interpretation and feedback.

Mothers and fathers are literally present in the life of our young clients and thus liable to exert explicit and implicit pressures on the therapist and the therapeutic process (Godfrind, 1996; see also Schowalter, 1985; Anastasopoulos & Tsiantis, 1996; Holder, 1996; Sandler, 1996). Even the ghostly presence of carers, those emotionally absent or lost through adoption or bereavement (Freiberg, Andelson, & Shapiro, 1975) and the child's institutional environment (Schowalter, 1985) can influence transferential processes.

It is vital, therefore, that the therapist reflects on the parental fantasies, projections, or unresolved wounding, as well as on her own feelings that are evoked when, for example, she identifies or competes with a parent (Schowalter, 1985). Somatic awareness provides extra support in this process: it allows the therapist to understand not just how it used to be for the client to be cared for (Bollas, 1987) but how it still may be for them in the present moment.

The second difference stems from the general discussion in the field of child psychotherapy about whether to interpret countertransference or not. Although Schowalter (1985) argues against it, I think a more nuanced approach may be useful. In the end, this is what our clients need from us—that we contain their unbearable feelings, find ways to return them in a digested, transformed, and more bearable form. I present the main principles of such a framework below, integrating arguments offered by Ekstein and Wallerstein (1956), Alvarez (1996), and Music (2018).

Alvarez (1996) says that interpreting countertransference with children relies on the therapist's capacity to consider the impact of her feedback, namely how the child may react to it, disregarding what the therapist intended. Depending on the child's needs and degree of vulnerability, she suggests, the therapist may choose from the following three options.

One, she can decide to give back the part the child projected and reflect on it together, providing the child is psychologically strong enough and can make use of it (Alvarez, 1996). Ekstein and Wallerstein (1956) are useful in expanding this option. They argue that, depending on the strength of the child's ego, the therapist must choose whether she stays in the primary process, and thus interprets within the metaphor created by the child through art or play, or reaches out to the secondary process by linking to the client's reality. Two, the therapist may decide to hold the client's painful experience, if returning it has the potential to drain the child of energy (Alvarez, 1996). Three, she may actively enact an affect that the child is not yet capable of feeling but needs to experience to thrive (Alvarez, 1996). Music (2018) gives concrete examples of what the latter may include, referring to neglected clients who, like Flora, come across as deadened and need their aliveness to be addressed in the first place. To split off their distress, they inhibit all feelings, so the therapist first needs to model for them how these affects look, sound, and feel, to make the work on dissociated parts possible.

Alvarez argues that the therapist in the latter scenario serves the role of "almost an auxiliary id, carrying the patient's sense of being alive" (1996, p. 117). It links to Orbach's concept, presented earlier, of the auxiliary body that the therapist provides to contain her client's basic aliveness before any deeper processing can take place (2004, 2012).

Figure 2.2 integrates the main aspects of working with somatic countertransference in adult therapy with the discussion of its specific nature in work with children. I suggest that the process of managing embodied countertransference in child psychotherapy is generally similar to adult work, flowing from pre-awareness to awareness to containing to intervention. Also, some of the methods adult therapists use to somatically attune to their clients can be easily implemented in work with children. Or perhaps I should say many of them have been in use there already, especially in gestalt work (Oaklander, 1978, 1997, 2006), simply without the label of somatic countertransference.

Nonetheless, managing embodied communication in child psychotherapy differs in two respects. First, the stage of containing is messier and in need of stronger holding thanks to the therapist's immediate engagement in her client's process and the third-party transferential influence of the carers. Second, the child psychotherapist must assess the impact of countertransference-based feedback and decide where to locate it (Alvarez, 1996): hold it in herself, return it to the client—and if so, on which level, primary or secondary—or enact it on the child's behalf (Alvarez, 1996; Ekstein & Wallerstein, 1956; Music, 2018). This is not to say that adult therapists spill out their interpretations, but to emphasise the imperative nature of this choice in child psychotherapy.

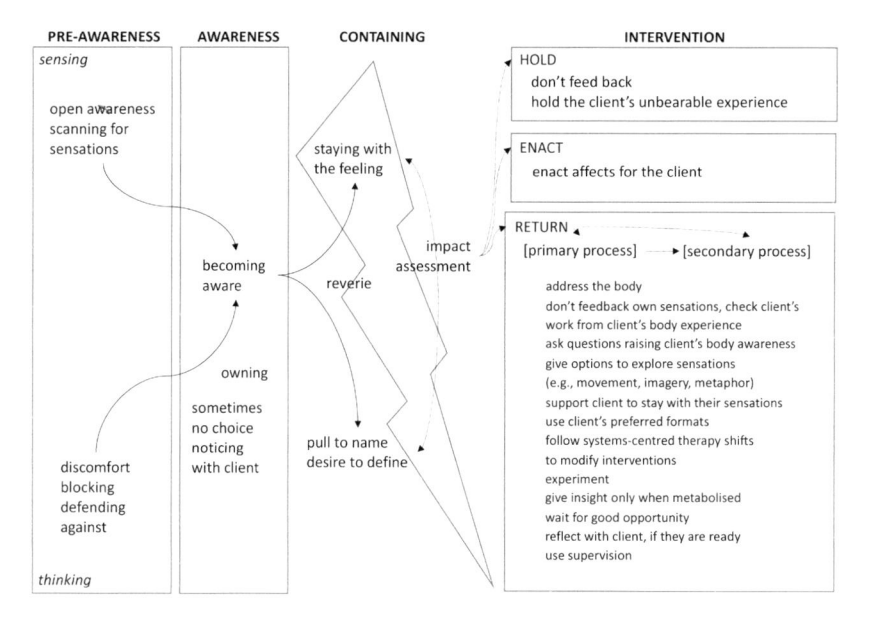

PRE-AWARENESS	AWARENESS	CONTAINING	INTERVENTION
sensing			**HOLD** — don't feed back; hold the client's unbearable experience
open awareness scanning for sensations		staying with the feeling	**ENACT** — enact affects for the client
	becoming aware	reverie	**RETURN** — [primary process] → [secondary process]
		impact assessment	address the body
	owning		don't feedback own sensations, check client's
			work from client's body experience
	sometimes no choice noticing with client	pull to name desire to define	ask questions raising client's body awareness
			give options to explore sensations (e.g., movement, imagery, metaphor)
discomfort blocking defending against			support client to stay with their sensations
			use client's preferred formats
			follow systems-centred therapy shifts to modify interventions
			experiment
			give insight only when metabolised
			wait for good opportunity
			reflect with client, if they are ready
thinking			use supervision

Figure 2.2 Stages of managing somatic countertransference (SCT) in child therapy

Case study: the scales of integration

Two winged horses were her favourites—East Asian Qianlima, who was so exceptionally elegant and fast that no human was allowed to ride her, and impossibly majestic and always white Pegasus, who carried Zeus's thunderbolts. For weeks and weeks, Flora drew different variants of these two to show me how it felt when she was "fine". They could also be discontented sometimes when something did not feel right, clapping their wings then, their noble faces frowning and their hooves up. She could not say what it was that made them feel this way, however.

A few months into our work, Flora drew a baby Pegasus. Curled in fear as his wings were tiny and not strong enough to fly in escape, he was alone in his lair, attacked by the Chimera, a hybrid, fire-blowing monster whose body was a composite of different animals: a lion with a goat's head and a snake's tail. I thought then that Flora was possibly integrating the fear of her mother, who felt patchy in her unpredictable pattern of absence and dominance. I also remembered how Flora was called Spike as a child, after that baby dragon who hiccupped fireballs, and wondered if she was getting ready to meet her own anger at last. It was too early to feed back, but I felt very satisfied with my capacity to link my client's symbolism to possible meanings.

The following session started as usual. Flora lightly sketched a typical silhouette and went on to add detail. By then, I was used to her sometimes putting more care into the head or the legs, while other times the wings, eyes, or hooves stood out. I learnt to look at it as if it was a map of her body and inner parts that felt more alive, but trying to feed it back to her was predictably met with "I don't know" or silence. But this time, something was different. She was adding tiny scales around the wings' roots.

The next twenty minutes felt like agony. Flora kept painstakingly drawing one lilac scale after another, one lilac scale at a time, adding lilac shading here, lilac shading there. Scaling trickled from the creature's shoulders down to its belly, then to its knees, finally to its rear. Only the head and hooves were free of it. All this time, I was sitting in my chair, feeling my right shoulder involuntarily twisting and pulling me upwards and back. It felt blunt, persistent, unbearable. I could not control it, in the same way, I realised, that I could not control the psoriasis that spread all over my body, except my face, hands, and feet, when I was a teenager. Like Flora's lilac scales. A sense of disgust filled me, similar to how I felt about myself all those years ago. Not normal, but different, deformed.

Yet I kept breathing, pressing my feet against the floor, quietly observing my sensations, and deciding to bridge my "back then" with Flora's "here and now". When she finished, I commented on how different her winged horse looked this time and wondered how it was for her to draw this hybrid look. Flora took a deep breath and, suddenly speaking so fast she was swallowing the ends of her words, she said that it was a Chinese Tianma who had dragon scales and could sweat blood. And that there were other flying horses she hated because they were deformed, made of mixed-up, unmatching parts. Hindu Uchchaihshravas, snow-white but with seven heads. Islamic Buraq with long ears and a human face. And, finally, a proper chimera, Greek Hippalektryon, half-horse and half-rooster. Not only did she know these complex words but also taught me how to spell them.

I thought about the scales in the context of skin defences (Bick, 1968), the fear of one's skin being poked or intruded upon by the other trying to enter their system, like Flora's mother, to control or to merge, and the related need to swell, coarsen, and thicken to prevent it. How the carer, if not attuned, can be felt as one who either abandons or enwraps and entraps.

It surely made sense, but I decided to stay with the original sense of deformity my shoulder still radiated and enact it as a possible feeling. It was risky, considering how close it was to my adolescent experience. Using my light and playful tone of voice to up-regulate her by lifting the affects in the room at the same time, I told Flora that "—Oh gosh …", what she said made me remember how terribly awkward I felt sometimes when I was her age, my body growing in ways I thought awfully weird, as if different parts had their own life, and if she ever experienced anything similar. I wanted to convey that she was not alone. For the first time, she did not shrug off my linking. She quietly said that she hated how she was towering above other girls at school, but especially her shoulders, thin and protruding, and how this made her want to hide and initially avoid PE, then school altogether.

Trust your gut

Countertransference in child psychotherapy is a paradox. On the one hand, the therapist has no choice but to rely on countertransference's psychosomatic signalling to understand the child's inner and outer relational experience (Schowalter, 1985; Anastasopoulos & Tsiantis, 1996; Trowell, 1996). On the other, it is more intense, direct, and physical than in adult therapy and thus more difficult to process and contain. Adding to this Stone's (2006) finding that most of us therapists tend to dissociate sensory information that our environment provides for the sake of exploring our inner reality, as I initially did until my body hiccupped the ball of disgust, it seems urgent therefore to include reflection on somatic countertransference in child psychotherapeutic training and supervision.

Flora's autistic defences most likely came up in response to insecure attachments she formed owing to the ruptured bond with her mother and general family dynamics. Yet it was meeting her where she was with her adolescent worries about her looks and how her body felt that made for the shift in our work. Without trusting my guts—that is, somatic countertransference—I could have missed it, trapped in my cognitive smugness, in a way, repeating the original harm. In the months following that sickening session, she told me she liked word games, and we played them for weeks. Then came astrology, Flora telling me all she knew about her constellation and mine. Then she became excited about personality types and kept testing us both using different questionnaires. In the next few months, she talked about her new friendships, crushes, heartbreaks, and not being sure if she wanted to study art, as her sister had, or psychology. Although her ways remained rigid and uncanny, she was back from her frozen exile, able and willing to relate. But that is another story.

References

Abbate, G. M. (1964). Child analysis at different developmental stages. *Journal of the American Psychoanalytic Association*, *12*(1), 135–150.

Alvarez, A. (1996). Different uses of the countertransference with neurotic, borderline, and psychotic patients. In: J. Tsiantis, A. Sandler, D. Anastasopoulos & B. Martindale (Eds.), *Countertransference in Psychoanalytic Psychotherapy with Children and Adolescents* (pp. 111–124). London: Karnac.

Anastasopoulos, D., & Tsiantis, J. (1996). Countertransference issues in psychoanalytic psychotherapy with children and adolescents: A brief review. In: J. Tsiantis, A. Sandler, D. Anastasopoulos & B. Martindale (Eds.), *Countertransference in Psychoanalytic Psychotherapy with Children and Adolescents* (pp. 1–36). London: Karnac.

Athanasiadou, C., & Halewood, A. (2011). A grounded theory exploration of therapists' experiences of somatic phenomena in the countertransference. *European Journal of Psychotherapy & Counselling*, *13*(3): 247–262.

Benveniste, D. (2005). Recognizing defenses in the drawings and play of children in therapy. *Psychoanalytic Psychology, 22*(3): 395–410.

Bick, E. (1968). The experience of the skin in early object relations. *International Journal of Psychoanalysis, 49*: 484–486.

Bion, W. R. (1962). *Learning from Experience*. London: Maresfield Library.

Boehmer, M. W. (2010). "Communication by impact" and other forms of non-verbal communication: A review of transference, counter-transference and projective identification. *African Journal of Psychiatry, 13*(3): 179–183.

Bollas, C. (1987). *The Shadow of the Object: Psychoanalysis of the Unthought Known* (30th anniversary edition). London and New York: Routledge.

Booth, A., Trimble, T., & Egan, J. (2010). Body-centred counter-transference in a sample of Irish clinical psychologists. *Psychologist, 35*(12): 284–289.

Brothers, D., & Sletvord, J. (2022). *Embodied Psychoanalytic Revisioning of Theory*. Live webinar. 15 July. Confer, https://www.confer.uk.com/event/concepts.html?utm_medium=email&utm_source=newsletter&utm_campaign=concepts

Carleton, J. A. (2009). Somatic treatment of attachment issues: Applying neuroscientific and experimental research to the clinical situation. Online article. Viewed 16 August 2018, http://www.jacquelineacarletonphd.com/text/pdfs/somatictreatmentofattachmentissues.pdf

Case, C. (2005). *Imagining Animals. Art, Psychotherapy and Primitive States of Mind*. London: Routledge.

Casement, P. (1985). *On Learning from the Patient*. London: Routledge.

Dosamantes-Beaudry, I. (2007). Somatic transference and countertransference in psychoanalytic intersubjective dance/movement therapy. *American Journal of Dance Therapy, 29*(2): 73–89.

Egan, J., & Carr, A. (2008). Body-centred countertransference in female trauma therapists. *Eisteacht, 8*(1), 24–27. Online article. Viewed 8 August 2018, https://www.researchgate.net/publication/235779891_Body-centred_countertransference_in_female_trauma_therapists, n.p.

Ekstein, R., & Wallerstein, J. (1956). Observations on the psychotherapy of borderline and psychotic children. *The Psychoanalytic Study of the Child, 11*(1): 303–311.

Field, N. (1988). Listening with the body: An exploration in the countertransference. *British Journal of Psychotherapy, 5*(4): 512–522.

Fisher, J. (2017). *Healing the Fragmented Selves of Trauma Survivors: Overcoming Internal Self-Alienation*. New York: Routledge.

Fonagy, P., & Allison, E. (2012). What is mentalization? The concept and its foundations in developmental research. In: N. Midgley & I. Vrouva (Eds.), *Minding the Child: Mentalization-Based Interventions with Children, Young People and their Families* (pp. 11–34). London: Routledge.

Ford, G. (1999). *Contented Little Baby Book*. New York: Random House.

Fordham, M. (1987). *The Self and Autism*. London: Karnac.

Forester, C. (2007). Your own body of wisdom: Recognizing and working with somatic countertransference with dissociative and traumatized patients. *Body, Movement and Dance in Psychotherapy*, 2(2): 123–133.

Freiberg, S., Andelson, E., & Shapiro, V. (1975). Ghosts in the nursery: A psychoanalytic approach to the problems of impaired infant–mother relationships. *Journal of the American Academy of Child Psychiatry*, 14(3): 387–421.

Godfrind, J. (1996). The influence of the presence of parents on the countertransference of the child psychotherapist. In: J. Tsiantis, A. Sandler, D. Anastasopoulos & B. Martindale (Eds.), *Countertransference in Psychoanalytic Psychotherapy with Children and Adolescents* (pp. 95–110). London: Karnac.

Godsil, G. (2018). Residues in the analyst of the patient's symbiotic connection at a somatic level: Unrepresented states in the patient and analyst. *Journal of Analytical Psychology*, 63(1): 6–25.

Gubb, K. (2014). Craving interpretation: A case of somatic countertransference. *British Journal of Psychotherapy*, 30(1): 51–67.

Hartung, T., & Steinbrecher, M. (2018). From somatic pain to psychic pain: The body in the psychoanalytic field. *The International Journal of Psychoanalysis*, 99(1): 159–180.

Holder, A. (1996). Reflections on transference, countertransference, session frequency, and the psychoanalytic process. In: J. Tsiantis, A. Sandler, D. Anastasopoulos & B. Martindale (Eds.), *Countertransference in Psychoanalytic Psychotherapy with Children and Adolescents* (pp. 51–68). London: Karnac.

Lemma, A. (2014). The body of the analyst and the analytic setting: Reflections on the embodied setting and the symbiotic transference. *The International Journal of Psychoanalysis*, 95(2): 225–244.

Luyten, P., & Fonagy, P. (2015). The neurobiology of mentalizing. *Personality Disorders: Theory, Research, and Treatment*, 6(4): 366–379.

Margarian, A. (2015). Somatic countertransference: A Chinese perspective. *Psychoanalysis and Psychotherapy in China*, 1: 63–77.

Martini, S. (2016). Embodying analysis: The body and the therapeutic process. *Journal of Analytical Psychology, 61*(1): 5–23.

Music, G. (2018). Neglect and its neglect: Developmental science, psychoanalytic thinking, and countertransference vitality. In: C. Bonovitz & A. Harlem (Eds.), *Developmental Perspectives in Child Psychoanalysis and Psychotherapy* (pp. 73–95). London: Routledge.

Oaklander, V. (1978). *Windows to Our Children: A Gestalt Therapy Approach to Children and Adolescents*. Moab, UT: Real People Press.

Oaklander, V. (1997). The therapeutic process with children and adolescents. *Gestalt Review, 1*(4): 292–317.

Oaklander, V. (2006). *Hidden Treasure: A Map to the Child's Inner Self*. London: Karnac.

Ogden, P. (2020). Personal communication. Understanding and addressing hopelessness & helplessness through the lens of sensorimotor therapy. Online webinar with Pat Ogden and Bonnie Goldstein. 11 April. Sensorimotor Therapy Institute.

Ogden, P., & Fisher, J. (2015). *Sensorimotor Psychotherapy: Interventions for Trauma and Attachment* (Norton Series on Interpersonal Neurobiology. Cam edition). London: W. W. Norton.

Orbach, S. (1995). Countertransference and the false body. *Winnicott Studies: The Journal of The Squiggle Foundation, 10*: 3–13.

Orbach, S. (2004). What can we learn from the therapist's body? *Attachment & Human Development, 6*(2): 141–150.

Orbach, S. (2012). There is no such thing as a body. *Psychotherapy Excellence*. Online article. Viewed 16 August 2018, https://www.psychotherapyexcellence.com/blog/read-listing/2012/november/there-is-no-such-thing-as-a-body

Orbach, S., & Carroll, R. (2006). Contemporary approaches to the body in psychotherapy: Two psychotherapists in dialogue. In: J. Corrigall, H. Payne & H. Wilkinson (Eds.), *About a Body: The Embodied Psychotherapist* (pp. 63–82). Hove: Brunner-Routledge.

Payne, P., Levine, P. A., & Crane-Godreau, M. A. (2015). Somatic experiencing: Using interception and proprioception as core elements of trauma therapy. *Frontiers in Psychology, 6*(93): 1–18.

Raczynska, M. (2019). The practice of somatic countertransference: Creating the context for using in in child psychotherapy. Unpublished manuscript.

MA Dissertation, MA in Integrative Child and Adolescent Psychotherapy and Counselling. London: Terapia and Middlesex University.

Samuels, A. (1985). Countertransference, the "mundus imaginalis" and a research project. *Journal of Analytical Psychology, 30*: 47–71.

Sandler, A.-M. (1996). Some problems in transference and countertransference in child and adolescent analysis. In: J. Tsiantis, A. Sandler, D. Anastasopoulos & B. Martindale (Eds.), *Countertransference in Psychoanalytic Psychotherapy with Children and Adolescents* (pp. 69–88). London: Karnac.

Schellinski, K. (2013). When psyche mutters through matter: Reflections on somatic countertransference. In: E. Krehl (Ed.), *Copenhagen 2013: 100 Years On: Origins, Innovation, and Controversies*. Proceedings of the 19th Congress of the International Association for Analytical Psychology. Daimon Verlag: Am Klosterplats. Viewed 14 September 2018, https://bit.ly/2UmonJi, n.p.

Schore, A. N. (2001). Effects of a secure attachment relationship on right brain development, affect regulation, and infant mental health. *Infant Mental Health Journal, 22*(1–2): 7–66.

Schore, A. N. (2009). Right brain affect regulation: An essential mechanism of development, trauma, dissociation, and psychotherapy. In: D. Fosha, D. J. Siegel & M. Solomon (Eds.), *The Healing Power of Emotion: Affective Neuroscience, Development and Clinical Practice* (pp. 112–144). New York: W. W. Norton.

Schore, A. N. (2014). The science of the art of psychotherapy. Masterclass with Allan Schore. 26 September. Terapia Centre, RAF Museum, London.

Schowalter, J. E. (1985). Countertransference in work with children: Review of a neglected concept. *Journal of the American Academy of Child Psychiatry, 25*(1): 40–45.

Shaw, R. (2004). The embodied psychotherapist: An exploration of the therapists' somatic phenomena within the therapeutic encounter. *Psychotherapy Research, 14*(3): 271–288.

Siegel, D. (1999). *The Developing Mind: Toward a Neurobiology of Interpersonal Experience*. New York: Guilford Press.

Stern, D. N. (1985). *The Interpersonal World of the Infant*. New York: Basic Books.

Stone, M. (2006). The analyst's body as tuning fork: Embodied resonance in countertransference. *Journal of Analytical Psychology, 51*(1): 109–124.

Thomson-Salo, F. (2018). *Engaging Infants: Embodied Communication in Short-Term Infant–Parent Therapy*. London: Karnac.

Trowell, J. (1996). Thoughts on countertransference and observation. In: J. Tsiantis, A. Sandler, D. Anastasopoulos & B. Martindale (Eds.), *Countertransference in Psychoanalytic Psychotherapy with Children and Adolescents* (pp. 37–50). London: Karnac.

Tsiantis, J., Sandler, A., Anastasopoulos, D., & Martindale, B. (Eds.) (1996). *Countertransference in Psychoanalytic Psychotherapy with Children and Adolescents*. London: Karnac.

Vulcan, M. (2009). Is there any body out there? A survey of literature on somatic countertransference and its significance for DMT. *The Arts in Psychotherapy*, 36: 275–281.

Winnicott, D. W. (1953). Transitional objects and transitional phenomena: A study of the first not-me possession. *International Journal of Psychoanalysis*, 34: 89–97.

Winnicott, D. W. (1968). The squiggle game. *Voices: The Art and Science of Psychotherapy*, 4(1): 98–112.

Wolstein, B. (Ed.) (1988). *Essential Papers on Countertransference*. New York: New York University Press.

CHAPTER 3

The absent other: reflections on the absence of male integrative child and adolescent psychotherapists

Jamie Butterworth

Addressing the elephant in the room

I became aware of the elephant in the room on the first evening with my training cohort. As I looked around the group, I realised I was the elephant; the solitary male out of nineteen eager trainees. Over the following four years, I would wrestle with my insecurities and feelings of alienation around being a man in a profession that is dominated by women. I also became aware that the training was structured around psychosocial and psychodynamic concepts that reinforced this sense of alienation for me.

During my training, I spoke with other male trainee child and adolescent psychotherapists, and I discovered that my experience was not unique. However, I realised that despite the obvious gender disparity in the profession, there was no research or discussion as to why. This led me to think about the barriers that might be holding men back from working therapeutically with children, and to consider the implications of more male integrative child and adolescent psychotherapists.

"I was expecting a lady, I don't want to see a man!" nine-year-old Lenny announced when I arrived at his classroom to pick him up for our first session. He looked me up and down silently, and I felt like an unwanted Christmas present, one that is examined from different angles with despondent curiosity before being discarded.

Lenny's experience of men had not been a positive one. He had not known his father, who left shortly after he was born. His mother had other partners during Lenny's early childhood; however, most of them had been abusive, and there was a history of domestic violence. For the past two years, Lenny and his mother had lived with his maternal grandmother; a caring, compassionate, and stable figure in both of their lives, but who had also experienced domestic violence. Lenny's experience of men had been at best elusive and disappointing, and at worst, abusive and violent. The influence of abusive, violent men was trans-generational, profoundly scarring his family's relationship with masculinity.

I had arrived excited about our journey together, standing in the doorway greeting Lenny with a smile. But for Lenny, I was a less than ideal travelling companion representing something reprehensible. Lenny's internal working model or internal blueprint of men was firmly established through his personal experience and the experiences of his mother and grandmother. In that moment, there was very little I could do to convince him that I would be any different.

Lenny took off back into the classroom and slumped into his chair, burying his head in his arms. I felt rejected and wanted to take myself back to the therapy room to hide myself away. However, I did not run away, and I waited patiently in the doorway, remaining available for Lenny, hoping that he would realise that I was different. Perhaps by not disappearing down the corridor back to my room, I had already begun to challenge Lenny's internal working model and taken a tentative step on a long journey towards forming trust.

Lenny's initial surprise and suspicion on discovering he had a male therapist was not unfounded. The British Association of Counsellors and Psychotherapists (BACP) surveyed 5,740 of their members in 2021 and less than 4 per cent of those surveyed identified as a male therapist working with children under the age of eighteen. Although the survey only accounts for around 10 per cent of the organisation's members, they concluded that the figure probably represented the wider picture (O'Donnell, J. Personal Communications, 22 March, 12 April, 14 April 2022). The Association of Child Psychotherapists (ACP) reported in 2022 that only 15 per cent of their members were male (Lorefice, Z. Personal Communications, 13 April 2022). Meanwhile, the United Kingdom Council for Psychotherapists (UKCP) reported that only 22 per cent of their 9,000 members were male but disclosed that they had not surveyed their child and adolescent members to establish the gender disparity (Dunne, E. Personal Communications, 23 March 2022).

Based on the responses from the three major professional bodies in the UK, it is undeniable that there is a lack of male therapists in the profession. During my research for this chapter, it also became apparent that there is scarce research on the impact of gender disparity amongst child and adolescent psychotherapists. Furthermore, there is insufficient research on the potential implications on the therapeutic outcomes for children and adolescents working with male therapists. With so many fathers and male role models absent from children's lives, male child and adolescent therapists can offer a unique opportunity to model a version of maleness and masculinity that differs from the child's experience. Furthermore, an increase of men working in nurturing roles with children may help to challenge outdated gender stereotypes that are still prevalent in our society.

I believe that there are complex sociocultural barriers preventing men from entering the profession, and these hurdles are constructed from our assumptions, attitudes, and misconceptions towards masculinity and gender roles. These deep-rooted assumptions, attitudes, and misconceptions fortify the work with children, and these fortifications can appear an ominously insurmountable barrier for men. Whilst the child and adolescent psychotherapy profession has a primary task to be inclusive, I feel there is an unconscious process, a basic assumption mentality, that undermines this primary task. The basic assumption mentality defends the system from anxiety (Stokes, 1994, p. 19–20). In this case, the anxiety is around men working with children, or men perhaps invading a place that feels sacred and safe for women. As Vega Zagier Roberts points out, a basic assumption activity "is driven by the demands of the internal environment and anxieties about psychological survival" (1994, p. 31). Many of those in the profession, both clients and therapists, have suffered abuse at the hands of men or the oppressive patriarchal system; thus, it makes sense that the system would be driven by an unconscious desire to keep men out.

As play therapist David Le Vay (2016) points out, these negative assumptions about men's motivation for working with children have been churned up by the media. He argues that child abuse has become a precious media commodity feeding a growing anxiety around the welfare of children. This has led to a culture of suspicion around men working with children, where we are perceived as abusers. Le Vay writes,

> This … is the real tragedy of a contemporary society saturated with increasingly lurid, disturbing … stories of child abuse that litter the scandalised post-Savile landscape like hidden IEDs, ready to blow up in men's faces at any moment if they put a foot wrong. (2016, p. 40)

Perhaps Le Vay's words appear overdramatic for some, but for me, they are poignant, and convey the sense of impediment I have felt, and the degree of hypervigilance I have had to maintain. This idea of being hypervigilant and tiptoeing carefully around potentially explosive situations is, of course, how those who have been abused feel, and it could also be seen as arising out of the transference between us and our clients and female colleagues.

One aspect of the work with children and young people that is extremely sensitive for male therapists is perhaps eroticised or sexualised transference. I remember being terrified about the possibility of this form of transference manifesting in my work with young people. When it happened with a girl who had been sexually abused by her father, I was mortified. The child would arrive to our sessions dressed inappropriately and would dance in a sexualised manner. I would literally turn away and felt nauseated, and after our sessions I would be consumed by shame. Initially, I was too ashamed to take my experience to supervision for fear my supervisor would chastise me. Of course, my feelings of shame and fear around disclosing to my supervisor were in the countertransference. However, my fear of this erotic or sexualised transference and my need to evade it, was also, I believe, based on my fear of putting myself in a position of vulnerability; something men are conditioned to avoid at all costs.

Neglected daughters and dangerous wolves

The culture of suspicion and perception of men as incapable or abusive when it comes to children is deeply woven into the tapestry of our Western culture. One of our first interactions with such stereotypes comes in the form of traditional fairy tales, most notably those of Charles Perrault. Two of Perrault's most famous fairy tales are "Cinderella" and "Little Red Riding Hood", both of which depict two different representations of men that I believe still consciously and unconsciously influence Western cultures' perceptions of men in relation to children.

In Cinderella, after the death of his first wife "who had been the best person in the world" (Hannon, 2001, p. 450), Cinderella's impoverished father welcomes into his home a wealthy but evil woman and her equally abhorrent daughters, and in doing so becomes "the agent of his daughters' disgrace" (Hannon, 2001, p. 946). Cinderella, out of devotion to her father, demurs to the abusive newcomers out of fear of her father's displeasure (ibid.). Perrault depicts Cinderella's father as weak and not concerned about endangering his daughter's welfare in exchange for social and economic gain (ibid., p. 947). The father is portrayed as being ill-equipped to take care of Cinderella, and worse still, complicit in the stepmother's abuse of the child. The story of Cinderella illustrates a familiar pattern of the father who is emotionally distant and weak, and, in this instance, focused on economic gain and social standing. Meanwhile, the child's mother is emotionally powerful and idolised, returning symbolically as the fairy godmother.

Other familiar patterns of masculinity are addressed in Perrault's "Little Red Riding Hood". Here we witness the antagonist, the wolf, seducing the young girl and eventually devouring her. Red Riding Hood arrives at her grandmother's house and is coerced by the wolf to undress and get into bed with him. After the now familiar exchange where Red Riding Hood begins to realise that she is not in bed with her grandmother, the wolf eats her (Hannon, 2001, p. 746). Perrault ends the tale with a chilling moral:

> One sees here that young children
> Especially pretty girls,
> Polite, well taught, and pure as pearls,
> Should stay on guard against all sorts of men
> For if one fails to stay alert, it won't be strange
> To see one eaten by a wolf enraged.
> I say a wolf since not all types are wild,
> Or can be said to be the same in kind.
> Some are winning and have sharp minds.
> Some are loud or smooth or mild.

> Others appear just kind unriled.
> They follow young ladies wherever they go,
> Right into the halls of their very own homes.
> Alas for those who've refused the truth:
> Sweetest tongue has the sharpest tooth.
>
> (Ibid., p. 747)

The hunter is another masculine stereotype portrayed in both Perrault's version of the story and the Brothers Grimm adaptation. The hunter represents the rescuing father figure, he who is responsible and strong (Bettelheim, 1976, p. 172). The fairy tale appears to illustrate the contradictory nature of maleness: "The selfish, asocial, violent, potentially destructive tendencies of the wolf versus the unselfish, social, thoughtful, and protective propensities of the hunter" (ibid.). Bruno Bettelheim points out that fairy tales have nothing to do with the individual's external life but much more to do with their internal problems, which seem incomprehensible and therefore unsolvable (1976, p. 25). I believe that the story of Little Red Riding Hood might illustrate our unconscious struggle to integrate these two polarised aspects of masculinity, the "wolf" and the "hunter", representing the unconscious processes that defend the work with children from men. Our reluctance to address and think about this problem, or a basic assumption mentality, runs the risk of reinforcing anxieties and mistrust in men, blocking the possibility that a man can be different from these deeply entrenched stereotypes. When we think about the story of Little Red Riding Hood, who is more memorable, the wolf or the hunter?

The mummy-daddy

I vividly remember a conversation between a friend of one of my children and his mum, while we were out on a play date together. The child turned to his mum and described me as a "mummy-daddy". It seemed incomprehensible that a daddy could embody the qualities of a mummy, so to overcome this dichotomy, he rather superbly invented a whole new subgenre for me as a "mummy-daddy". This situation highlights how language and meaning can also create potential barriers for men who wish to enter child psychotherapy or any other nurturing work with children. For example, if we take the verb *to mother*, it is defined as "to treat a person with great kindness and love and try to protect from anything dangerous or difficult" (Cambridge Dictionary Online). However, the verb *to father* is defined as, "to become a father of a child by making a woman pregnant" (ibid.).

Mothering implies a state of nurture and care, whereas fathering is a functional, biological process; the language we use defines or enforces our gender roles. If a man transcends his gender role and acts in nurturant manner, we will say he is "mothering" (Chodorow, 1978, p. 11); there is no masculine verb that describes a nurturing father. The term "mothering" is therefore associated with being a woman, and as Roger Horrocks (1994) asserts, in our society "the male has to distance himself from femaleness and femininity, in order to prove that he is male" (p. 33). This suggests that men need to avoid displays of femininity, such as "mothering", as they potentially threaten the male's sense of masculinity and position of power.

This belief is deeply entrenched in Western culture—as Paul Verhaeghe (2011) points out, monotheistic religions propose the concept of "One Man" (p. 82). The installation of God the Father links one sex to power, which immediately designates the other sex inferior (2011, pp. 82–83). Images of God or the Father and Son exert a masculine tyranny and morality (Horrocks, 1994, p. 15), whereas representations of femininity, such as the Virgin Mary, depict an approachable, human figure who is emotional and intuitive (1994, pp. 43–44). These qualities, which we perhaps associate with psychotherapeutic work with children, are therefore seen as feminine characteristics and perceived to be subordinate to the characteristics of masculinity, which exert power and control.

Working in an emotional and nurturing capacity with children could therefore be regarded by men as emasculating, freezing men out of psychotherapeutic work with children and contributing to a systemic belief that women are more nurturing than men (O'Sullivan & Chambers, 2012, p. 6). However, this is a social construction, with no biological evidence to support this belief. Although there is some evidence that male hormones may partially inhibit maternal, nurturant behaviour, there is no overall effect on whether men are capable of nurturing. Men can adequately care for children and feel just as nurturant as biological mothers (Chodorow, 1978, p. 29). There has been an enormous amount of research into the differences between the cognitive and emotional capacities of men and women (Connell, 2020, p. 21). Psychological differences between the sexes are either non-existent or significantly small. All have been culturally exaggerated and are much smaller than the social differences that have been justified by the belief in psychological differences between the sexes, such as unequal incomes, unequal responsibilities in childcare, and access to social power (ibid.). Furthermore, there is no anthropological or evolutionary evidence that supports the notion that men cannot be nurturant. Sarah Blaffer Hrdy (2009) explains that observations of some hunter-gather societies have shown that men spend a considerable amount of time in arm's reach of their infants, often hugging, kissing, nuzzling, or simply holding them throughout the day (2009, p. 128).

What does the cultural exaggeration of psychological differences teach children about men? Furthermore, what are boys internalising about masculinity? Chimamanda Ngozi Adiche writes:

> We stifle the humanity of boys. We define masculinity in a *very* narrow way. Masculinity is a hard, small cage, and we put boys inside this cage. (2014, p. 26)

The patriarchal system oppresses women, but it also imprisons men, and the consequence of this emotional incarceration can be seen in the staggering figures around male suicide in the UK. The Office of National Statistics reports that 74 per cent of the total registered suicides in 2021 in the United Kingdom were those of men (ONS, 2021). Anthony Clare points out that these high suicide rates are "the tip of the iceberg" and asserts that men are "too emotionally constipated and too proud to admit their feelings are out of control" (2000, p. 3). Masculinity therefore becomes identified with being alone and relinquishing relationships; it is associated with being tough and censoring emotions. From an early age, young boys are internalising this toxic soup of masculinity and developing what Robert Stoller (1985) suggests is a defensive armour against femininity that shields against manifesting and revealing feminine attributes that they possess such as tenderness, affection, and free expression of feeling (p. 183). Stoller continues:

"The first order of business being a man is: don't be a woman" (ibid.). Meanwhile, girls are internalising that boys are emotionally straightjacketed and relationally unavailable.

Training

Training to become a therapist is an intrinsically relational and exceptionally emotional process. It involves us sitting with uncomfortable feelings and experiencing moments of raw vulnerability. Considering what I have discussed above, is it any surprise that so few men enter the field of child psychotherapy? We have been conditioned to shy away from our emotions, to be lone wolves rather than building and sustaining strong relationships with others.

As a male trainee, I often found myself wondering where I fitted in and was overwhelmed at times with feelings of not belonging. This sense of being marginalised is not uncommon for male trainees within the field, with many often feeling that they do not have a voice or place within the profession (Michel, Hall, Hays, & Runyan, 2013, p. 480). Again, these feelings can be attributed to issues I have discussed above; however, I also felt that the training content itself minimised the father's influence in child development and overlooked the unique challenges men face on training courses.

Much of what we studied felt mother-centric, and the position of the father was often seen as auxiliary, providing emotional and physical support for the mother. In terms of the relationship with the child, men are seen through the lens of the primal family triangle where they facilitate the development of the infants capacity to see themselves in relationship with others (Britton, 1998, p. 42). Furthermore, we are also seen as essential components in the establishment of the same-sex identification in our male offspring as they separate from their primary identification with the mother (Le Vay, 2016, p. 41). If the father identifies as stereotypically masculine, the boy will therefore identify with all the aspects of masculinity that have a stranglehold on our society and perpetuate masculine dominance and feminine subordination. I feel we should be more critical of these outdated notions around the role of the father.

During my training, I felt the father's role was again depicted as functional and distant, a sentiment that was at odds with my own experience as a parent, where I have been a nurturing presence in my children's lives. This sense of being an outsider manifested as a struggle to integrate into my training group, and I found myself consciously and unconsciously withdrawing from my peers both physically and emotionally. This was perhaps a socialised defensive response that shielded me from experiences of vulnerability. I noticed how this defensive response would emerge in the therapy room during times of vulnerability. An example of this can be seen in the following case study from a session with Lenny, two years into our work together.

Case study: Lenny

Lenny grabbed the blanket and a cushion, "I'm going to sleep now, I'm tired"; he yawned and stretched his arms high above his head, before building a bed on two chairs. "Can you tuck me in?" he asked. "How would you like me to tuck you in, Lenny?" I replied. Lenny said he wanted me to tuck the blanket under his feet and pull it right up to his head, which made him look like a swaddled infant.

"Bottle, baby wants bottle!" Lenny cried out. I handed Lenny a pretend bottle and he sucked on it contentedly, a smile tentatively crept across his mouth and then established itself. He looked like the cat that had got the cream. "Oh, baby looks so happy all tucked up in its bed with a bottle." Lenny regressed further, "Ga ga ga goo!" he responded. The bottle was then replaced by a thumb, and baby fell asleep. I sat on my chair, a short distance away from Lenny.

Suddenly he burst into a primal wail: "Wah! Wah! Wah!" I did not know what to do. I felt unsafe and concerned that a member of staff might look through the window and consider our play inappropriate. However, there was another part of me that wanted to rush to Lenny's side and soothe him. I sat for a moment with these polarised feelings.

There was something for me around the inappropriateness of being near a vulnerable young child, like the erotic or sexualised transference I previously described. With Lenny, it felt as if my instinctive response to care for him was being inhibited by my social conditioning; it was not my place to soothe the baby, and if witnessed by someone else, it might be seen as inappropriate. However, in terms of my client's needs, sitting at a distance felt like I was colluding with his father who had abandoned him.

Eventually, I returned to Lenny's side, and for the rest of the session I moved back and forth, attending to him when he needed me. This could be described as a maternal transference, but as with mothering, it overlooks the possibility that a father, or a male therapist, can provide compassion and tenderness. It also discounts the prospect that perhaps in the transference the child is seeking the unmet paternal, rather than maternal, love or attachment.

One of the biggest hurdles I faced during my training was the infant observation. Maternity is synonymous with womanhood, and the atmosphere around pregnancy is predominantly female (Jackson, 1998, p. 84). Unlike female trainees, male trainees often face prejudice when searching for a baby and mother to observe. Men are treated with suspicion, and mothers often instinctively refuse to have a male observer (ibid.). When I was looking for a baby to observe, I approached a local mother-and-baby group leader to advertise on her Facebook group. I created a flyer with details of what the observations entailed and the contacts for my training organisation. I also added a photo of myself. By being as transparent as possible, I hoped to alleviate any fears around my credibility or ulterior motives. The group leader was keen to help, but suggested I add a photo of me with my children, because she believed it would alleviate any fears that I was "a pervert". I was devastated and did not follow her advice, and I eventually found a wonderful family who welcomed me into their home. As a white, middle-aged, heterosexual male, experiencing being a minority and prejudice is not such as bad thing. It is by no means comparable to other minority groups; however, this illustrates the underlying fear that men have an ulterior motive and the prejudices we face.

A bridge over troubled water

According to Aristophanes … in the ancient world of legend there were three types of people … people weren't simply male or female, but one of three types: male/male, male/female or female/female. In other words, each person was made of the components of two people.
—(Murakami, 2012, p. 40)

Carl Gustav Jung proclaimed that "No man is so entirely masculine that he has nothing feminine in him. The fact is, rather, that very masculine men have—carefully guarded and hidden—a very soft emotional life often incorrectly describe as feminine" (2003, p. 87). We have disavowed an aspect of the self that is inherent in both sexes. We all possess these traits, regardless of our sex; they have, as Jung points out, been incorrectly categorised.

As a male therapist, I feel as if I have been through a lengthy process of integration and am coming to a place where I can accept all aspects of myself. I accept and am happy with the parts that are labelled by society "masculine" and "feminine" in the knowledge that these are not attributes of sex or gender, but are simply characteristics of being human. Art therapist Michael Franklin (2007) suggests that male therapists can be "Middle Men", straddling masculinity and femininity and avoiding collusion with the masculine stereotype. In doing so, we restructure the masculine stereotype and project out into the world something different (Franklin, 2007, pp. 4–9). Franklin asserts that "the liberating potential inherent in the conceptualization of the middle man is the movement from complex forms of subjugation to a new vision of masculine identity that is systemically aware" (2007, p. 9). Franklin states that the emancipation from the masculine stereotype and movement towards a new masculine identity shifts us from a position of alienation to social engagement (ibid.).

How does this translate into the therapy room? I have worked with boys who, through projective play and role-playing, have symbolically murdered "the father" in the room. One perspective is that this represents oedipal dynamics and the child's unconscious desire to usurp the father's position in the family. However, many of the boys I have worked with have experienced oppressive, elusive, abusive, or absent fathers; the cause of which, as discussed above, can be traced to the social construct of masculinity. With this in mind, I am also curious whether their murderous desires and need to control represent the child's experience of masculinity, which has controlled and imprisoned them since birth.

As a male therapist, I have the unique opportunity to model an alternative version of manhood, and this idea of an alternative is key. Men are often called upon to be role models for boys, but the expectation is that we will model the very traits that reinforce gendered ideologies and normative masculine identity such as being authoritarian and disciplinarian (Bhana, Moosa, Xu, & Emilsen, 2022). There have been numerous occasions where I have been referred a boy in a school setting who is disruptive or aggressive. When I have met with their teacher or the special educational needs co-ordinator (SENCO), they have voiced relief that the child has a male therapist. These boys often have absent fathers, and there is a perhaps a belief that the lack of an authoritarian male figure in their lives is the reason for their presentation. As a male therapist, I feel the expectation is that I will fill the void and provide a disciplinarian father figure for these boys. However, this simply reinforces the gendered stereotype and affirms the boys' masculinity. Most of these boys need a man who is available, consistent, and nurturing rather than a prison warden. Furthermore, this idea that boys need men who model stereotyped gender normative traits reinforces heteronormativity and overlooks diverse family structures such as those of same-sex parents (Bhana, Moosa, Xu, & Emilsen, 2022).

The notion that, as a man, I am best placed working with troubled boys can be frustrating. I have worked with far fewer girls, but those I have worked with have all similarly had absent fathers. As with the boys, there is an opportunity to model an alternative experience of manhood. We can also model an alternative for parents, especially fathers who are struggling to emotionally connect with their children.

Case study: Jessica

Jessica was a sixteen-year-old girl who lived with her father. Her mother had died suddenly when she was fourteen, and since her death, the once-vibrant, assertive, and social teenager had withdrawn, spending most of her time in her room. She was referred to our service when her father noticed that she had self-harmed. In our first session together, she explained that her father had never shown any outward emotional response to her mother's death. Like Jessica, he had withdrawn, he did not speak about her mother, he did not cry; life just continued. She told me it was like living in an old black-and-white movie; the colour from their lives had drained away. Her father provided for her, he went to work, she was clothed, fed, and had a roof over her head, but she experienced him as cold, emotionless, and elusive. Together we thought about the self-harming, something that had only happened on that one occasion, and Jessica conceded that it was the only way she could get her father to see her pain as well as providing her with an outlet for her anguish.

I worked with both Jessica and her father, and eventually her father was able to access therapy for himself, and they briefly engaged in family therapy. Over time, the relationship between father and daughter was repaired, they were able to grieve openly together, and both began to build relationships outside of the family home. The father attended widowers' groups and Jessica began to build friendships at school.

My therapeutic approach has always centred around the reparative actions of the therapeutic relationship. It is not what I do, more how I am with my clients. One of the key aspects of my work is the concept of "containment" (Bion, 1962) or "holding" (Winnicott, 1990), which Lavinia Gomez describes as "trying to reach towards the notion that the therapist's actions matter less than the state of mind they come with" (2004, p. 7). The therapist's emotional openness, presence, and ways of responding lead the client to accept themselves more fully (ibid.).

During my work with Jessica and her father, I often wondered what it was like for them to experience a male therapist who could contain and provide emotional openness; characteristics our society does not attribute to masculinity. For Jessica, in the transference, perhaps I became the father she desired, one who would hear her despair, sit with her anguish, and allow her to cry and be angry. For her father, perhaps my openness and empathetic presence modelled an alternative experience of manhood and, through our relationship, he was not only able to repair his relationship with his daughter and grieve the loss of his wife, but also able to repair the damage that a lifetime of introjecting a toxic form of masculinity had created.

Changes

As I have proposed, the social construction of gender plays a significant role in preventing men from entering the field of child and adolescent psychotherapy. Culturally exaggerated notions around men's incompetency with regard to children's emotional welfare, and stereotyping men as abusers, stir up a cultural whirlwind of fear and negativity. A world with more men in nurturing roles, whether it be in child psychotherapy, as primary childcare providers, or in early years and primary education, will show a new generation that these rigid stereotypes are not biological mechanisms that divide men and women into polarised camps. The traits we are so quick to separate into masculine or feminine are, in fact, attributes of both sexes and intrinsically human. Gender is no longer binary; with so many children and young people migrating from the poles, gender is rapidly becoming a spectrum, and as a profession we need to adapt to this change. We have a narrow window of opportunity with children when it comes to their gender socialisation; by the age of ten, children have already introjected restrictive norms about socially accepted gender conduct (Heise et al., 2019, p. 2441). If we are going to challenge restrictive gender norms, gender diversity needs to be represented in the therapy room.

Unarguably, there is gender disparity amongst child and adolescent psychotherapists, and in these few pages I have attempted to illustrate some of reasons why men might be deterred from working with children. These ideas have arisen from my experience as a trainee and as a therapist. My hope is to open a conversation, not only about what inhibits men from working with children, but also the changing landscape of gender in our society.

References

Bettelheim, B. (1976). *The Uses of Enchantment: The Meaning and Importance of Fairy Tales*. London: Penguin.

Bhana, D., Moosa, S., Xu, Y., & Emilsen, K. (2022). Men in early childhood education and care: On navigating a gendered terrain. *European Early Childhood Education Research Journal, 30*(4): 543–556.

Bion, W. R. (1962). *Learning from Experience*. London: Karnac.

Blaffer Hrdy, S. (2009). *Mothers and Others: The Evolutionary Origins of Mutual Understanding*. London: The Belknap Press.

Britton, R. (1998). *Subjectivity, Objectivity and Triangular Space*. In: *Belief and Imagination: Explorations in Psychoanalysis*. London: Karnac.

Cambridge Dictionary Online. https://dictionary.cambridge.org/ (last accessed 15 December 2022).

Chodorow, N. (1978). *The Reproduction of Mothering: Psychoanalysis and the Sociology of Gender*. London: University of California Press.

Clare, A. (2000). *On Men: Masculinity in Crisis*. London: Arrow.

Connell, R. W. (2020). *Masculinities*. Cambridge: Polity.

Franklin, M. (2007). Contemplations on the middle man: Anima rising. *Journal of the American Art Therapy Association*, *24*(1): 4–9.

Gomez, L. (2004). Humanistic or psychodynamic: What is the difference and do we have to make a choice? *Self and Society*, *31*(6): 5–19.

Hannon, P. (2001). Heroes and Heroines in Perrault. In: J. Zipes (Ed.), *The Great Fairy Tale Tradition: From Straparola and Basile to the Brothers Grimm*. London: W. W. Norton.

Heise, L., Greene, M. E., Opper, N., Stavropoulou, M., Harper, C., Nascimento, M., & Zewdie, D. (2019). Gender inequality and restrictive gender norms: Framing the challenges to health. *The Lancet*, *393*: 2440–2454.

Horrocks, R. (1994). *Masculinity in Crisis*. London: Macmillan.

Jackson, J. (1998). The male observer in infant observation: An evaluation. *International Journal of Infant Observation*, *1*(2): 84–99.

Jung, C. G. (2003). *Aspects of the Feminine*. Abingdon, UK: Routledge.

Le Vay, D. (2016). Reflections on Gender: The Male Play Therapist. In: D. Le Vay, & E. Cuschieri (Eds.), *Challenges in the Theory and Practice of Play Therapy*. Abingdon, UK: Routledge.

Michel, R. E., Hall, S. B., Hays, D. G., & Runyan, H. I. (2013). A mixed methods study of male recruitment in the counselling profession. *Journal of Counselling and Development*, *91*: 475–482.

Murakami, H. (2012). *Kafka on the Shore*. Dublin: Vintage.

Ngozi Adiche, C. (2014). *We Should all be Feminists*. London: Fourth Estate.

ONS (Office for National Statistics). https://www.ons.gov.uk/ (last accessed 11 October 2022).

O'Sullivan, J., & Chambers, S. (2012). Men working in childcare: Does it matter to children. London Early Years Foundation. www.leyf.org.uk

Stokes, J. (1994). The unconscious at work in groups and teams: Contributions from the work of Wilfred Bion. In: A. Obholzer, & V. Zagier Roberts (Eds.), *The Unconscious at Work: Individual and Organisational Stress in Human Services*. Hove, UK: Routledge.

Stoller, R. (1985). *Presentations of Gender*. London: Yale University Press.

Veiri Cenerini, M., & Messina, D. (2019). A "strong enough" father: Observations from groups for expectant and new fathers. *Infant Observation*, *22*(2–3): 147–164.

Verhaeghe, P. (2011). *Love in a Time of Loneliness*. London: Karnac.

Winnicott, D. W. (1990). *The Maturational Processes and the Facilitating Environment: Studies in the Theory of Emotional Development.* Abingdon, UK: Routledge.

Zagier Roberts, V. (1994). The organisation of work: Contributions from open system theory. In: A. Obholzer, & V. Zagier Roberts (Eds.), *The Unconscious at Work: Individual and Organisational Stress in Human Services.* Hove, UK: Routledge.

Part II

Race and cultural identity

CHAPTER 4

Meet them where they are: integrative psychotherapy with refugee children and young people

Evania Inward

Introduction

The terms "refugee" and "asylum seeker" are often loaded with political agendas and meaning. Draconian government policies and populist media can drive narratives of illegality, fearmongering, polarising and inciting judgement along racial, national, cultural, and religious lines, which can affect social perceptions of host communities, exposing refugee children to continuing traumas of racism, discrimination, and systemic, economic hardships (Reed, Fazel, Jones, Panter-Brick, & Stein, 2012).

Even if afforded entry to a "safe" country, refugee children are extremely vulnerable, and unknown numbers of children "disappear" (Townsend, 2022), vulnerable to abuse and sexual or domestic slavery. Some children arrive alone or lose their family or carers along the route to safety, labelled unaccompanied refugee minors (URMs) or unaccompanied asylum-seeking children (UASCs) (UN General Assembly, 2005). Schwartz and Melzak (2005, p. 295) suggest, "All refugee children are psychologically unaccompanied". Working with refugee children means automatically working with sociopolitical and human rights issues whether they, or we, are aware or not. Political, legal, immigration-based, racial, and economic lived experiences will be in the child's internal world and in the therapy room. Blackwell asserts that, "all psychotherapy is a political activity, and the idea of therapeutic neutrality is inherently problematic" (2005b, p. 35).

In 2020, one in four refugees to the UK were children; the majority, aged up to 17, came from refugee camps and directly from countries of origin, including Syria, Yemen, Eritrea, Somalia, Sudan, Afghanistan, Vietnam, Iraq, Iran, Albania, Ethiopia, and more (Home Office, 2021; Refugee Council, 2020; UNHCR, 2018). Considering refugee children and adolescents as one "client group" could be construed as reductionist and stereotyping.

Beyond PTSD: widening "trauma" definitions and interventions

There is little doubt about the devastating complex mental health difficulties experienced by refugee children and young people (Bronstein & Montgomery, 2011; Fazel, Reed, Panter-Brick, & Stein, 2012; Frounfelker et al., 2020; Melzak, McLoughlin, & Watt, 2018). In addition, each refugee child will also be at a different stage in their asylum, immigration, and settlement process, which will affect their security, status, and safety in the host country. Bronstein and Montgomery describe a "triple trauma paradigm" (2011, p. 44), where refugee children may have multiple, cumulative traumatic experiences during their escape, flight, and post-migration stressors. Refugee child mental health and therapy needs will vary and may not fit into any one diagnostic category.

The current, dominant assessment and treatment of "trauma" for refugee children is psychometric and biomedical, based on DSM-5 criteria (APA, 2013), where children must meet diagnostic thresholds for post-traumatic stress disorder (PTSD). Alayarian (2009, 2015) agrees there may be universal physiological symptoms, but also finds deep traumatic grief, psychosomatic illnesses, academic difficulties, and developmental delay and regression, sometimes due to parents' mental health difficulties. She suggests the way DSM diagnostics is a deficit-model, reducing refugee experiences and their deep impact to symptoms, can be over-pathologising and can actually undermine children's resilience and adaptability (ibid., 2009, p. 152). Alayarian also warns that disregarding sociopolitical contexts and background cultures risks "defective conceptualisation and misdiagnosis" (ibid., 2009, p.155).

Melzak (2017, pp. 369–378) also widens trauma definitions, describing how refugee children can be deeply impacted in a range of different ways, including internal confusion, shock and rage, fragmentation, conflicts, dualities, and "developmental stuckness". Blackwell (2005b, pp. 49–51) finds refugees can suffer deep intrapsychic overwhelm, where "normal defensive structures are unable to cope … high levels of anxiety related to annihilation, engulfment, disintegration and destructiveness … a powerful sense of abandonment, helplessness … [and] psychic numbing where parts of Self shut down."

As psychotherapists, we might expand our clinical thinking for refugee child clients, carefully considering the relevance and impact of our approach and modalities, what we offer such clients, and what our own and the child's own therapeutic aims might be. In this chapter, we meet two refugee children and consider the importance and benefits of explicitly considering six "dimensions" of lived experience: political, economic, cultural, religious or spiritual, interpersonal, and intrapsychic (Blackwell, 2005b, 2007). These multilayered factors can significantly impact refugee children's internal processes, mental health, and the therapeutic relationship, yet can be omitted, minimised, or misunderstood.

Ali, sixteen, from Afghanistan

"Hello Miss."

Large, almond-shaped, deep-brown eyes and a mop of hair came into view around the side of the door and stared directly at me, unblinking and with trepidation.

"Hello and welcome! Please do come in!" I replied with a smile, gesturing with warm and friendly intention.

The rest of a young man's thin face and tall, thin body moved slowly into full view, and he stood back, remaining in the doorway.

"Umm, I am to meet you, I think?" He held up a note in the air.

"Hello, you must be Ali?" I asked. I took proactive interest in the newly arriving refugee children coming into the school, and communicated with safeguarding staff, who identified Ali as a "conflict refugee".

They had no idea of what conflict, nor from what country he originated, nor even what language he spoke. I already had a sense of his potential isolation, becoming invisible or lost in the system.

I noticed Ali's direct, watchful gaze on me as he came into the room and sat gingerly down on the edge of his seat, as if ready to leave. I felt the dynamics of power and powerlessness in the room already, potentially at different levels: adult–child, teacher–student, authority–applicant, immigration official–asylum seeker.

My job was to help him feel safe, here and now. First, confirming how we might best communicate verbally and nonverbally.

"Ali, welcome, it is so nice to meet you, I am Evania, and I work here at the school to support children. Can you understand me? Would you like an interpreter?"

"Oh no! I not like interpreter! I must learn English if I here in UK."

I heard his drive and determination, perhaps a need for independence or self-reliance. However, if children prefer speaking in mother-tongue languages, the temptation to use family or community members must be avoided, and instead invest in trained, professional interpreters that understand and hold ethical boundaries of confidentiality and accurate translation. I was mindful that interpreters are a third person in the therapy room and can be a tricky dynamic, even if on a screen or phone; training in how to work with them is beneficial. We can ask our client if they prefer a same-gender or same-culture therapist, or not, as some children may even feel mistrust, guilt, shame, or pain to talk in their own language (Alayarian, 2009). We must not assume.

In setting the therapeutic frame with Ali, I explicitly named the possibility of short-term work, and clarified my role, explaining what I could and could not be to him. Ali spoke of his future hopes for life in the UK, and we discussed who else might support him with different parts of his journey. Ali did not think about himself in need. He was proud and dignified; he had brought himself to safety alone, and operated mainly in the adult position. We set initial goals for our meetings through pictures and diagrams, and he chose to come fortnightly at first. My offering him flexibility and space could avoid therapy becoming too intrusive or triggering for him.

I put what I knew about Ali on the table.

"I understand that you are a refugee and have come here to the UK. Do you have people who support you?"

"Why you do this? *Why* you do this job?"

Naming Ali as a "refugee" (Siegel, 2010) activated his defences but brought the issue into the conscious here-and-now, where it could be addressed. Ali needed to see my motives, to assess my authenticity, so I had to decide how much to disclose of my personal self.

"Of course you need to know who I am and why I do this, and you are right to check who I am. Everyone has an agenda, even me. I do not do this just for the money. We all are human, have wounds and hurt, and sometimes need help from others. I care deeply that children have someone to help them."

Ali softened in his body and sat back in the chair, connecting with my response.

"Everyone they always do things for money only. I don't trust anyone. Always the money. I hate this."

I glimpsed deep hurt and mistrust within Ali. As with many refugee children, he may have needed to be wary and mistrust others for physical and psychic survival. He might be hypervigilant and have high ability in reading body language, communications, and intentions. Being authentic, open, and honest is crucial with refugee children.

I reminded Ali that he need not tell me anything he did not wish to, but that to understand some legal terminology might help him to understand the process to gain leave to stay in the UK. Ali welcomed my invitation to sit together at the computer to work out the meanings and relevance of some of the legal terms and his rights as a young unaccompanied migrant child. Beginning with Ali's real world, his here-and-now political and economic needs, built a cornerstone of a warm, trusting, safe therapeutic relationship.

Refugee children often fear and mistrust mental health workers as representing authority or the state, perhaps with dubious intentions, motives, and future actions (Horlings & Hein, 2017). Thus, there is a potential we may activate psychological dualities and conflicts from past into present through the transference.

I imagined innumerable authority figures and institutions Ali might have encountered in his sixteen years, in his home country, his family, his community, and those persons who have caused him to flee, the traffickers who smuggled him, the immigration authorities he met in his country of safety. I held in mind Ali's potential projections onto me, who I might represent to him in the transference. His cultural background had given him limited access to speaking with females; how did it feel to him to speak to me now? Did Ali see me as an authority figure, someone who could help him gain or ruin his chances of refugee status? Did I also unconsciously represent white colonial power? Again, naming such differences opened up a curiosity and a space for exploration and dialogue.

Reflecting on my own possible projections, transferences, and countertransference I brought into the therapeutic relationship with Ali, with a horrific past and uncertain future, so alone in the world, I could touch despair quite easily. But I knew my role was to meet him where he was at right now—to hold compassion and hope for safety and healing.

Establishing internalised safety

Clinical supervision is essential from the assessment and conceptualising stages. In Ali's case, we felt that he was still in crisis, his nervous system and whole being was in survival mode. Traditional psychotherapy is not possible in this state; the first stage is to establish an internalised sense of safety (Herman, 1992). I built safety into the fabric of our therapeutic relationship from contracting, offering him freedom and choice, his right to not discuss overwhelmingly painful topics that might arise, inviting him to directly say no, question, or challenge me. Ali unconsciously tested this out on many subsequent occasions, which I believe empowered him to develop trust and safety within the therapeutic relationship.

Ali held deep existential fear of the consequences of being denied refuge and being deported back to Afghanistan or elsewhere to an unknown country.

"If I am deported back home I will die, maybe before I am sent." I heard a suicidal undertone and worked with the school's safeguarding processes and Ali around this.

Ali used many sessions searching for meaning in his existence, questioning why he was he born, why he survived when many others died (survivor guilt is common), what his life purpose might be. We used art and symbolism to depict his journey from present to future. Ali did not want to draw anything about his past, about which he said, "It is gone, it not exists for me, I must think *only* about the future, this is all that matters now."

Noting a strong psychic defence (Freud, 1966), I respected it as such. This therapeutic relationship was new and the long-term nature of psychodynamic psychotherapy required a much deeper and secure therapeutic frame. I remained child-led, focusing on resourcing him, elaborating and expanding on his hopes and dreams and internal protective factors.

Ali described how he lived for the future but could not visualise anything except darkness. Offering him art materials, he used a thick black marker to scribble across the page, chaotic, confusing, and scary. I invited him to bring light or colour into the picture, and he drew a small yellow flame. I wondered with him what or who he could see alongside him now a fire was alight. Could this fire provide warmth and light?

"I want my family to be here with me by this fire as we were before. But I do not know if they are even in this world now."

Ali had forgotten to forget, and became silent, dissociated, and frozen, which I wondered might be a familiar state to Ali, to numb and protect against deep pain, anxiety, or distress. I invited him to return to the safe external world in the present moment, to know he was safe in a now-familiar room with me. I invited him to wiggle his toes in his shoes, feel the solid ground beneath his feet, the chair he sat upon, the sunlight streaming through the window onto his face, and the fresh air coming easily through his breath.

When he had fully regulated, he was interested in how I had brought him back so quickly, and confirmed he would "zone out" for much longer periods. Offering refugee children grounding, co-regulation, and psychoeducation around how and why their brain, nervous system, and body react to overwhelming painful experiences (Porges, 2007; Porges & Dana, 2018; Rothschild, 2000; Siegel, 2010; Van der Kolk, 2014) can help them develop self-understanding and self-compassion around their normal human reactions to abnormal, traumatic experiences (Maté, 2011).

Somatic presentations and cultural idioms of illness and distress

Ali preferred to stay in the cognitive, verbal realm, interested in scientific and medical language about nervous system dysregulation, nightmares, and visual and emotional flashbacks, but rejected any references to "feelings" or mental or emotional health. I wondered if it was culturally stigmatising for him as a young Muslim man from the Middle East to talk about or express emotions outwardly. Western psychotherapy might even consider "disorders" such as alexithymia, but Ali sought to understand his symptoms on a somatic and, to some extent, a spiritual or supernatural level.

Mindful of differences of cultural idioms and explanations of distress, "parts of self" (Schwartz, 2013) enabled Ali to consider his whole well-being. Gesturing with my hands, I offered, "We can hurt in our mind [I held my forehead], in our heart [I placed my hand over my chest], in our body [I put my hands on my stomach], or in our soul, spirit, or higher self [I gestured to the top of my head, the crown chakra]."

I would often notice Ali's shifting physiological states and would invite him to notice his somatic, sensory realm to deepen his self-connection. Ali offered, "I have pain in my head. I have this in the night so I can't sleep. And I have pain here. [Ali pointed to his upper stomach.] But this is my pain, I must carry on, I am lucky, this is nothing, my family, my people, they have worse."

Somatisation is common in many non-Western cultures. Refugees from non-Western origins may present with more medically unexplained physical or somatic symptoms and chronic pain than Western clients, but not always with visible wounds, meaning they often go unexplained and undiagnosed (Wylie et al., 2018). Refugee children from non-Western cultures often experience stress in the body and may seek help for these physical symptoms rather than, or before, emotional difficulties (Isakson, Legerski, & Layne, 2015). Rohlof, Knipscheer, and Kleber (2014) identified autonomic hyper-arousal causing chronic pain, neuro-endocrinological and stress sensitivity, musculo-skeletal, gastro-intestinal, genito-urinary, cardio-vascular and respiratory symptoms, sleep disturbances, and other physical deconditioning. They also found tortured refugees had greater somatic pain and proposed the direct role of culture in somatising symptoms and relating to the nature and severity of trauma. I encouraged Ali to visit the GP, aware that somatisation can be a source of misunderstanding, and to ensure his symptoms were followed up medically to exclude the possibility of other organic pathology or disease.

I felt for many months an internal disconnect in Ali, his focus on basic survival, learning English, how to get a job and earn money. Perhaps it was necessary for him to maintain emotional distance. Ali was alone in the world; the only reliable anchor was himself. He often insisted, "I have no problems, I am fine, I am lucky. I do not need anything."

Of course, Ali needed strong defences, he had needed these highly functional, self-protective adaptations, survival skills, and coping mechanisms that had enabled him to live through and escape possible genocide in his land, to travel alone with human traffickers across continents, to navigate borders and immigration authorities, and to be sitting here, speaking a new language and studying for exams. I felt inspired, in awe of this young person. Ali was not powerless. It was important to help him connect with and further develop his existing skills, strengths, resilience, and resources (internal and external), to empower him and develop his sense of agency by uncovering new avenues of possibility, connection, and recovery.

Social, cultural connection

I became acutely aware of Ali's rigidity in his holding the observing, adult position, his rationalising focus on the future and distancing from any present state of feeling, pleasant or unpleasant. I was concerned that friendships, family, or community connections held no obvious importance to him. I noted the omission of his past as a whole. Understandably, he avoided pain and trauma, but I wondered why he rejected his heritage, belonging, and identity too. He did not want to attend mosque, nor to speak his mother tongue. Ali was keen to assimilate to his new Western home, but might he experience some cultural grief and loss? Might opportunities to speak his mother tongue allow him some respite from constant internal translation? Or might it trigger painful repressed/suppressed pain from his homeland? Could attending the *masjid* link him in with a supportive *umma* community, nourishing faith or existential healing? Blackwell (2005b, p. 44) describes the importance of the interpersonal dimension: "Immediate family, extended family, friends and colleagues provide a major dimension of personal identity … the context within which (their) sense of self is formed and maintained."

My wondering was met at first with Ali's polite appreciation. "It's ok Miss, don't worry about me." Despite the brave adult persona and self-reliance, I considered a potentially trapped and lonely inner child hidden behind, who might like to meet others, play, and feel free sometimes. I decided to give him choice, so researched and printed out a list of same-culture and same-language refugee voluntary community groups. Ali's face lit up with an open-mouthed grin when I presented him with the contacts.

"Is this real? All these people, they are from my country? How come you do this! How come you find this for me?"

Ali began to speak more often of "his people", although not of his lost family or past experiences in his homeland. He spoke of his community being an ethnic and religious minority, and I saw his internal life force awakened in the room. "His people" seemed central to his identity, his belonging, his upbringing, his philosophy, values, and beliefs, roots of his core Self, and he was pleased to share them with me.

I asked Ali if he experienced any racism or name-calling from his peers at school. Ali revealed he had been verbally abused, isolated, and discriminated against by boys at school. He shared his perception of racism in wider society and the UK government's immigration and foreign office policies and international military interventions. Ali told me how he knew racism from Afghanistan, as he and his people faced rudeness, hatred, and suspicion and could not get good jobs. Ali was a smart and politically aware young man. However, feeling so grateful to be in the UK, he had not felt safe enough to speak about racism publicly. Racism is a most powerful, difficult, and provocative subject, one that can be all too easy for therapists to avoid, minimise, or dismiss. Refugee children might not otherwise bring the subject up unless the therapist is proactive and compassionately curious about the child's experiences.

Lønning and Kohli note:

> when memory is both a wound and an evocation, and forgetting can be an analgesic, anaesthetic, or an act of suppression, a balance needs to be struck between three aspects of memory: remembering, remembering to forget, and forgetting to remember … The challenge is to use the past to salvage a future and to not drown in a flood of rampant and disarrayed memories. (2022, p. 242)

Ali sometimes felt unsafe remembering, but delighted in invitations to reconnect to his collective community belonging and identity. Genuinely interested in his cultural background and ancestral lineage, I invited him to show me the mountains he had described to me on Google Earth. Giving him control of the computer, he only wished to explore the map from a distance, to show me an overview of cities, the "political map-view", for to zoom into his village felt too close to bear. Melzak, CEO of the organisation Baobab Young Survivors in Exile, suggests (in conversation, December 2021) that explicitly inviting young refugees to explore geographical maps of their country of origin and allowing space to discuss sociopolitical issues can bring context and meaning to their exile, regardless of if they had prior knowledge or were politicised themselves. These simple interventions may help refugee clients further understand and integrate their experiences within individual, contextual, and collective experiences of their people.

I consciously cultivated a safe "intercultural space" (BenEzer, 2012), where Ali came to know that I genuinely embraced human difference, not just the tolerance or curiosity that can contribute to "othering" of a client. After a few months, it seemed enough trust and containment in the therapeutic relationship had developed for Ali to safely remember more positive memories of his homeland. He described "his mountains" in Afghanistan, the differing seasons, and the colourful flowers that grew at different times of year there. I found opportunities to invite him to recall and immerse himself in the vivid sensory and body memories of when he had been young, safe, and happy in his mountains. He might choose to visit these internalised safe places (Rothschild, 2006a) whenever he wanted. We discussed how he might bring the mountain colours and flowers into his life, and Ali spoke of his joy visiting a local florist, a visceral and sensory present moment experience (Stern, 2004) of his homeland.

It was useful to gain a basic knowledge of Afghanistan. Once he knew I was not prying or linked to authority, Ali seemed delighted when I showed genuine interest in his cultural background, or when I knew just a few Arabic words and Islamic ways of life. We had many inter-religious, spiritual, existential, and political discussions in which I hoped he could explore his developing intercultural sense of Self from a safe distance.

After fifteen sessions, Ali wanted to tell me some of the story of his exile. He told me he had to flee because men and boys in neighbouring area had been killed. His family paid people-smugglers to get him out before the killers came to their area. He had a long overland journey with "many terrible people" and arrived in the UK by boat, alone. He did not know where his parents and sisters were now but hoped they were alive.

In his narrative, I heard a well-versed script he might have repeated so many times to many officials. No embellishment of narrative, little emotion, just headlines of perhaps what he thought I should know.

Our curiosity around the children's refugee "stories" do not necessarily help them; we must tread carefully and ensure we stay child-led to respect their internal and external safety. I did not wish to intrude unnecessarily into the depths of Ali's intrapsychic world so early on and with no assurance of long-term therapy, careful not to open any deep wounds, which may cause him to become re-traumatised. Instead, outside of the therapy room, I researched further into "his people", the Hazara in Afghanistan, and realised the high probability that originating from a politically oppressed religious minority, Ali might have directly experienced lifelong oppression, extreme poverty, and structural, systemic discrimination, racial violence, and the killing, rape, torture, and enslavement of his people over decades by governments, Taliban, and Isis.

I stayed alert to the potential of my own minimising or misunderstanding the level of racial trauma that Ali might have experienced. As a white Western woman, I wondered if I could ever truly know or understand his experiences or his internal world. However, I could offer my full attention, presence, containment, holding, and authentic empathy. I could "bear witness" to his experiences, which Blackwell (1997) notes important when crimes and abuses by perpetrators have not been brought to justice.

At first, I felt detached and numb, aware of an internal voice saying "it can't be real" and resistance to believe the extreme evil of people. This momentary dissociation led to guilt and questioning of how I might reflect "appropriate" containment and empathy. What survival skills and psychic defences must Ali have to endure unimaginable horrors and not fall into suicidal depression?

We must understand and work with our own unconscious defences as refugee children may reveal unspeakable, unbearable experiences. How do we stay with extreme countertransference difficulties and triggering of our unconscious defences and resistances? (Alayarian, 2009,

p. 150) We may be conscious of our privilege, or see the links between our national and colonial histories of oppression, slavery, neglect, collaboration with international arms dealing, and warfare against these children. Some refugee children may have been forced or groomed to be perpetrators of murder, torture, rape, and violence—but they are also victims.

I awoke on occasion from nightmares, flooded with distorted images of death, destruction, brutality, torture, murder. The impact of secondary, vicarious trauma on therapists is real and to be taken seriously; it is not simply hearing and taking in another's suffering—the process of containment can feel almost an energetic exchange. Therapists also risk becoming exhausted, desensitised, or demotivated, as our own nervous systems are bombarded with traumatic stories and unconscious countertransferences. As well as our clients, trauma can become stuck in our bodies (Van der Kolk, 2014), so self-care might include somatic movement and physiological release, rest, mindfulness, connection, playfulness, and adequate clinical supervision (Rothschild, 2006b; van Dernoot Lipsky & Burk, 2009). Every therapist will know how hard these balances are, but working with refugee children, the risk is higher.

Uncertain future: economic realities

Many refugee children will have been affected by extreme poverty and destitution at some point (Blackwell, 2007). Some will have been abandoned, faced violence living on the street, or forced into child labour or trading sexual "favours" for food and shelter (Alayarian, 2009, p. 147).

"I want to help my people. I want to send them money, they have no food, no home, no place, I am lucky."

I glimpsed perhaps Ali's own past experience of hunger and poverty, beyond what I have experienced or could imagine. It was clear that Ali's economic, material, and financial realities significantly impacted his mental health. As a refugee child, his psychic vulnerabilities were compounded by uncertainty of immigration status, unstable housing, being a looked-after child in foster care, and, for his near future, he would be leaving care, self-reliant again. Kazdin (2006, cited in Isakson et al., 2015) suggests psychotherapists should support "clinically significant change in real world metrics that are relevant to clients". We might include clients' preferences, hopes, and outcomes and whatever is in "the best interests of the child" as an integral part of our treatment plan.

So I reflected how I might widen my therapeutic agenda and role with this child, to support the strengthening of his holding environment (Winnicott, 1965), and building his social support networks. I offered to assist Ali to find out who else might help him navigate UK systems and services. He smiled grimly and nodded, "I had so many problems when I came, I did not have good papers so they did not believe I was not adult."

Age assessments of older adolescent refugee children without paper-based evidence can be extensive and they risk being termed adults and having services withdrawn. In line with the therapeutic aim to establish safety and security, I found external, specialist legal and community-based resources, and, with Ali's permission, contacted a key worker at the local authority. I also gave him contacts for specialist legal centres and some refugee youth voluntary sector organisations who might provide further clinical care, casework, advocacy, and other support for Ali—if not now, when he left foster care as an "adult".

Mental health services in isolation cannot meet the needs of refugee children; the wider context is critical in exacerbating or preventing further mental health problems. The World Health Organization's layered system of care (Inter-Agency Standing Committee, IASC, 2007) prioritises refugee children's economic and social conditions to prevent further traumatisation and compounding psychiatric/psychological disorders. Refugee children need help to find advocates and caseworkers, navigate social care needs and local pathways, and make recommendations and referrals across services. Child and adolescent psychotherapists are in a unique position to hold the different aspects of children's lives, including their economic situations. We are integral in participating in, if not building a multidisciplinary team around the child (TAC) and liaising with professionals to meet the multilayered needs of refugee children. Isakson et al. (2015) recommend including caregivers, psychiatrists and psychotherapists, primary health-care workers, child welfare and caseworkers, teachers, refugee resettlement agencies, juvenile justice advocates, and refugee community and religious leaders where appropriate.

Depending on our capacity and motivations, psychotherapists can also be advocates and campaigners for refugee children (Horlings & Hein, 2017); and Frounfelker et al. (2020) suggest there could be more proactive dialogue between researchers/psychotherapists and policymakers, immigration officials, or local communities.

It turned out that our therapeutic relationship was ruptured prematurely by Ali moving school, but we were able to have a few weeks to review the work we had done, to think together about what the ending meant, what was next for him, and to mitigate some feelings around abandonment or mistrust. Ali was able to reflect on a "good enough" experience of a white, Western, non-Muslim female therapist and told me he felt a little more able to trust professionals to help him. I felt we had built trust based on our differences, not despite them. I hoped he had internalised some sense of safety and connection when he had seemed so alone and disconnected, and that he found spaciousness and hope for his future.

Adaku, seven, from Nigeria

A small-framed, thin African child, Adaku was referred by her primary school for appearing to be anxious, withdrawn, and sad. "She hardly speaks at all, and she won't tell me if anything is wrong," her class teacher told me. Although the school had an idea the family had immigrated from Africa, very little was known about Adaku's sociocultural background or flight to Europe. Adaku's school had no idea about the depth of trauma she and her family had experienced.

My understanding around Adaku's traumatic early years and refugee experience came from working reflectively with her mother, Chinwe. Born in rural Nigeria, Adaku was the fifth child of seven, with four older sisters and two younger brothers who were born in quick succession after Adaku. Whilst having many children was thought of as a "blessing" culturally, life for Adaku's family in Nigeria was hard; they were cattle famers/herders who struggled with drought, hunger, and poverty and were dependent on their kinship system and wider community.

When Adaku was three years old, decades of ethnic and religious conflict reached their village, and young men affiliated with Boko Haram burned down their church and many houses. The gangs kidnapped young boys, including Adaku's cousin, and killed her uncle by cutting his throat. Some women and girls were raped in the village. Adaku's parents and two other adults fled with the children. The family had experienced horrors, loss of loved ones, their home, their land and livestock, their community, and, ultimately, their homeland. Adaku's early life was one of basic survival, terror, and grief, unsatiated hunger, poverty, and homelessness. If not in conscious memory, many of these experiences would lie latent in unconscious neural networks, in her nervous system and body, and she might be experiencing transgenerational trauma through her parents' distress, their unconscious interactions, projections, and displaced emotional flashbacks. And although they now had refugee status with indefinite leave to remain in the UK, their housing was unstable, having been evicted and moved around filthy and inadequate private-rented accommodation in a deprived area.

In conceptualising Adaku's case, DSM-5 (APA, 2013) lists separate criteria for children under six years, but Alayarian (2009, p. 152) notes how young refugee children can present differently and may not present with clear PTSD symptoms, but rather with manifestations that are less visible and easily missed in young children, such as generalised fears, separation anxiety, developmental delays or regressions, attachment issues, avoidance, or pre-occupation with symbols and words that seem unrelated to trauma. She recommends individualised, in-depth assessment, and longer-term holistic therapies that encompass childhood and developmental traumas, attachment, and involving wider systems of family/carers and community.

I wanted to meet Adaku and be fully present for her and who and where she was as a seven-year-old child, here and now. Although I had introduced myself to her around the school, in our first therapy session, Adaku walked solemnly into the room, her head bowed, with no eye contact. She looked nervous as she sat on the chair, a foot tapping rhythmically against the chair leg. Adaku said nothing, her mouth pursed shut, but although she remained silent, I saw her whole body, especially her feet, communicating loudly, her anxiety palpable in the room.

Adaku had shining dark brown skin, her hair braided tightly against her head, running into little plaits at the back of her bowed neck, and her uniform neat and tucked in, her socks pulled up to her knee. She appeared physically fragile and small to me compared to her classmates, her arms and legs thin and bony. I wondered how well she ate and grew. In the countertransference, I felt unusually very consciously aware of my size and height compared to Adaku's tiny frame and her being so polite and inhibited, her apparent need to please me, mixed with a tangible sense of her fear and confusion. She had no reference point as to what she was doing in this room with this white woman and did not speak nor question anything, even when I explicitly invited her to ask me anything. In addition to feeling safe, a therapeutic aim was to find sense of power, sense of Self, and voice.

My contracting with children and adolescents always includes naming and rebalancing or equalising of the power differential in the therapeutic relationship from the start, in an age-appropriate way.

"You have not done anything wrong, Adaku! I am here to help you, but I am not the boss or the teacher or an expert in you! How can I possibly know what it is like to be you, Adaku? Only you know what it is like to be you inside."

Adaku nodded but stayed staring at the floor; but she was listening. I continued.

"As long as you are safe and I'm not worried about you being hurt or harmed, whatever you draw, do, or say in here is private. I will not be telling your parents or teacher or friends, although you can talk to anyone about whatever you want, okay?"

Adaku looked up, as if to check my face for truth—this part was relevant to her. As she glanced up briefly, I saw fear and vulnerability but also depth and hope in her round, brown eyes.

I wondered about how safe Adaku felt if she did not feel able to speak or interact. Although she may have political safety in having refugee status, and had some immediate family around her, her somatic state conveyed "unsafe" to me. Was her silence protective? I wondered what she might need from therapy and me. Working child-led, I allowed Adaku's process to unfold slowly through her choice of integrative, creative, art, play, and sand-tray therapies.

Adaku stood back and touched nothing in the room as I showed her around the sand-tray, figurines, toys, and art materials in the room. Only when I explicitly invited her to take something, in silence she took an A4 paper and lead pencil and started drawing clouds and birds. I checked she was ok with where I sat, that she wanted me to sit next to her, and paid full attention to tracking her unconscious process and allowing the therapeutic relationship to form. She worked in silence; I sensed it was comfortable but was careful not to abandon her by offering narrative around key elements of her drawing every so often. Over the first few sessions, I felt spaciousness in her silence, and she worked slowly, methodically, every pen and brush stroke purposeful and careful. Every now and again, she would glance up to see if I was still watching her, still present; she was experiencing being seen and heard.

As she felt more comfortable, she stopped seeking permission to explore or use materials, and began to use larger pieces of paper, more and brighter colours, and her diagrammatic line drawings transformed into more fluid, colour-filled paintings of sky, clouds, land. But no people. I invited her to name a large painting she had spent four sessions doing.

"Free," Adaku whispered.

In the first few weeks of therapy, Adaku seemed desperate to play with everything in the room, as if she would not get to use them again. Like much else in her life, coming from a poor and displaced refugee family, good things do not last. Her projective play with dolls, black and white interacting together, suggested her own difficulties and differences of lifestyle with peers at school. She used various figurines in the sand-tray, deeply buried snakes symbolising unknown or unconscious threats, swords, and other weapons for protection, shoes and feet for escape and freedom (I believe they walked for weeks during their flight out of Nigeria). I noted she began to take her shoes off in the therapy room as she became more comfortable.

Adaku began to express herself more freely in her movement; her feet, toes, and movements would tell me how she felt that day more than her words. Over time, I saw her sadness and anxious energy shift; she would dance and skip, her feet would flick, and she would spin in circles around the room. I saw the power and gift of providing a neutral, non-judgemental, and intermediate space to play (Winnicott, 1971). Through nonverbal, creative, expressive therapies and play in the therapy room, Adaku could experience some free expression and communicate her inner world, her experiences, and her unique socio-cultural experiences and perspectives. The quality and tone of her play and exploration became less frantic, and with this relaxing, she began to seek my interaction with her to play games, with some minimal talking. Staying fully in metaphor, we explored themes of bad luck and skill, strategies, trust, and mistrust. She was finding her voice through play.

Cultural identity and belonging

It appeared Adaku had not learned, nor had space to say, how she felt, so communicating her feelings was a new experience. I hoped through therapy she might experience some connection to herself and gain new perspective about her unique cultural, religious identities, growing up a "British Nigerian" child.

Adaku liked dressing up and draped materials over me to be her "fashion model" and told me she wanted to be a fashion designer.

"I love TV! We watch Nigerian TV all the time. But I like Netflix, but Mum and Dad hate American TV, so I sneak downstairs to watch it. Don't tell them will you, they will be angry." Adaku constantly checked out the therapeutic boundaries of confidentiality, the neutral, non-critical space she needed to find her voice and the free space to explore the different cultural realms she lived in.

She had once watched "RuPaul's Drag Race" on her older sister's mobile phone and was confused but fascinated in men dressing as women. Despite her young age, she asked me questions about gender and sexuality. She told me "gay people" would be killed in her country and that her parents said it was "an abomination to God". I found her family's homophobia extremely hard to even hear coming from such a small child. It was a challenge to sensitively acknowledge her family's cultural and religious values whilst being authentic and conveying to Adaku human rights and values of equality and empathy. I wondered how it was for Adaku to navigate, transition between her different cultural worlds now and over her lifetime, and how I might adapt our work together to incorporate Nigerian-African perspectives. Integrative approaches such as play, sand-tray, and art therapy enabled a creative space into which Adaku could bring whatever arose in this regard.

Culture relates to every level of lived experience, a "symbolic universe", a "matrix of representation, enactment, communication and meaning … the internal structuring of individual mental life" (Blackwell, 2005b, p. 38). Culture is central to identity and belonging, influencing how we view ourselves, others, and the world around us. Few validated assessment tools exist to assess and measure the sociocultural or religious dimensions of refugee children's lives, but there is clear understanding that culture plays a role in trauma and healing (Kirmayer, Rousseau, & Measham, 2011).

There is debate about whether using therapists' "cultural consultants" or "cultural competency" is either desirable or possible (Kleinman & Benson, 2006). To avoid stereotyping, categorising, or othering, perhaps a subjective, anthropological, ethnographic approach (Siddique & Dominguez, 2021) is more relevant to refugee clients in the therapy room.

Likewise, as child psychotherapists, we can reflect on our own cultures, values, and potential unconscious biases and assumptions about our clients and guard against cultural differences becoming "a huge and unmanageable gap … or becoming entirely absent" (Blackwell, 2005b, p. 69). Exploring and working through client–therapist differences can help build trust and shared understanding between client and therapist and "establish a conversation not between cultures, but among human beings" (Kohrt, Maharjan, Timsina, & Griffith, 2012, p. 105).

Parent, family, and systemic work

Considering developmental and relational traumas (unrelated to refugee experience) and, where possible, reflective work with parents and carers can be essential, especially with younger children. So as a usual part of the consent, assessment, and referral process, and as part of Adaku's therapy, I met with Adaku's mother Chinwe every half term, "to think together". I invited both parents, but Dad never came; he was always working one of his three jobs.

With a good grasp of English, standing tall and proud, wearing traditional African colours, Chinwe seemed at first glance to be a wealthy, middle-class woman. Although she had given written consent, she wanted to know how therapy could change Adaku's behaviour and make her listen and learn better, and was initially not concerned with Adaku's mental or emotional state.

"She is a naughty girl sometimes, she must be obedient and learn the rules. We are lucky to be in this country and she has to work hard to show God that she is grateful and she will then be a success for us. We raise her in the good Christian and African way, she must respect her elders, learn these things and God will bless her."

Adaku's name also had particular meaning to the family—"one who brings wealth to the family"—so, from birth, potentially lived with unconscious projections, hope, and burden. Much of the work with Chinwe centred around developing mentalizing capacity, empathy, and aspirations for Adaku for herself as a young child, beyond the needs of the family. Chinwe was able to describe her own upbringing and harsh expectations and understand that her own cultural transition to the UK went deeper than fashion and environment.

As often happens, I heard a parent's defensive position, and a potential "authoritarian parenting style" (a Western concept). I also felt compassion for Chinwe and understood that with so much traumatic grief and loss, and wanting so desperately to return to her homeland, Mum held on tightly to what she could from their religious and cultural heritage, identities, and practices. Culturally, Chinwe's village did raise the children together, and the importance of family, community, and cultural collective far outweighed individual need. I held in mind if referral to more specialist systemic, family interventions may be beneficial in addition to my working with Adaku (Woodcock, 2000; Slobodin & de Jong, 2015).

I kept safeguarding and the best interests of Adaku firmly in the forefront of my mind as cultural and religious views came up. At one meeting, Chinwe told me: "Adaku gets headaches, but we have a nice pastor in my community, we are going to ask him to deal with her bad behaviour, we are worried about bad spirits."

I became more concerned as Chinwe's approach to obedience and discipline felt more like punishment through isolation and shaming, and, although undisclosed, I suspected smacking or other physical chastisement. Potentially a child protection issue, I opened up discussion with Mum and the designated safeguarding lead (DSL) and the need to involve the GP about Adaku's medical needs. The school developed a "team around the child" approach where we were able to actively monitor and navigate Adaku's health and well-being whilst respecting the family's cultural and religious beliefs. Compassionate, reflective parenting work can be critical to navigating cultural practices that cross the lines of safeguarding, emotional, and physical abuse. As with any child, attachment issues and parental mental health needs are essential to consider with parents and carers of refugee children. This can be the key to change in the child's life.

I reflected with Mum, too, about Adaku's minimal eating, low weight, and tiny frame. Mum at first linked her weight loss to "spiritual illness", and she hoped Adaku had the potential to be a healer. I raised another cause for concern with the DSL and thought with Mum about the potential of eating disorders, which is not a commonly diagnosed disorder in Africa but too high a risk to dismiss as cultural or religious beliefs.

Chinwe developed enough trust to tell me more about their religious beliefs, which incorporated a mix of traditional African spirituality in four interacting layers of mind-vitality, body-vitality, body, and inner spirit, integrated with Christianity. Adaku also showed me her sense of fearing supernatural forces in her play, projecting through the figurines in the sand-tray, dark figures and "spirits" that terrified her. Therapy can provide a safe place to express children's religious experience. Demazure, Gaultier, and Pinsault (2018) found refugee children can experience "possession and trance symptoms", sorcery, and ghosts, and proposed children who were still developing and constructing coping and defensive strategies might avoid or suppress emotions and "fall back" on spiritual and religious beliefs to help them cope.

Ensuring Adaku felt grounded and could find a "safe place" in the therapy room from the spirits, it was important to check both in and out of metaphor the potential of psychosis, how she experienced these spirits. Adaku was not always plagued by them; it was part of the familial, sociocultural narrative. Faith can provide positive, protective factors, existential understanding, and meaning to experiences (e.g. "karma"). Blackwell (2007) notes religious beliefs have specific significance to many of our clients, whether in political, sociocultural, or psychological terms, giving strength, resilience, or meaning to their experiences. Fennig (2021) describes how indigenous faith and healing practices can be used either as specific methods or systematically integrated within psychotherapy. For example, prayer and meditative practices have been shown to enhance behavioural activation, cognitive restructuring, and emotional regulation (Hinton & Jalal, 2014, cited in Fennig, 2021).

Religion and politics often seem to activate defences of avoidance or ridicule in British culture, or are not spoken of for fear of intrusion or offence. Blackwell (2005a, p. 17) notes therapists may resist or minimise religious belief systems as "quirks … inhibitions, prohibitions or delusions", rather than "sources of revelation and inspiration". We might wonder about our own "neutrality", assumptions, and biases, and how we implement humanistic core conditions in this regard.

Working with both Adaku and Mum, my mind switched constantly between trying to understand and empathise from Adaku's cultural and religious perspective and my Western perspective drawn from integrative child psychotherapy training, attachment in a large family, my developmental age, developmental trauma, sibling position and rivalries. I also knew I had Westernised projections and hopes for Adaku to be recognised, appreciated, and that she might live as the unique, individual child she is. In supervision, I grappled with uncomfortable feelings and biased thoughts around the differences in my own and her parents' parenting style, and their cultural values of "strength" being work, academic achievement, and financial wealth.

This was my task in working with our cultural and religious differences, to traverse and contain, to hold compassion, warmth, and empathy for Mum, whilst encouraging those same qualities to be passed on to Adaku, separating our behaviours from the emotional and psychological needs of both Adaku and her family. Mum's fears and suffering were being displaced onto Adaku, almost as if Adaku was to be the "carrier" of the family's past and thus their "healer".

Over the months, as Mum got to know me and understood that I was not there to judge her or her child, her defences softened and revealed her own childhood traumas and my naming of "transgenerational trauma" and "collective trauma" (Hübl & Avritt, 2020). These concepts captured Mum's interest and helped her to understand how Adaku might be carrying some of Mum's own experiences and that Chinwe might actively begin her own process of recovery and healing, as she accepted my signposting to local adult and refugee therapeutic and support services.

Alongside a free, playful therapy space for Adaku, the reflective work with Mum felt essential, and led to the school leading a wider "team around the child" approach, which provided long-term support for Adaku, her parents, and her siblings.

Reflections

Working therapeutically with refugee children and adolescents requires us to explicitly acknowledge and embrace multilayered realms of difference. Only when we endeavour to meet the child where they are at, where they are from, and with what they have experienced, might we begin to come to know each child, their needs, and how we might support them best.

Blackwell's six dimensions of refugee lived experience (2005b, 2007) is a credible, relevant lens and practical framework within which integrative child and adolescent psychotherapy may work more inclusively with these diverse and vulnerable children. This multilayered approach makes explicit the often hidden, sensitive, or seemingly overwhelming issues and wider contextual factors for both refugee client and therapist that require exploration within therapy settings—factors that may otherwise be misunderstood or missed entirely.

What and how psychotherapists assess, conceptualise, and treat refugee children and adolescents will vary depending on theoretical modality and clinical practice approach and the aim and agenda of therapy. No one intervention has yet been found to be more efficacious or superior to another. In fact, different interventions may lend themselves to different outcome measures of success or progress. Child and adolescent psychotherapists have a responsibility to regularly reflect honestly on our own agendas and aims for interventions or research with refugee children. Are we stuck on a particular modality, approach, or intervention? Do we unconsciously have political or ideological positions about the child's background situation? Do we seek authority or validation of our position or knowledge? We might continue to reflect on why we do our job, when and why we offer interventions, and assess if they are helpful and empowering to refugee children from diverse backgrounds and experiences.

If we scratch the surface of our own schools and communities, we will find many refugee children and young people from varying contexts and backgrounds already among us. Many have lived through complex, traumatic experiences, some still unsafe, without a permanent family to take care of them or without certainty of making their home here. Many children suffer in silence with devastating grief and loss, complex, multilayered trauma, fear and isolation. Very few will ever reach our therapy rooms unless we reach out.

References

Alayarian A. (2009). Children, torture and psychological consequences. *Torture*, *19*(2): 145–156.

Alayarian, A. (2015). *Handbook of Working with Children, Trauma, and Resilience: An Intercultural Psychoanalytic View*. London: Karnac.

American Psychiatric Association (APA) (2013). *Diagnostic and Statistical Manual of Mental Disorders: DSM-5-TR*. Washington, DC: American Psychiatric Association.

BenEzer, G. (2012). From Winnicott's potential space to mutual creative space: A principle for intercultural psychotherapy. *Transcultural Psychiatry*, *49*(2): 323–339. https://doi.org/10.1177/1363461511435803

Blackwell, D. (1997). Holding, containing and bearing witness: The problem of helpfulness in encounters with torture survivors. *Journal of Social Work Practice*, *11*(2): 81–89. https://doi.org/10.1080/02650539708415116

Blackwell, D. (2005a). Psychotherapy, politics and trauma: Working with survivors of torture and organized violence. *Group Analysis*, *38*(2): 307–323. https://doi.org/10.1177/0533316405052386

Blackwell, D. (2005b). *Counselling and Psychotherapy with Refugees*. London: Jessica Kingsley.

Blackwell, D. (2007). Oppression and freedom in therapeutic space. *European Journal of Psychotherapy & Counselling*, *9*(3): 255–265. https://doi.org/10.1080/13642530701496856

Bronstein, I., & Montgomery, P. (2011). Psychological Distress in refugee children: A systematic review. *Clinical Child and Family Psychology Review*, *14*(1): 44–56. https://doi.org/10.1007/s10567-010-0081-0

Demazure, G., Gaultier, S., & Pinsault, N. (2018). Dealing with difference: A scoping review of psychotherapeutic interventions with unaccompanied refugee minors. *European Child & Adolescent Psychiatry*, *27*(4): 447–466. https://doi.org/10.1007/s00787-017-1083-y

Fazel, M., Reed, R. V., Panter-Brick, C., & Stein, A. (2012). Mental health of displaced and refugee children resettled in high-income countries: Risk and protective factors. *The Lancet*, *379*(9812): 266–28. https://doi.org/10.1016/s0140-6736(11)60051-2

Fennig, M. (2021). Cultural adaptations of evidence-based mental health interventions for refugees: Implications for clinical social work. *The British Journal of Social Work*, *51*(3): 964–981. https://doi.org/10.1093/bjsw/bcaa024

Freud, A. (1966). *The Ego and the Mechanisms of Defence.* London: Routledge. https://doi.org/10.4324/9780429481550

Frounfelker, R. L., Miconi, D., Farrar, J., Brooks, M. A., Rousseau, C., & Betancourt, T. S. (2020). Mental health of refugee children and youth: Epidemiology, interventions, and future directions. *Annual Review of Public Health*, *41*(1): 159–176. https://doi.org/10.1146/annurev-publhealth-040119-094230

Herman, J. L. (1992). *Trauma and Recovery.* London: Pandora.

Home Office (2021). https://www.gov.uk/government/collections/immigration-statistics-quarterly-release https://www.gov.uk/government/statistical-data-sets/asylum-and-resettlement-datasets, https://www.gov.uk/entering-staying-uk/refugees-asylum-human-rights

Horlings, A., & Hein, I. (2017). Psychiatric screening and interventions for minor refugees in Europe: An overview of approaches and tools. *European Journal of Paediatrics*, *177*: 163–169. https://doi.org/10.1007/s00431-017-3027-4

Hübl, T., & Avritt, J. J. (2020). *Healing Collective Trauma: A Process for Integrating Our Intergenerational and Cultural Wounds.* London: Macmillan.

Inter-Agency Standing Committee (2007). *IASC Guidelines on Mental Health and Psychosocial Support in Emergency Settings.* Geneva: IASC, Inter-Agency Standing Committee.

Isakson, B. L., Legerski, J. P. & Layne, C. M. (2015). Adapting and implementing evidence-based interventions for trauma-exposed refugee youth and families. *Journal of Contemporary Psychotherapy: On the Cutting Edge of Modern Developments in Psychotherapy*, *45*(4): 245–253. https://doi.org/10.1007/s10879-015-9304-5

Kirmayer, L. J., Rousseau C., & Measham T. (2011). Sociocultural considerations of trauma and PTSD. In: D. M. Benedek & G. H. Wynn (Eds.), *Clinical Manual for the Management of PTSD* (pp. 415–444). Washington: American Psychiatric Press.

Kleinman, A. M., & Benson, P. L. (2006). Anthropology in the clinic: The problem of cultural competency and how to fix it. *PLoS Medicine*, *3*(10): 294. https://doi.org/10.1371/journal.pmed.0030294

Kohrt, B. A., Maharjan, S. M., Timsina, D., & Griffith, J. L. (2012). Applying Nepali ethnopsychology to psychotherapy for the treatment of mental illness and prevention of suicide among Bhutanese refugees. *Annals of Anthropological Practice*, *36*(1): 88–112. https://doi.org/10.1111/j.2153-9588.2012.01094.x

Lønning, M. N., & Kohli, R. K. (2022). Memories, mementos, and memorialization of young unaccompanied Afghans navigating within Europe. *Journal of Refugee Studies*, *35*(1): 242–261. https://doi.org/10.1093/jrs/feab074

Maté, G. (2011). *When the Body Says No: The Cost of Hidden Stress*. Toronto: Vintage Canada.

Melzak, S. (2017). Building seven bridges with young asylum seekers living in exile in the UK (Part 1). *Psychodynamic Practice*, *23*(3): 235–248. https://doi.org/10.1080/14753634.2017.1335227

Melzak, S., McLoughlin, C., & Watt, F. (2018). Shifting ground: The child without family in a strange new community. *Journal of Child Psychotherapy*, *44*(3): 326–347. https://doi.org/10.1080/0075417x.2018.1556316

Porges, S. W. (2007). The polyvagal perspective. *Biological Psychology*, *74*(2): 116–143. https://doi.org/10.1016/j.biopsycho.2006.06.009

Porges, S. W., & Dana, D. (2018). *Clinical Applications of the Polyvagal Theory: The Emergence of Polyvagal-Informed Therapies*. New York: W. W. Norton.

Reed, R. V., Fazel, M., Jones, L., Panter-Brick, C., & Stein, A. (2012). Mental health of displaced and refugee children resettled in low-income and middle-income countries: Risk and protective factors: Review. *The Lancet*, *379*: 250–265. https://doi.org/10.1016/s0140-6736(11)60050-0

Refugee Council (2020). Children in the asylum system, May 2019. https://www.refugeecouncil.org.uk/wp-content/uploads/2019/06/Children-in-the-Asylum-System-May-2019.pdf

Rohlof, H., Knipscheer, J. W., & Kleber, R. J. (2014). Somatization in refugees: A review. *Social Psychiatry and Psychiatric Epidemiology*, *49*(11): 1793–1804. https://doi.org/10.1007/s00127-014-0877-1

Rothschild, B. (2000). *The Body Remembers: The Psychophysiology of Trauma and Trauma Treatment*. London: W. W. Norton.

Rothschild, B. (2006a). *The Body Remembers Casebook: Unifying Methods and Models in the Treatment of Trauma and PTSD*. London: W. W. Norton.

Rothschild, B. (2006b). *Help for the Helper: The Psychophysiology of Compassion Fatigue and Vicarious Trauma*. London: W. W. Norton.

Schwartz, R. C. (2013). *Internal Family Systems Therapy*. New York: Guilford.

Schwartz, S., & Melzak, S. (2005). Using storytelling in psychotherapeutic group work with young refugees. *Group Analysis*, *38*(2): 293–306. https://doi.org/10.1177/0533316405052385

Siddique, S., & Dominguez, V. R. (2021). Anthropology in the consulting room: An interview with Salma Siddique by Virginia R. Dominguez. *American Anthropologist*, 123(1): 179–183. https://doi.org/10.1111/aman.13531

Siegel, D. J. (2010). *The Mindful Therapist: A Clinician's Guide to Mindsight and Neural Integration*. New York: W. W. Norton.

Slobodin, O., & De Jong, J. T. (2015). Family interventions in traumatized immigrants and refugees: A systematic review. *Transcultural Psychiatry*, 52(6): 723–742. https://doi.org/10.1177/1363461515588855

Stern, D. N. (2004). *The Present Moment in Psychotherapy and Everyday Life*. New York: W. W. Norton.

Townsend, M. (2022, October 22). Asylum seekers: Home Office accused of "catastrophic child protection failure". *The Guardian*. https://www.theguardian.com/uk-news/2022/oct/22/uk-asylum-seekers-home-office-accused-of-catastrophic-child-protection-failure

United Nations General Assembly (UNGA) (2005). Assistance to unaccompanied refugee minors: Report of the Secretary-General. www.unicef.org/protection/files/CRCGC6_EN.pdf

United Nations High Commissioner for Refugees (UNHCR) (2018). Global trends: Forced displacement in 2017. Report, Geneva. www.unhcr.org/dach/wp-content/uploads/sites/27/2018/06/GlobalTrends2017.pdf

Van der Kolk, B. A. (2014). *The Body Keeps the Score: Brain, Mind, and Body in the Healing of Trauma*. New York: Penguin.

Van Dernoot Lipsky, L., & Burk, C. (2009). *Trauma Stewardship: An Everyday Guide to Caring for Self While Caring for Others*. Oakland, CA: Berrett-Koehler.

Winnicott, D. W. (1965). *The Maturational Processes and the Facilitating Environment: Studies in the Theory of Emotional Development*. Connecticut: International Universities Press.

Winnicott, D. W. (1971). *Playing and Reality*. New York: Basic Books.

Woodcock, J. (2000). Refugee children and their families: Theoretical and clinical perspectives. In: K. Dwivedi (Ed.), *Post Traumatic Stress Disorder in Children and Adolescents*. London: Whurr.

Wylie, L., Van Meyel, R., Harder, H., Sukhera, J., Luc, C., Ganjavi, H., Elfakhani, M., & Wardrop, N. (2018). Assessing trauma in a transcultural context: Challenges in mental health care with immigrants and refugees. *Public Health Reviews*, 39(1). https://doi.org/10.1186/s40985-018-0102-y

Specialist contacts and resources supporting refugee children and adolescents—psychotherapy, clinical care, and multi-disciplinary support

Amna Refugee Trauma Initiative https://amna.org/

Anna Freud Centre https://mentallyhealthyschools.org.uk/risks-and-protective-factors/vulnerable-children/refugee-asylum-seeker-children/

Asphaleia https://www.asphaleia.co.uk/

Baobab Centre for Young Survivors in Exile https://baobabsurvivors.org/

Barnardos https://www.barnardos.org.uk/what-we-do/helping-families/children-seeking-asylum

Childline https://www.childline.org.uk/info-advice/bullying-abuse-safety/your-rights/child-refugees-and-asylum-seekers/

Children and Families Across Borders https://www.cfab.org.uk/

The Children's Society https://www.childrenssociety.org.uk/what-we-do/our-work/young-refugees-migrants

Freedom from Torture https://www.freedomfromtorture.org/

Helen Bamber Foundation https://www.helenbamber.org/

Migrant Help https://www.migranthelpuk.org/what-we-do

Nafsiyat Intercultural Therapy Centre https://www.nafsiyat.org.uk/

Red Cross https://www.redcross.org.uk/get-help/get-help-as-a-young-refugee-or-asylum-seeker

Refugee Council https://www.refugeecouncil.org.uk/our-work/children/

Refugee Effective Partnership—list of refugee community support organisations http://reap.org.uk/useful-websites-for-refugee-groups/support-organisations-young-refugees-children/

Refugee Therapy Centre https://refugeetherapy.org.uk

Solace (Yorkshire) https://www.solace-uk.org.uk/

UK Trauma Council https://uktraumacouncil.org/research_practice/refugee-asylum-seeking-resources

Waterloo Community Counselling https://waterloocc.co.uk/multi-ethnic-counselling-service/

YoungMinds https://www.youngminds.org.uk/professional/resources/supporting-refugee-and-asylum-seeking-children/

Young Roots https://www.youngroots.org.uk/

Medical and health care

Doctors of the World https://www.doctorsoftheworld.org.uk/

Legal, asylum, and immigration

Association of Visitors to Immigration Detainees https://aviddetention.org.uk/
Asylum Aid https://www.asylumaid.org.uk/
Asylum Support Appeals Project https://www.asaproject.org/
Coram Children's Legal Centre Advocacy Service https://coramvoice.org.uk/get-help/alwaysheard/
Coram Legal Centre Migrant Children's Project https://www.childrenslegalcentre.com/about-us/what-we-do/migrant-childrens-project/
Just for Kids Law https://www.justforkidslaw.org/
Rainbow Migration (LGBTQ+) https://www.rainbowmigration.org.uk/
Safe Passage https://www.safepassage.org.uk/

Further resources

The Fostering Network https://www.thefosteringnetwork.org.uk/advice-information/looking-after-fostered-child/looking-after-unaccompanied-asylum-seeker-children
National Education Union https://neu.org.uk/media/1936
UK Council for International Student Affairs https://www.ukcisa.org.uk/
UNICEF https://www.unicef.org/migrant-refugee-internally-displaced-children
United Nations High Commission for Refugees (UNHCR) https://www.unhcr.org/handbooks/ih/age-gender-diversity/refugee-children-and-youth

Campaigns

Amnesty International https://www.amnesty.org.uk/refugee-asylum-seeker-migrant-human-rights
Human Rights Watch https://www.hrw.org/topic/refugees-and-migrants
Migrant Rights Network https://migrantsrights.org.uk/
Refugee Action https://www.refugee-action.org.uk/
Save the Children https://www.savethechildren.org/us/what-we-do/emergency-response/refugee-children-crisis

CHAPTER 5

Unveiling racial trauma in the practice of the integrative child and adolescent psychotherapist

Audrey Adeyemi

Introduction

In this chapter, I present two case studies: the case of fourteen-year-old Missy and that of seven-year-old Ike. Both young people are referred by their prospective schools for weekly forty-to-fifty minute sessions. In both cases, I gain insight into the difficulties they face surrounding racial/ethnic identity through an acculturation framework (Berry, 2006, 2007). I chose this framework because it regards the phenomena between two or more ethnocultural groups interacting with each other and the strategies used to adapt to living with diverse racial, ethnic, and cultural groups (Berry, 2006, 2007). Acculturative stress is a feature of acculturation when the process becomes problematic due to the social and psychological adaptations that must occur (Berry, 2006, 2007).

The four acculturation strategies that can be adopted relate to the preference for maintaining heritage culture and/or preference for maintaining proximity to the dominant ethnocultural group (Berry, 2006, 2007). Figure 5.1 shows the four acculturation strategies of non-dominant groups.

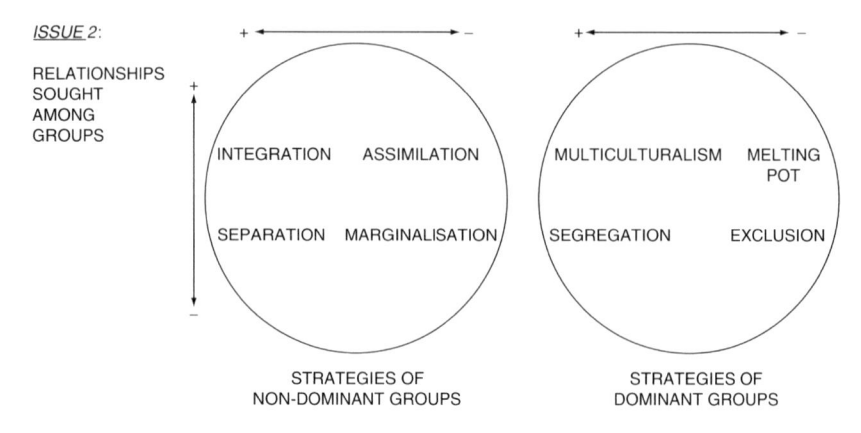

Figure 5.1 Acculturation strategies in ethnocultural groups and in the larger society

By using this framework, I identified that the obligation to choose acculturation strategies can be stressful, particularly when ethnic or racial identity is emerging. Ethnic identity becomes salient in adolescence (Evans, Copping, Rowley, & Kurtz-Costes, 2011; Rogers, Scott, & Way, 2014). How the outside world perceives specific ethnocultural groups becomes pertinent (Erikson, 1968), and young people from non-dominant groups begin to question their ethnic identity and how that shapes their sense of self. Racial and ethnic identity development signals an awareness of belonging to a racial or ethnic group and the extent to which that is central to a core identity (Phinney, 1990; Wakefield & Hudley, 2007; Quintana, 2007).

The acculturation experiences of young people from black, Asian, and minority ethnic (BAME) communities will likely be different than those from other ethnocultural groups due to the historical ways in which people with brown skin from Africa or the Caribbean have been negatively perceived. They may become vulnerable to racist projections through projective identification (Klein, 1996) and begin to feel intellectually inferior based on existing feelings of inferiority originating from structural racism. Psychological processes such as those stemming from racial difference induce acculturative stress.

Racial and ethnic identity can have more salience than gender identity in spaces where acculturation takes place, compared to an ethnically or racially homogenous society (Phinney, 1990) where gender identity may have more primacy. Acculturative stress born from a feeling of not belonging and feeling racially inferior can be buffered by a strong feeling of ethnic or racial pride (Hope et al., 2021; Okeke, Howard, Kurtz-Costes, & Rowley, 2009; Oyserman, Kemmelmeier, Fryberg, Brosh, & Hart-Johnson, 2003; Robinson, 2000; Seaton & Iida, 2019; Sellers, Copeland-Linder, Martin, & Lewis, 2006; Utsey, Chae, Brown, & Kelly, 2002; Wakefield & Hudley, 2007; Wong, Eccles, & Sameroff, 2003).

As in the cases of Missy and Ike, some children may attempt to obscure their "blackness" and cultural differences through modifications of speech, appearance, or behaviour to belong and find acceptance within a white hegemonic society. "Splitting" (Klein, 1996) is a defence mechanism that becomes mobilised to feel more white and less black, given that "blackness" has been denigrated historically. Fundamentally, successful acculturation such as the integration and assimilation approach denotes "proximity to white people" (Liu et al., 2017, p. 143) and being "racially innocuous" (ibid.).

Missy

Fourteen-year-old Missy is referred to me by the school due to their concerns about her academic performance. In the year preceding the sessions, her grades have changed from straight As to Cs, and she has become withdrawn and less sociable with her peers. Missy agrees to therapy as she is worried about her future beyond school. I am not aware of Missy's cultural background at the point of referral, just her age, school year, and reason for referral. My sessions with Missy take place in the morning during the first period, in a small room in a quiet part of the school.

When I meet Missy, I notice her brown complexion, hair, and features which indicate she is mixed-race. She arrives five minutes early and I gently ask her to wait until the allotted time. At the appointed time, I open the door and look out to see that she is sitting by the door reading a book. I usher her in and ask what she is reading. It's an astrology book. She moves slowly, puts her book back in her bag, and stands up.

She attempts to smile and enters looking nervous, but then stops and looks around the room curiously. Her bushy, curly hair is held back in a bun, but I notice the volume of her hair and that her school blazer seems too big, although beneath she appears slim. Her big, brown eyes look at me enquiringly, as if she is trying to figure me out. I immediately feel the urge to guide and protect her, unsure if I am experiencing maternal countertransference triggered by the troubled look in her eyes or if my maternal urges have been triggered.

I invite her to take a seat on the floor cushions or the chair, and she chooses the chair. I start the session as I do, explaining what I know about her referral and her expectations for therapy. Missy explains that she is worried about her motivation and is struggling to concentrate on lessons and homework. She is not sure why she is feeling demotivated except that she is experiencing school as stressful and feels the need to relax and not constantly worry about grades. As she speaks about not knowing why she feels as she does, there are moments she stops to think and reflect, as if she is focusing on understanding what has been taking place in her life. I enquire about changes that may have occurred during the last two years and there are none that she recalls. As she is not consciously aware of what has triggered the changes, I wonder what her unconscious difficulties are.

I invite Missy to tell me more about her family and offer her the option to draw a family tree. Missy wants to draw one using pen and paper. She includes her parents, brother, aunt, and cousins from her father's side. There is more information about the aunt's side of the family, including cousins, their partners' names, as well as their children. This side of the family comes to life on the page compared to the information about Missy's mother's side. I ask what she would like to tell me about her father, mother, brother, and aunt.

As she explains family life, she keeps her head down, looking at the page. She enjoys spending time with her aunt and visits when she can, as her home is bigger and her parents cannot accommodate them all when they visit. I note a longing in her tone as she speaks about spending time with her aunt, and I say it sounds as if she is missing them, to which she nods. At this stage, I explain the therapeutic contract and ask if she would like to add to it. She says, "So you won't tell my parents what I tell you?" I confirm the confidentiality rule unless she raises a safeguarding concern. I also explain that beyond the initial assessment, she is free thereafter to use the materials in the room and/or to talk about what is on her mind. I ask what materials she is drawn to, and she says she likes to draw and paint.

I reflect upon the session and think about the family tree she has drawn. I wonder what her aunt and that side of her family represent and why she spoke scantily about home life. It seems as if home life is distinctly different from her aunt's home, in the absence of information about it. There were moments when she seemed relaxed and others when she withdrew from eye contact and seemed uncomfortable. I think about her appearance and the discordance between her big blazer and her small frame and how her big, curly hair has been tied back. She has bright enquiring eyes and a quiet, gentle tone, looking younger than her fourteen years. She is articulate, but appears passive, shrinking. I wonder whether she favours one side of her racial heritage. She has not mentioned the racial or cultural origins of her family, and I did not ask, perhaps because the inquiry felt forbidden. I think about getting-to-know activities that could provide insight into her life.

In the following sessions, I learn about Missy's interest in astrology and spending time with her aunt and cousins. I find out she is a Virgo and that she enjoys cooking Caribbean food with her aunt and cousins.

She often speaks about the Grenadian foods she enjoys, and I sense she wants me to know about that side of her. Is she communicating a cultural aspect of her Grenadian heritage that is important and gives her identity?

In supervision, we discuss Missy's attachment to her Grenadian side and the apparent absence of information about her Irish side. There appears to be an ambivalence between home life and life with her aunt with whom she experiences connection and cultural enrichment. She appears to seek a "cultural home" (Vivero & Jenkins, 1999), a place of belonging and receiving a "cultural identity" (Vivero & Jenkins, 1999). Perhaps this is missing at home, creating a defensive reaction of disavowal and possible resentment within Missy (Bokanowski, 2018).

I think about my racial/cultural identity and the anchor it provided as an adolescent black, British/African female. The West African cultural traditions my parents instilled at home grounded me during my racial/cultural identity struggles. How might Missy feel without a sense of belonging at home?

In the following sessions, themes around belonging and difference emerge. Missy begins to talk about the difficulties in school and at home. She becomes visibly upset and angry during a session after I mention the changes that have occurred in her performance at school. She looks at me and holds a scared, defiant stare. I feel destabilised by it, as I have not seen any anger or rage in her until that moment. I am unsure whether I should stay with her feeling or soothe it, but I sense the gravity in her expression, and so I ask if she can share what she would say to her mother and father if they were in the room with her now. Tears come and she begins to sob. As she sobs, I sit near her, saying that it is okay to cry and that if anything is needed, such as a hug or to hold her hand, she can ask. She asks me to hold her hand as her tears flow, and I wait for her to stop and wipe her eyes. They are swollen and red, but the heaviness has disappeared from the room. Missy begins telling me about her home life, and over several sessions I learn a great deal about Missy and her life.

The racial trauma

Missy explains that her parents have an unhappy marriage. They met after her father's first wife died. Her mother's Irish family did not accept her marriage to a black, Grenadian man, and she is ostracised by all but a few of her nieces. The sacrifices each has made to be together has put an enormous strain on their relationship. Missy feels split between the two sides and begins to consider how this division affects her feelings towards her mixed-race heritage. There is a deprivation of practices that allow her to experience cultural or racial pride at home and construct a coherent narrative about her cultural and racial identity. She notices she is struggling with a sense of familial and societal belonging.

The session that reveals Missy's feelings about belonging and acceptance aligning with feelings towards her racial and cultural heritage follows an exercise called "the shape I am in" (Gammage, 2021). I hope this exercise offers Missy the space to project onto paper the "phantasies" (Klein, 1923, p. 437) she has about her phenotypic characteristics and for us to explore that. I ask her to draw an image of herself and provide skin-tone crayons to choose her skin colour. She depicts herself as a small figure with lighter brown skin than her own and with big, curly, brown hair that covers most of the page. I look at the drawing for a while, as the incongruent nature of her image absorbs me. She laughs and says she looks ridiculous in her drawing and wonders why she has drawn herself in such a way. I say that I notice the hair and that it takes up much of the page. She laughs again and says her hair is always in the way. On both occasions when she laughs, I experience a bodily sensation as if something unpleasant and disowned is being forced into me (Segal, 1954). I suddenly feel awkward and aware that her drawing has elicited a defensive reaction that I am identifying with (Klein, 1996).

I am curious about why she says her drawing is ridiculous and ask her to elaborate on that theme. She becomes reflective but unsure of why she has drawn herself that way. I ask her to speak as the drawing. I ask her to introduce herself, to which she replies, "Hello, I'm the weird, mixed-race girl, with no friends." I feel immense sadness and notice Missy becomes limp and looks exhausted. I draw attention to her body language and she looks up with watery eyes and says loudly, "No one gets me!" I feel that she is perhaps furious at me for not getting her and I gently enquire. She says, "I thought you would understand what it is like to be me because you look like me." I feel her outrage that I do not get her. She looks pained and I ask her if she is referring to us both having brown skin. She nods and says, "I guess you would understand, but we never talk about it." I am pleased yet taken by surprise by her honesty, and consider why skin colour has not entered the room until now. I ask what being brown means for her and she explains in detail the difficulties she experiences feeling accepted in most places. The lack of a clear sense of her ethnic/racial identity at home has impacted her life at school, as she feels alone in this regard and does not want anyone to know her struggles.

She is dealing with "acculturative stress" (Berry, 2006, 2007) brought on by the inability to integrate her cultural and racial identities, and coping by withdrawing herself from the systems that are not providing the cultural and racial identity enrichment she needs. The symptoms of her acculturative stress include withdrawal from school, avoidance of friendships, having negative thoughts, feeling misunderstood, having a distorted view of herself, and confusion caused by her unconscious desire to be more like her Irish side yet finding solace in a culture that belongs to people with darker skin. I think about "cultural homelessness" (Vivero & Jenkins, 1999, p. 6), which creates a sense of "wanting to be at home but not knowing where home is or how it feels" (Vivero & Jenkins, 1999, p. 13), and her anxious resistant attachment style (Bowlby, 1998), which I have observed in the way she seeks proximity to me. I wonder how the two be linked.

I reflect on Missy challenging me about skin colour. I believe in defining people by their character, not their skin colour (Tikkanen, 1963). However, navigating life as a person with brown skin brings challenges that people with white skin do not have, and racism in its many guises continues to cause psychological damage to those who do not have the buffer of ethnic/racial pride (Hope et al., 2021; Okeke, Howard, Kurtz-Costes, & Rowley, 2009; Oyserman, Kemmelmeier, Fryberg, Brosh, & Hart-Johnson, 2003; Robinson, 2000; Seaton & Iida, 2019; Sellers, Copeland-Linder, Martin, & Lewis, 2006; Utsey, Chae, Brown, & Kelly, 2002; Wakefield & Hudley, 2009; Wong, Eccles, & Sameroff, 2003). I am bothered by my blindness to it because it feels as if I have colluded with the silence about race. The Race Commission Report (Commission on Race and Ethnic Disparities, 2021) gaslit the lived experiences of many BAME communities by stating that the UK is not structurally racist, failing to acknowledge the unconscious racial bias and racial microaggressions that people from these communities frequently experience. Such dogma has created an illusion that race and racism have vanished. Conversations about race are often emotionally triggering, and silence is a coping mechanism that maintains the status quo (Graham & Robinson, 2004).

Missy is perhaps coping with her racial/ethnic identity struggles by withdrawing—in parallel with the avoidance and silence around the family conflict. The absence of her ethnic/racial identity on the referral form also echoes the silence around race.

Missy's withdrawal may also relate to the onset of puberty, the biological changes and psychic struggles (Frankel, 1999) that occur during adolescence. Dependency away from the family begins during the second individuation process (Blos, 1970) in adolescence, which can be an ambivalent and unsettling experience whilst navigating intersecting identities of race, gender, and class (Carbado, Crenshaw, Mays, & Tomlinson, 2013).

I recognise as well that psychodynamic theory has dominated my clinical thinking and I have internalised a "white psychotherapist": this means psychotherapy shaped by white Europeans who have typically given scant consideration to race, culture and identity politics.

In the following session, I explore what both of us having brown skin means for Missy, and she shares her desire to have someone who looks like her, who is confident, happy, and smart. Missy is striving to have such qualities and lacks a person who emulates that. She needs a mother, confidante, and friend, and I wonder how I can enable her to see those qualities within herself.

In one session, I invite Missy to try mirroring exercises in which we take turns copying what the other is doing or saying, closely following tone, delivery, and expression. She enjoys this and wants to do it in subsequent sessions. I also give Missy opportunities to express her interest in astrology and food, which she keenly takes up using the drawing materials, Play-Doh, and sand-tray. I watch with interest and enthusiasm, which I hope will allow her to experience a "grandiose self" (Kohut & Elson, 1987, pp. 72–73).

Missy attempts "focusing" (Gendlin, 1978) in another session to explore her feelings and sensations related to being withdrawn. She notices tension around her shoulders and a ball of tension in her stomach which feels prominent. She explains the size of the knot and how it looks. I ask if the knot could speak, what it would say. She mentions it is scared and I ask what she would like to say to the knot, to which she replies she would like to hold it and tell it not to be scared. She notices the knot feels different once she has spoken to it, and I begin to understand how fear has played a role in her withdrawal. I also observe Missy's capacity to love and protect herself.

She begins to understand the challenges she faces regarding integrating her ethnic and cultural identities. She begins to speak more openly about racism in her family and society and her struggle with belonging within herself, at home, and in the world. I think about what is present within the "collective shadow" (Brewster, 2020; Jung, 1969; Kimbles, 2021) of this family, the racism, the death of her father's first wife, the sadness, and the extent to which these collective struggles have impacted her. There is also potentially the unconscious guilt, perhaps shame, about being the product of a marriage marred by racial conflict.

I describe to Missy my observations of her acculturative stress and the likelihood of it contributing to her feelings about not belonging or feeling accepted. We think about experiences when she is with the group; with her aunt and cousins compared to being outside of the group. She acknowledges the safety of being part of this group and the feeling of security it gives her. I invite her to do an exercise where she draws or collects objects that have value, and I ask her to imagine how she would feel if I removed or treated them with mockery. She recognises she would feel sad and angry, and I compare that to how it might feel being disconnected from herself and her identity. The analogy resonates with her.

Missy recognises her internal struggles are ongoing, but the sessions allow her to establish the significance of ethnic and racial identity in promoting self-esteem and the resources she has at her disposal to support her through a critical stage in her development.

Ike

Seven-year-old Ike is referred due to his persistent disruptive behaviour in school. He is not maintaining long-term relationships with peers and has occasionally been involved in physical altercations. He is described as hyperactive with attention deficit hyperactivity disorder (ADHD) traits. The school's concern level is high. I read the referral with a sense of urgency.

I speak to Ike's parents before my first meeting with him. They are from Ghana and have lived in the UK for fifteen years. The school informed me that they were reluctant to give their consent for Ike to receive therapy. I imagine they have a distrust due to a perceived cultural scepticism within some West African cultures towards mental health and the stigma attached to it (Meechan, John, & Hanna, 2021; Pieterse, 2018). Ike's mother tells me he has always struggled to listen and behave himself. His father is frustrated that taking him to church and prayers has not worked. I again experience a sense of urgency. As I listen, I realise that my belief system is dissonant with theirs and ponder the difficulties Ike is living through. I think about their struggle to comprehend his behaviour, the school information about him, and how I feel as I listen, and I imagine Ike's own dissonant experiences. They have not completed the ADHD assessment forms, as they do not want any labels put on him.

In my first session with Ike, I immediately notice his composure. He looks strong, hypervigilant, curious, and looks at me with a smile. He is dark-skinned and athletic. He looks at me only briefly, struggling to maintain eye contact. He asks my name, where I come from, how long the session is, and about the materials in the room. I introduce myself and say that he has so many questions to ask and that I can hear how curious he is and that he seems excited to be in the room. He nods energetically but his eyes are darting around and he seems to be distracted by what he sees. He moves around the room checking the materials, and asking how to use them. As I explain, he seems distracted by the next object and appears to lose interest in my explanation. I instinctively want to slow Ike down but my hypothesis about dissonant experiences is on my mind and I try to attune (Stern, 2000) by matching my affect and voice with his excitement. My only agenda is to explain the safety and confidentiality rules to him, but I am struggling to keep his attention. He appears more excited when he finds an Iron Man action figure and explains in detail an episode from a Marvel hero show that he has recently seen. He is articulate and his face shows a range of affect as he explains the episode. After I explain the rules of therapy, following several attempts to get his attention, I ask if he understands these rules and he laughs. I say, "You seem to find the rules funny", to which he replies, "Yeah, because they are not rules". I ask him to explain what rules mean to him and he quotes some of the Ten Commandments. I playfully suggest we name them something else and ask for his ideas. He tells me to name them in a disinterested voice.

I am feeling exhausted and bewildered by the end of the session. Ike is like a butterfly, and as I follow him tentatively around the room, I feel the need for grounding. I wonder how to provide a contained therapeutic space (Finlay, 2016) whilst accommodating his need for expression.

The next two sessions involve me trying to gain information about Ike's world through words, drawings, and role play. It is difficult for him to stay with my ideas to inquire more about him, and it is difficult for him to stay focused for a long time. He appears to be in a flight/fight state, and I feel unable to reach him. I spend time in supervision thinking about my countertransference to shed light on how that informs me about his internal world. I discuss my anticipation before our meetings and how I might engage with him and have a dyadic experience rather than one where I am following him around the room feeling lost. I realise that Ike may also be experiencing his world in the same way I experience him. I become aware of my need to find a connection with him. I feel confused about whether that need belongs to me or him.

I moderate my desire for connection and focus on what emerges in the sessions. Ike gravitates towards the action figures and appears to enjoy role play with them. He sits and becomes two or three characters and the plot often involves his characters conspiring to beat the bad guys. Through this projective and role play (Jennings, 1995), he appears to be expressing his desire to have special powers. In one session, I ask him about the special powers he would like and he says to change the way he looks. I ask him to tell me how he wants to look and he replies he wants floppy hair and to look like the boys in his class. I pause for a while before enquiring how they look. He explains they have white skin and look the same and he has brown skin and then looks at me directly and says, "I don't like that." I maintain eye contact and ask what would happen if he looked different. He says sadly, "People would like me." I ask what people he is referring to and he replies, "People at school." I enquire further about "the people" and it appears that it's everyone at school. I notice a jabbing knot in my stomach as he speaks. I show Ike my embodied expression of how I imagine he feels and I ask him to show me how being unliked feels. He pulls a face. I ask what his face is showing me and he says it's his mad face. I ask who else knows about the way he feels and he looks down and shrugs his shoulders. I ask how he would feel about me speaking to his parents and the school about the difficulties he has just disclosed and he says, "Okay." This is the first time I feel an authentic connection with him.

His parents are aware the school lacks diversity, but they believe it is a good school and encourage him to behave well. I explain that he appears to struggle with cultural or racial differences and a sense of belonging. Ike has expressed wanting to be white before, but they tell him to be proud of where he comes from. I enquire about the extent to which Ike embraces Ghanaian culture. He loves the food, but they mention his behaviour not aligning with their cultural values. On further inquiry, I learn that he does not behave like "a good Ghanaian boy" because he is stubborn and does not do as he is told. I ask about his interests and he spends more time pursuing family activities such as visiting grandparents, shopping, and church.

The school explains Ike's behaviour as disruptive due to his failure to take turns when answering questions, difficulty knowing when to be quiet in class, and losing his temper when he is unhappy. They have not noticed that he feels different, but he pronounces words differently sometimes and the kids laugh.

I feel unsettled after the contact with his parents and school because they are revealing to me that Ike is not liked or loved for who he is, and I wonder what he has internalised. If he has not received adequate attunement (Stern, 2000) and validation, is his behaviour emotional rather than attributable to ADHD? I wonder what is it that makes Ike feel different? Is this difference felt at home as well as at school? I think about how to explore the theme of "othering" (Frosh, 2002; Wright, 2010) for the next session.

Ike listens carefully while I invite him to imagine one of the action figures is from a place where people have different faces, eat different food, and sound different. The figure visits a place where everybody else is different. I wonder what the figure might feel like. I allocate ten minutes for this activity due to his attention difficulties and he seems keen to try. We imagine different scenarios for the figure such as going to the shops and meeting people. The figure has a desire for connection with the pretend people it meets and is curious about where they live, what food they like, and what their favourite TV show is. The figure seems excited but ends up on Ike's lap and becomes quiet. I pick up another figure and I say that it seems that Ike's figure is looking for someone to talk to. Ike's figure replies, "Yes," excitedly, and my figure matches the curiosity and excitement level of his figure. I ask his figure what it is like to have someone to talk to and it replies happily, "I have someone who is like me." I ask how the figure is like him and he says, "They are friendly to me." Ike remains focused on the activity for ten minutes and then, once over, I ask if there are times when he wished people were friendlier to him. He looks at me directly and says, "Yeah," with resonance. I ask him how often he feels this way and he says sadly, "Most of the time." I am moved by his integrity.

In supervision, we reflect on this session and how Ike appears to be seeking connection, belonging, and understanding, and has possibly internalised shame and worthlessness. Is his emotional state being masked by behaviours at home and school which are seen as disruptive and challenging? We hypothesise that he is not experiencing group belonging at home and has "phantasies" (Klein, 1923, p. 437) about being white. There is tension surrounding his anguish about his physical appearance and the way he is perceived culturally by his parents. Moreover, I wonder what may have been projected onto him by his teachers as a minority brown-skinned boy who struggles to conform to their standards and whether he has been scapegoated as the bad black boy. We speculate about his transference towards me and I realise in some sessions I embody the guide in an archetypal sense (Jung, 2004), and I wonder if that is symbolic of the superpower he wants me to possess. I imagine his parents' religious belief system about Ike needing to be saved by God has contributed to a failure complex and I might represent for him the person who is going to save him. Perhaps he is yearning for his parents' approval?

I think about ways to bring integration experiences into our sessions to help Ike see and talk about what makes him similar and different so that he can begin to feel validated and integrate his different parts. We do this through activities such as making a coloured sand jar. I ask Ike to choose up to five colours that represent him. They can represent his physical characteristics, interests, people who are important to him, and any other attributes he chooses. He marvels at his creation, enjoying the patterns and laughing joyfully at it. In another session, we discuss what he would look like as an action hero. He is excited and curious as he wonders about his superpowers. I ask him to think about the superpowers he would use at home and in school. I provide comic magazines to create collage pictures of himself as a superhero. He sits absorbed in this activity and appears calm, his vigilance eases.

I speak to Ike's parents about using "racial socialisation" (RS) messages to provide positive messages about race that boost his self-esteem (Metzger, Anderson, Are, & Ritchwood, 2020, p. 3). I offer thoughts about his emotional needs and signpost them to sites that offer insights about attention deficiency and ways to support him. I give them space to reflect upon how Ike might feel unable to meet their expectations whilst struggling to assimilate at school. I explain that Ike's struggle to fit in at school is a symptom of acculturative stress, which can be psychologically harmful (Berry, 2006, 2007).

I have a difficult conversation with his teacher about how unconscious racial bias can result in black boys being more harshly disciplined than their white peers over similar behaviour, due to the negative stereotypes that exist about black boys in education (Blair, 2001; Carlile, 2012; Crozier, 2005; Demie, 2019; Gillborn, Rollock, Vincent, & Ball, 2012; Wright, Weekes, McGlaughlin, & Webb, 1998) and in the media (Moore, Jewell, & Cushion, 2011). I am also aware of the adultification of black children, which results in them being treated as adults rather than children when they make mistakes, violating their rights to fair treatment and adequate safeguarding (Davis & Marsh, 2020; Goff, Jackson, Di Leone, Culotta, & DiTomasso, 2014). I hope to impart wisdom rather than show judgement. I explain Ike's sense of alienation and we think of ways to facilitate ways for him to be part of the group yet be proud of his difference.

I start to experience a relational shift as Ike begins to seek validation through mirroring and alter ego experiences (Kohut, 1987). We start to create a narrative around the toys together, and he begins to ask me to join in or watch him whilst he shows me his ideas for play. I feel motherly towards him as he starts to rely on my presence and engagement in the room. I wonder if he is eliciting these feelings in me because of his unmet needs.

I continue to see Ike for several months and he starts to become calmer, his behaviour improves at school, and his parents begin to understand his needs with continued psychoeducational signposting.

Conclusion

Missy and Ike were both struggling to reconcile their ethnic identities due to their unique family constellations, which included difficulties with acculturation at home, school, and beyond. Scant attention has been paid to the difficulties certain ethnocultural groups face trying to become a part of white British culture whilst attempting to successfully integrate their ethnic, racial, and/or cultural heritage. The cases of Missy and Ike show that the themes of belonging, acceptance, and fitting in apply to many ethnocultural groups. However, young people from BAME communities may experience further acculturative stress due to societal and structural anti-black racism and negative stereotyping.

The assimilation and integration acculturation strategies appear to involve less acculturative stress, although the assimilation strategy involves the most adaptations (Berry, 2006, p. 294) and, I imagine, a greater degree of unconscious or conscious disavowal of racial and ethnic heritage. The expectation for many ethnocultural groups in the UK is to partake in the white British culture, which for some means forfeiting their ethnocultural identities to benefit from belonging within white power-based societies. The ensuing acculturative stress may be traumatic for some who are constantly seeking belonging and acceptance and cannot find it. The constant and insidious effects of feeling displaced, like an outsider, can have serious psychological consequences, particularly when there is not a single direct cause for distressing feelings. Missy and Ike were both experiencing self-esteem and self-worth difficulties linked to their ethnic identity formation struggles and required space to explore them.

As a black, female child and adolescent psychotherapist, I have experienced similar racial and ethnic identity struggles, which have fortified my understanding of acculturative stress and how that intersects with structural and societal racism. It would not be prudent to assume an understanding of any client's identity struggles based on a homogenous group experience, as I realised with Missy. However, acknowledging that our racial and cultural experiences are in the room and our intersectional identities (Carbado, Crenshaw, Mays, & Tomlinson, 2013), particularly when the clients have different backgrounds, gives the client permission to talk openly about events related to their racial, ethnic, and cultural lives.

Fundamentally, Missy and Ike were not receiving positive racial socialisation (RS) messages (Metzger, Anderson, Are, & Ritchwood, 2021, p. 3), which bolster young people's resilience when coping with difficult events related to race and racism. Several studies in the United States have established that those who are more positively identified with their racial or ethnic group are significantly less likely to succumb to negative stereotyping and discrimination than those who are more negatively identified with their group (Hope et al., 2021; Okeke, Howard, Kurtz-Costes, & Rowley, 2009; Oyserman, Kemmelmeier,

Fryberg, Brosh, & Hart-Johnson, 2003; Robinson, 2000; Seaton & Iida, 2019; Sellers, Copeland-Linder, Martin, & Lewis, 2006; Utsey, Chae, Brown, & Kelly, 2002; Wakefield & Hudley, 2009; Wong, Eccles, & Sameroff, 2003). It was possible to offer systemic support to Ike's parents by informing them about the benefits of RS. In the case of Missy, I supported her with identifying the enriching and positive areas of her cultural life.

Establishing a culturally sensitive practice warrants an awareness of perspectives that are framed within a white normative cultural standard (Meechan, John, & Hanna, 2021) and becoming familiar with the racial, ethnic, or cultural background of the client. The client may already feel marginalised by their experiences beyond the therapeutic space; thus, it is essential to allow space and understanding for the world they inhabit and not to pathologise experiences that might be less familiar (Mintah, 2022). Supervision can be helpful with this process (McKenzie-Mavinga, 2009) to aid supervisees with "racial self-awareness" and an "anti-racist stance" (Pieterse, 2018, p. 207) in order to not perpetuate any further racial stress or trauma.

Over the last ten to twenty years, there has been an acculturative shift in the UK from a "melting pot" (Berry, 2006, p. 291) society where an assimilation approach was encouraged, towards "multiculturalism" (Berry, 2006, p. 291), where an integration approach is emerging, particularly in cities such as London. There has been a celebration of different cultures, which is now reflected in British culture. More recently, following the worldwide Black Lives Matter protests in 2020, there is greater awareness about the difficult, racialised experiences of BAME youth, and this has catalysed a movement to make them more visible in society, reflecting the diversity and strengths of such individuals, changing the narrative around how BAME communities are perceived, and, with hope, how BAME youth perceive themselves.

References

Berry, J. W. (2006). Acculturative stress. In: P. T. P. Wong, & L. C. J. Wong (Eds.), *Handbook of Multicultural Perspectives on Stress and Coping*. Boston, MA: Springer.

Berry, J. W. (2007). Acculturation and identity. In: D. Bhugra, & K. Bhui (Eds.), *Textbook of Cultural Psychiatry* (pp. 169–178). Cambridge: Cambridge

University Press. Available at: https://www.cambridge.org/core/books/abs/textbook-of-cultural-psychiatry/acculturation-and-identity/EC9F0ABA9650A3C75D0D9160750E54F3 (last accessed 22 December 2022).

Blair, M. (2001). *Why Pick on Me?: School Exclusion and Black Youth*. Stoke-On-Trent: Trentham Books.

Blos, P. (1970). *Young Adolescent*. New York: The Free Press.

Bokanowski, T. (2018). *On Freud's "Splitting of the Ego in the Process of Defence"*. Abingdon, UK: Routledge.

Bowlby, J. (1998). *A Secure Base*. London: Routledge.

Brewster, F. (2020). *The Racial Complex: A Jungian Perspective on Culture and Race*. Abingdon, UK: Routledge.

Carbado, D. W., Crenshaw, K. W., Mays, V. M., & Tomlinson, B. (2013). Intersectionality: Mapping the movements of a theory. *Du Bois Review: Social Science Research on Race*, 10(2): 303–312. doi:10.1017/s1742058x13000349 (last accessed 17 December 2022).

Carlile, A. (2012). An ethnography of permanent exclusion from school: Revealing and untangling the threads of institutionalised racism. *Race Ethnicity and Education*, 15(2): 175–194. doi:10.1080/13613324.2010.548377 (last accessed 10 October 2022).

Commission on Race and Ethnic Disparities (2021). The report of the Commission on Race and Ethnic Disparities. [online] GOV.UK. Available at: https://www.gov.uk/government/publications/the-report-of-the-commission-on-race-and-ethnic-disparities (last accessed 15 November 2022).

Crozier, G. (2005). "There's a war against our children": Black educational underachievement revisited. *British Journal of Sociology of Education*, 26(5): 585–598. doi:10.1080/01425690500293520 (last accessed 10 October 2022).

Davis, J., & Marsh, N. (2020). Boys to men: The cost of "adultification" in safeguarding responses to Black boys. *Critical and Radical Social Work*, 8(2). doi:10.1332/204986020x15945756023543 (last accessed 10 October 2022).

Demie, F. (2019). The experience of Black Caribbean pupils in school exclusion in England. *Educational Review*, [online] 73: 55–70. Available at: https://www.semanticscholar.org/paper/The-experience-of-Black-Caribbean-pupils-in-school-Demie/050a56ee54f3c9c952e631c3e8b38314d54b987c (last accessed 23 December 2022).

Erikson, E. H. (1968). *Identity: Youth and Crisis*. New York: W. W. Norton.

Evans, A. B., Copping, K. E., Rowley, S. J., & Kurtz-Costes, B. (2011). Academic self-concept in Black adolescents: Do race and gender stereotypes matter? *Self and Identity*, [online] *10*(2): 263–277. doi:10.1080/15298868.2010.485358 (last accessed 12 October 2022).

Finlay, L. (2016). *Relational Integrative Psychotherapy: Engaging Process and Theory in Practice.* Oxford: John Wiley.

Frankel, R. (1999). *The Adolescent Psyche: Jungian and Winnicottian Perspectives.* London: Routledge.

Frosh, S. (2002). The Other. *American Imago*, [online] *59*(4): 389–407. Available at: https://www.jstor.org/stable/26304845 (last accessed 23 December 2022).

Gammage, D. (2021). The shape I am in (teaching notes) Terapia, 11 August.

Gendlin, E. T. (1978). *Focusing.* New York: Bantam Books.

Gillborn, D., Rollock, N., Vincent, C., & Ball, S. J. (2012). "You got a pass, so what more do you want?": Race, class and gender intersections in the educational experiences of the Black middle class. *Race Ethnicity and Education*, *15*(1): 121–139. doi:10.1080/13613324.2012.638869 (last accessed 11 September 2022).

Goff, P. A., Jackson, M. C., Di Leone, B. A. L., Culotta, C. M., & Di Tomasso, N. A. (2014). The essence of innocence: Consequences of dehumanizing Black children. [online] *Journal of Personality and Social Psychology*. Available at: https://pubmed.ncbi.nlm.nih.gov/24564373/ (last accessed 18 November 2022).

Graham, M., & Robinson, G. (2004). "The silent catastrophe": Institutional racism in the British educational system and the underachievement of Black boys. *Journal of Black Studies*, [online] *34*(5): 653–671. Available at: https://www.jstor.org/stable/3180922 (last accessed 18 September 2022).

Hope, E. C., Brinkman, M., Hoggard, L. S., Stokes, M. N., Hatton, V., Volpe, V. V., & Elliot, E. (2021). Black adolescents' anticipatory stress responses to multilevel racism: The role of racial identity. *American Journal of Orthopsychiatry*, *91*(4): 487–498. doi:10.1037/ort0000547 (last accessed 14 August 2022).

Jennings, S. (1995). *Dramatherapy with Children and Adolescents.* London: Routledge.

Jung, C. G. (1969). *Structure and Dynamics of the Psyche. Vol. 8.* R. F. C. Hull (Trans.), H. Read, M. Fordham, G. Adler, & W. McGuire, (Eds.).

The Collected Works of C. G. Jung. Bollingen Series XX. Princeton, NJ: Princeton University Press.

Jung, C. G. (2004). *On the Nature of the Psyche.* London: Routledge.

Kimbles, S. L. (2021). *Intergenerational Complexes in Analytical Psychology: The Suffering of Ghosts.* Abingdon, UK: Routledge.

Klein, M. (1923). The development of a child. *The International Journal of Psychoanalysis,* [online] 4: 419–474. doi:https://pep-web.org/browse/document/IJP.004.0419A?page=P0419 (last accessed 22 November 2022).

Klein, M. (1996). Notes on some schizoid mechanisms. *The Journal of Psychotherapy Practice and Research,* [online] 5(2): 160–179. Available at: https://pubmed.ncbi.nlm.nih.gov/22700275/ (last accessed 22 December 2022).

Kohut, H., & Elson, M. (1987). *The Kohut Seminars on Self Psychology and Psychotherapy with Adolescents and Young Adults.* New York: W. W. Norton.

Liu, W. M., Liu, R. Z., Garrison, Y. L., Kim, J. Y. C., Chan, L., Ho, Y. C. S., & Yeung, C. W. (2019). Racial trauma, microaggressions, and becoming racially innocuous: The role of acculturation and White supremacist ideology. *American Psychologist,* 74(1): 143–155. doi:10.1037/amp0000368 (last accessed 15 November 2022).

McKenzie-Mavinga, I. (2009). *Black Issues in the Therapeutic Process.* Houndmills: Plagrave Macmillan.

Meechan, H., John, M., & Hanna, P. (2021). Understandings of mental health and support for Black male adolescents living in the UK. *Children and Youth Services Review,* 129: 106192. doi:10.1016/j.childyouth.2021.106192 (last accessed 10 September 2022).

Metzger, I. W., Anderson, R. E., Are, F., & Ritchwood, T. (2020). Healing interpersonal and racial trauma: Integrating racial socialization into trauma-focused cognitive behavioral therapy for African American youth. *Child Maltreatment,* 26(1): 17–27. doi:10.1177/1077559520921457 (last accessed 10 September 2022).

Mintah, R. (2022). Speaking the unspeakable unbreakable, exploring black women's experiences of disclosing sexual violence. Community Trauma Conference, Black Women Trauma and Mental Health. London 30 October 2022.

Moore, K., Jewell, J. G., & Cushion, S. (2011). Media representations of black young men and boys: Report of the REACH media monitoring project. [online] Available at: https://www.semanticscholar.org/paper/Media-representations-of-black-young-men-and-boys%3A-Moore-Jewell/1f653e03dbc3959555c2882cc0af8247d983aa1d (last accessed 10 September 2022).

Okeke, N. A., Howard, L. C., Kurtz-Costes, B., & Rowley, S. J. (2009). Academic race stereotypes, academic self-concept, and racial centrality in African American youth. *Journal of Black Psychology*, [online] *35*(3): 366–387. doi:10.1177/0095798409333615 (last accessed 12 September 2022).

Oyserman, D., Kemmelmeier, M., Fryberg, S., Brosh, H., & Hart-Johnson, T. (2003). Racial-ethnic self-schemas. *Social Psychology Quarterly*, *66*(4): 333. doi:10.2307/1519833 (last accessed 12 September 2022).

Phinney, J. S. (1990). Ethnic identity in adolescents and adults: Review of research. *Psychological Bulletin*, *108*(3): 499–514. doi:10.1037/0033-2909.108.3.499 (last accessed 12 August 2022).

Pieterse, A. L. (2018). Attending to racial trauma in clinical supervision: Enhancing client and supervisee outcomes. *The Clinical Supervisor*, *37*(1): 204–220. doi:10.1080/07325223.2018.1443304 (last accessed 4 August 2022).

Quintana, S. (2007). Racial and ethnic identity: Developmental perspectives and research. *Journal of Counseling Psychology*, [online] *54*(3): 259–270. Available at: https://www.semanticscholar.org/paper/Racial-and-ethnic-identity%3A-Developmental-and-Quintana/222c0928a37cb065bace3491bc64760192f193ef (last accessed 22 December 2022).

Robinson, L. (2000). Racial identity attitudes and self-esteem of black adolescents in residential care: An exploratory study. *The British Journal of Social Work*, [online] *30*(1): 3–24. Available at: https://www.jstor.org/stable/23716276 (last accessed 4 August 2022).

Rogers, L. O., Scott, M. A., & Way, N. (2014). Racial and gender identity among Black adolescent males: An intersectionality perspective. *Child Development*, *86*(2): 407–424. doi:10.1111/cdev.12303 (last accessed 15 July 2022).

Seaton, E. K., & Iida, M. (2019). Racial discrimination and racial identity: Daily moderation among Black youth. *American Psychologist*, *74*(1): 117–127. doi:10.1037/amp0000367 (last accessed 10 September 2022).

Segal, H. (1954). A note on schizoid mechanisms underlying phobia formation. *The International Journal of Psycho-Analysis*, [online] *35*(2): 238–241. Available at: https://pubmed.ncbi.nlm.nih.gov/13162607/ (last accessed 23 December 2022).

Sellers, R. M., Copeland-Linder, N., Martin, P. P., & Lewis, R. L. (2006). Racial identity matters: The relationship between racial discrimination and psychological functioning in African American Aaolescents. *Journal of Research on Adolescence*, *16*(2): 187–216. doi:10.1111/j.1532-7795.2006.00128.x (last accessed 7 July 2022).

Stern, D. N. (2000). *The Interpersonal World of the Infant: A View from Psychoanalysis and Developmental Psychology.* New York: Basic Books.

Tikkanen, A. (2018). "I have a dream". Speech by King, 1963. In: *Encyclopædia Britannica* [online]. Available at: https://www.britannica.com/topic/I-Have-A-Dream (last accessed 12 December 2022).

Utsey, S. O., Chae, M. H., Brown, C. F., & Kelly, D. (2002). Effect of ethnic group membership on ethnic identity, race-related stress, and quality of life. *Cultural Diversity and Ethnic Minority Psychology, 8*(4): 366–377. doi:10.1037/1099-9809.8.4.367 (last accessed 10 August 2022).

Vivero, V. N., & Jenkins, S. (1999). Existential hazards of the multicultural individual: Defining and understanding. *Cultural Diversity and Ethnic Minority Psychology*, [online] *5*(1): 6–26. Available at: https://www.semanticscholar.org/paper/Existential-hazards-of-the-multicultural-defining-Vivero-Jenkins/12ae81b9620cc84e43371d0b018eed556b02d70c (last accessed 22 December 2022).

Wakefield, W. D., & Hudley, C. (2007). Ethnic and racial identity and adolescent well-being. *Theory Into Practice, 46*(2): 147–154. doi:10.1080/00405840701233099 (last accessed 12 July 2022).

Wong, C. A., Eccles, J. S., & Sameroff, A. (2003). The influence of ethnic discrimination and ethnic identification on African American adolescents' school and socioemotional adjustment. *Journal of Personality*, [online] *71*(6): 1197–1232. doi:10.1111/1467-6494.7106012 (last accessed 12 July 2022).

Wright, C. (2010). Othering difference: Framing identities and representation in black children's schooling in the British context. *Irish Educational Studies, 29*(3): 305–320. doi:10.1080/03323315.2010.498569.

Wright, C., Weekes, D., McGlaughlin, A., & Webb, D. (1998). Masculinised discourses within education and the construction of Black male identities amongst African Caribbean youth. *British Journal of Sociology of Education, 19*(1): 75–87. doi:10.1080/0142569980190105 (last accessed 12 July 2022).

CHAPTER 6

Understanding the trauma and implications of female genital mutilation (FGM) through child psychotherapy

Irene Mburu

Tohara (Kukeketa)

The topic of FGM is all too familiar to me because I grew up in a community that practised it. During my formative years as a young girl in Kenya, we were persistently bombarded with information about our culture and cultural practices that defined our community and set us apart from others. Most of the practices were positive and meant to instil good morals from a young age. However, one ritual that stood out was the FGM practice. At the time, older women would discreetly and nostalgically introduce the subject at every opportune moment. They would talk of girls who brought fame to their families because they went through the FGM procedure or shame for failing to do so. The girls were groomed and manipulated into embracing FGM. Furthermore, there was peer pressure, and continues to be, and fear of rejection for non-conformity, amongst the girls who are mostly illiterate and naive. International human rights bodies have highlighted the disadvantages of power control and the resultant inequalities due to the fact that the victims of FGM are nearly always minors, whose rights to protection, health, and a life that is free from torture and integrity are violated (WHO, 2008, p. 8).

The FGM procedure is regarded as a rite of passage from childhood to adulthood in many cultures (WHO, 1998, p. 2). It was, and still is, seen as the ritual that swiftly transforms and transitions young girls into maturity instantly, seemingly giving them a sense of graduating into a preferential class, and earning a position of respect in their community. At the top of the list is getting suitors for marriage (Ahmadu, 2001; Dellenborg, 2004; Shell-Duncan & Hernlund, 2001) and enjoying certain privileges. Marriage is held in high regard since it guarantees family/community continuity. Nonconformity to FGM is seen as the deal breaker. The FGM practice supposedly ensures that a girl's sexual urges and sensations are suppressed, thereby guaranteeing and preserving their virginity until marriage and thereafter, to be faithful to their spouse (Gruenbaum, 2006). The irony is, in a patriarchal society, some rules only apply to the females and not the males. It is outrageous that the girls are objectified as tools for others' pleasure and gratification.

There were, and still are, a lot of unknown and unspoken factors about FGM that are supposed to be discovered during the actual procedure. In the light of this, the victims have little or no understanding about the practice. They innocently go through the procedure for the sake of the family's status in the community and to avoid being labelled a social pariah. The young girls only realise the dire consequences after going through the procedure; too little too late, after the damage has been inflicted. Sadly, the description of FGM and the accompanying benefits do not really depict it for what it is, and the majority of the girls agree to it blindly. They are led rather like lambs to the slaughter.

Ironically, perpetrators of FGM are close family members (parents, relatives, caregivers), who should be protecting the young girls from harm (Berg, Denison, & Fretheim, 2010, p. 45). Fortunately, through the work of church missionaries, my family were amongst the minority who were more enlightened about the negative effects of FGM and gradually desisted from the practice. They were frowned upon and their uncircumcised girls were referred to as "kirigu", which means unclean, immature, and lacking in etiquette. This turn of events created a divide where sons were discouraged from marrying into families that did not practice FGM and vice versa. While wearing my therapist hat, I imagine the thought of being rejected by suitors, and the ensuing collateral damage to their social and family status in their respective community, is enough to coerce innocent girls into accepting FGM. They only learn about the plan the night before or early in the morning on the day of the event.

What is female genital mutilation?

Female genital mutilation (FGM) is also described as female genital cutting (FGC) or female circumcision (FC). The World Health Organization defines FGM as:

> an exercise that comprises all procedures involving partial or total removal of the external female genitalia or other injury to the female genital organs for cultural, social religious, or other non-medical reasons. (WHO, 2008, p. 4)

FGM is considered a violation of human rights and a form of child abuse (BBC, 2016; WHO, 2008, p. 8). It is very invasive and undertaken without the victims' consent since they are not "Gillick competent" (Smaranda, 1985). The barbaric "cutters" reuse unsterilised razor blades, scissors, and sometimes crude weapons such as sharpened stones, broken glass, or their long nails to cut and/or scrape off the flesh, without any form of anaesthesia.

"Female genital mutilation" was first coined by a feminist campaigner, Fran Hosken (1979, p. 368), and adopted by the United Nations Agencies (WHO, 2008, p. 22). It is a historical practice that dates back more than 2,000 years (Wilson, 2021, p. 54), and it is done for sociocultural reasons that vary from one ethnic group to another. The origin of FGM is shrouded in mystery, with some texts associating the practice to a Pharaonic ritual from Ancient Egypt, going back to 502–575 AD (Abusharaf, 2006, p. 2; Hadi, 2006, p. 106). Some of the factors that facilitate and maintain the practice of FGM include belief systems that are enmeshed in patriarchal family systems, historical cultural/traditional practices, religious beliefs, and myths associated with perceived health benefits (Berg & Denison, 2013; Berg, Denison, & Fretheim, 2010, p. 51; Johnson, 2005). The extent of the practice is reflected in the WHO (2016, p. 23) report which says that there are over 200 million girls and women living with the traumatic effects of FGM globally. Additionally, an estimated three million girls in Africa alone are at risk of being put through the FGM procedure annually before they turn fifteen years old.

FGM remains a difficult, emotive, and sensitive subject that bears the hallmarks of an immoral outdated practice. Conforming, by the said communities, gives them a sense of belonging. It is loved and loathed in equal measure, by those who are for and against. It is an inhumane practice that poses serious physical and mental health risks. Regrettably, the enablers of FGM completely disregard the welfare of the victims, who have no voice.

Four types of FGM have been identified, based on procedure and severity (Banks et al., 2006; WHO, 2008, p. 4). The specific type varies from one community to another. Somalia, for example, is said to be one of the countries where the most extensive and invasive type III of FGM (infibulation—narrowing of the vaginal opening with the creation of a covering seal) is practised. For the lucky few, this can be medically corrected via de-infibulation, whereby the sealed vaginal opening is cut open. Some synonyms of the word "mutilation" include explicit terms such as damage, disfigurement, vandalisation, desecration, maiming, and dismemberment.

> Mutilation emphasizes the gravity and harm and reinforces the fact that the practice is a violation of girls' and women's rights. (WHO, 2008, p. 33)

The above descriptions are extremely graphic and could provoke anxiety and fear in the target group. As a result, different cultures have their own choice of names which, in essence, attenuate the seriousness of the practice. For example, the Arabic/Swahili name for circumcision is *tahara*, meaning "to be purified". Sudan refer to it as *tahur* (cleansing or purification). In Egypt and Kenya, they use the derogatory terms *kirigu* and *nigsa* (unclean) to describe uncircumcised girls, while Mali and Mauritania consider the clitoris ugly and believe that cutting (*tizian*) is meant to "make it beautiful" (Erlich, 1986, p. 193).

This chapter focuses on the practice of FGM, inflicted on girls aged from birth to eighteen, and the consequences thereof. The aim is to draw the reader's attention to the mental and psychological health implications of FGM on the young person's quality of life.

FGM has been predominantly practised in Africa and a few countries in Asia, the Middle East, and South America. However, with increasing people migration, it is now a global concern, particularly in the West, since the said communities are keen to continue with their practices, to maintain the status quo. Data obtained from the 28-Too-Many and End-FGM-European-Network websites shows that, in 2011,

> over 600,000 girls residing in 32 European countries had experienced FGM, with the majority residing in the United Kingdom, France, Italy, Spain, Germany, the Netherlands and Sweden. Additionally, it was estimated about 190,000 girls under the age of 18 were at risk of FGM. The majority of those who had undergone FGM or were at risk of it originated from FGM-practising countries in Africa. (Europe, 2019)

The following material aims to draw attention to key pointers to be aware of and how the client might present.

Nuru

I was approached by Nuru's parents to offer therapeutic support to their fifteen-year-old daughter. A family friend had recommended the parents consider therapeutic support. The parents said Nuru was unduly anxious, defiant, easily lost her temper, and experienced panic attacks, mood swings, and nightmares. I later came to realise these symptoms were a mirror image of those portrayed by FGM victims (Reisel & Creighton, 2015). This was seriously affecting Nuru's quality of life, which also impacted on her family. The parents were very concerned, hence their decision to "try therapy". As one who grew up in a community that discouraged "washing your dirty linen in public", I imagined how difficult it might have been for the family to seek help from a third party.

Nuru's family had moved from an East African country to the UK approximately five years earlier when she was ten. Nuru had three younger siblings—two brothers and a sister—aged twelve, nine, and six years respectively. The family had made a big move into a new country when Nuru was at a critical developmental stage. This in itself might have been a traumatic experience: integrating in a new culture, acclimatising, joining a new education system, and forming new relationships.

Mwanzo

First meeting

Dad came across as well-educated. During our initial conversation, he disclosed that he worked in the city with a hedge fund company. He confirmed they were financially stable. Mum was a housewife and presented as docile and somehow passive, while her husband seemed to take charge of the conversations around family matters and decision-making. This was no surprise to me, as it is generally a common trait in traditional families. I remember in my countertransference how my mind wandered in pity as I visualised the all-too-familiar family dynamics that I witnessed during my formative years amongst my community and family; women and children being seen but not heard. Due to the power imbalance, the women, who would perhaps protect the girls, have no say (Johnson, 2005). Nuru's Mum only spoke briefly about Nuru's life story. At this point, Nuru's Dad looked at her as if giving her permission to talk. Her face lightened while talking about the happy and confident Nuru when she was little.

Dad seemed genuinely concerned, worried, and perhaps confused as he spoke about Nuru's challenges. He said Nuru was easily triggered, did not engage much at home, and preferred to spend most of her time in the bedroom. This made it very difficult for the family to engage in normal conversations or offer her the necessary support. Ironically, the parents said even at her worst of times, Nuru always adored and was protective towards her little sister. They were worried that despite their relentless efforts to engage and support Nuru, it seemed whatever they did was not good enough and wondered aloud about "what else can we do?"

I enquired when they first noticed the change in Nuru's mannerism. Both parents confirmed it started when she was about nine years and continued to deteriorate, particularly towards the end of summer term. I wondered if there were any major experiences or changes that they could recall happening in the family or specifically to Nuru around that time. Dad replied, "No, apart from the family visiting our extended family in our native country, in order to keep in touch with the wider family and our roots." I remember having a strong sense of cultural superiority and Dad intentionally striving to maintain the status quo. I was still curious about the timing of the triggers and the ensuing change. Dad looked straight into Mum's eye as she mumbled something but did not, only saying, "Uumm … uumm." I felt like Mum was holding something back. Dad seemed very nervous and uncomfortable as he interjected to say they were also at a loss about the triggers, hence their decision to seek therapeutic intervention. It was obvious he had high expectations of having Nuru fixed speedily.

As the meeting ended, Dad asked about my approach and wondered what areas we would be focusing on with Nuru. I informed him that our work would be child-led to give Nuru the autonomy to decide how to engage, either through talk therapy, play, or creatively. There was something unsettling about his enquiry, and I hoped he would not interfere by micro-managing Nuru. Was he concerned about something that Nuru might say/disclose, I wondered?

Second meeting

The trio attended the second meeting together. Nuru walked in, seemingly confident. She cut a slender figure, approximately five feet in height. She looked well-groomed, with dark hair that was partly covered in a traditional head scarf (hijab). I noticed Nuru's dressing style—T-shirt, a baggy tracksuit, and trainers. Dad had previously expressed his disappointment with Nuru's "rebelliousness" with her choice of clothing, with a cultural undertone. She sat directly opposite me, which was an ideal position to observe her verbal engagement and body language. I became aware of my thoughts around Nuru's style of dressing. Furthermore, matters of sexuality or body dysmorphia crossed my mind. I realised that in order for me to have an unbiased assessment, I needed to keep my inner conversation in check. Nuru sat quietly listening as Dad explained why they had come to see me. She seemed rather shamed and struggled to maintain eye contact. This observation was confusing and a contrast to my first impression of "confident Nuru", which made me even more curious. Once again, Dad dominated the conversation with Mum and Nuru looking subdued; power play was obvious.

These two meetings provided crucial background material that was useful in laying the foundation of our therapeutic work. I gathered more information during our subsequent review and reflective parenting sessions. Sadly, Mum struggled to engage in the beginning. Her contribution was minimal and low-key. She came across as one who lacked self-esteem, seemed shy, and often passively seeking her husband's approval before engaging. In my countertransference, I was harbouring a lot of anger towards Dad, who obviously seemed domineering, and sympathy towards Mum, who was only seen but not heard. This is a common occurrence in traditional families, and I wondered if Nuru felt seen or heard as a young girl. I imagined she was probably confused about the place of a child, or worse still, a female, in her culture versus life in a new culture that believed in equality and respect for all, regardless of gender. Regrettably, the silence and disempowerment of the women perpetuates the abuse. It would have been ideal to meet Mum alone, but I needed to wait for the right moment, since our work was just beginning.

Fortunately, three weeks later, I met with Mum alone, twice, while Dad was away on official duties. I suggested that she consider having some personal therapy, or better still, attend therapy with Dad as a couple. She seemed open to it but doubted if Dad would accept. I was not surprised when she later confided that Dad did not think it was necessary. However, he was happy for Mum to go ahead if she so wished. After a fortnight, Mum confirmed she was talking to a therapist and hoping to start therapy soon. This would later prove to be a huge boost to our work.

> Our work [...] is more effective when parent work is included in the overall structure of the treatment. (Novick & Novick, 2005, p. 1)

First session

During our first one-to-one session, Nuru came across as perceptive and articulate. Her physical and cognitive development seemed above average. She was proactive as we co-created the contract. We discussed the confidentiality clause at length, as well as scenarios that would lead to a disclosure. I hoped this gave her a sense of trust and safety within the therapeutic space.

Thereafter, I invited Nuru to introduce her family in the sand-tray. She chose figurines to represent each family member. She picked three dinosaurs of different sizes and shapes, a little dog, and two butterflies. She placed them in the middle of the sand-tray seemingly deep in thought about where to put them. This took a while before she made a move. I watched as the family took shape. At first, the butterflies and the little dog were placed together while the two little dinosaurs stood next to the big spiky dinosaur, just opposite the butterflies. She then took a step back, perhaps to have a better view of her family. I stood nearby, silently witnessing. She seemed dissatisfied and started moving them again. This time, the butterflies were kept together, and the little dog was alone in close proximity, while the three dinosaurs maintained their position a distance away. There was a clear divide between the butterflies and the dog versus the dinosaurs. She looked at the creativity one more time and said, "I'm done." I thanked Nuru and welcomed her to introduce me to her family. The introduction included a description of each figurine. "This is my Dad and brothers. The dinosaur is extinct and sometimes I imagine a world without men. This is my Mum, the dog is protective and faithful, just like her. The butterflies are me and my sister. They are multicoloured, beautiful, and delicate."

This was Nuru's snapshot of her perception of family. I pondered over the symbolism—the dinosaur seemed like a representation of the past which still has some influence on the present, while the butterfly was symbolic of stages of change in life. Nuru was accurate about the dog, possibly depicting the Mum who looks after the "butterflies". However, the image of the little dog, placed a distance away from the butterflies, made me wonder whether Mum was really capable of actively protecting the girls from the "three dinosaurs".

This exercise enabled Nuru to connect with the unconscious content of her internalised family through projective play. However, she resisted engaging more with the family, even when I wondered about her experience or the feelings that were coming up for her.

> Sand play evokes very deep realities. It cuts across many familial and cultural taboos as it activates the deep, primordial integrative forces of the psyche. (DeDomenico, 1995, p. x)

Instead, she spent the rest of the time exploring the characteristics of the different animals. This exercise was powerful and revealing in the sessions that followed.

> Sand play really is based on the self-healing of the patient [...] It is the experiencing of the process that heals. (Bradway & McCoard, 1997, p. 49)

Similarly,

> Sand play helps to connect with 'the small child' who cannot say 'where it hurts', brings healing and a higher level of consciousness. (Amman, 1991, p. xvi)

I hypothesised that Nuru was expressing her lived life metaphorically and connecting with aspects of self that were too painful or difficult to verbalise. Through the process of projecting into the sand-tray, Nuru's defences seemed to soften.

Tenth session

Nuru was now engaging spontaneously through play and creativity, evidence of a good rapport, through our shared experience. She spotted the story cubes box and inquisitively picked it, saying, "Can I open it?" She poured the cubes out and started scanning each with interest. While at this, I said, "Perhaps you can tell me a story; any story". She smiled and continued looking at the cubes. Shortly, she jokingly started, "Once upon a time there was a family who lived in a far-off country. One day, somebody was planning to attack the two sisters, but there was a camera near their house and they saw the enemy coming. Suddenly, the sisters got magical powers and flew across the bridge to the other side, and they were safe and lived happily ever after." I wondered about the two sisters flying across the bridge and it really felt like a metaphor of Nuru's personal life story. Maybe her adopted country was "across the bridge and safe".

> Children are capable of participating in their own healing process, growth and positive change through role play, enactment and pretend play. (Weber & Haen, 2005, p. 150)

(For dialogue, T stands for Therapist; C for Child)

T: Wow! How scary! And, what a happy ending for the sisters!
C: [*smile on her face*]
T: I know you have a little sister and wonder about your sense of safety.
C: Umm … [*frowns*] Umm … it's a scarrryyyy world …
T: Okay … what about the scary bit?
C: Like, I mean … ehh … like not being safe … especially for girls. [*face down with a prolonged frown*]

This was followed by a long silence. As we sat there in quiet, I became aware of a sharp pain that cut through my lower abdomen. I was convinced this was a countertransference experience. I told Nuru how my body reacted when she mentioned "the scary world". She confirmed she often experiences such pain when anxious. The themes of danger and finding ways to keep from harm's way continued. I was aware that Nuru and her little sister seemed to be most vulnerable. This was material for discussion in my next supervision. After consultation with my supervisor, we felt it was important to reflect and explore the material more and consider liaising with Nuru's teacher for safeguarding. It was a learning experience for both myself and my supervisor, whose knowledge on FGM was limited at the time. A BACP survey found that:

> In general, many counsellors and psychotherapists are lacking confidence in their awareness and understanding of FGM, including their safeguarding responsibilities. Only 10% had knowingly worked with survivors of FGM. (Jackson, 2017, p. 4)

Eleventh session

All the while, my assessment was ongoing. At this point in time, I felt Nuru was ready to engage with a timeline activity. During this session, she spoke fondly and positively about her early life experiences. However, there seemed to be an unusual memory loss or deliberate avoidance of her life story from her eighth to her tenth birthday, when they relocated to the UK. She nostalgically recalled her happy childhood and how glad she was when they left their country. She spoke about missing her girlfriends but there was no mention of family members.

I hypothesised there were some difficult memories that were too triggering and Nuru's way to escape was by burying them in the unconscious.

> Lack of recall is associated with the neglecting, rejecting and emotionally disconnected pattern of relationships. (Siegel, 2012, p. 123)

When I became curious about that gap, Nuru went into a long, thoughtful silence. Finally, she broke the silence with:

C: I don't want to talk about it.

As she responded, I noticed she shut her eyes tightly and grimaced like one who was either disgusted, in pain, or both. She coiled her body and put her hands over her lap. I named my observation and wonderings, but Nuru declined to say more. For the second time, I felt a tightening of muscles and sharp sudden pain cut through my lower abdomen.

Eighteenth session

Nuru usually announced her arrival with a "Hi" before sitting down on the chair. However, on this occasion, she came in and sat down without saying a word. I welcomed her and allowed her to settle before inviting her to choose a feeling/emotion on the card that resonated with her in the present moment. She pointed to the "annoyed face" but did not verbalise it.

T: Tell me more about the "annoyed face".
C: Uumm … It reminds me of Dad … It is annoying when he keeps talking about going home! He kept rubbing it in this whole weekend! I can't stand going back there again!
T: Sorry to interrupt; I just noticed how angry you are when you talk about going home, and I'm really curious what's going on for you right now.
C: I am really angry and no one listens to me! He doesn't understand!
T: I sense your anger for not being understood.

C: Yes, I hate going there! I can stay with my sister! My brothers call me the killjoy when I say I don't want to go!
(The sense of guilt and confliction about going or not was real.)
C: It is annoying, honestly! I hate the double standards.
T: What exactly do you mean when you say "double standards"?
C: Uumm … I mean … I mean, girls and boys …
T: What about them? I'm missing something here.
C: Umm … I don't know how to say it … I don't think you'd understand. [*Nuru fidgets and looks down*] It's really hard to talk about it.
(I often noted her uneasiness while trying to verbally engage and then almost certainly retracting. In my countertransference, I was harbouring shame and persecutory feelings, which brought a sense of inhibition.)
T: I'm listening and noticing how uneasy it is for you right now. It is okay to say as little or as much as you are happy to.
(I wished to demonstrate the ability to contain the difficult feelings and be empathic. A long silence followed. For a moment, Nuru seemed lost in thoughts. Shortly, she broke the silence with a big sigh and re-established eye contact. Her eyes were tearful.)
T: That's a big sigh and … I note you look upset.
C: [*silence*] … It's not faiiir!
T: I wonder what fairness and perhaps lack of it mean to you.
C: Umm … Is there fairness, really?
T: What do you think?
C: I don't think there is! It's not fair to be treated differently!
T: Differently?
C: Yes, so differently! [*followed by an extended silence*] Why, why, whyyyyy!!!! [*angry and agitated*]
T: I notice how upset you are right now as you reflect on being treated differently. I am also aware you used the words double standards earlier on and really curious about your feelings.
C: Not sure I even have feelings, you know … never mind!
(I was aware the last part of her "never mind" response, which was somehow dismissive, and I wondered aloud:)
T: Never mind?
C: Yes … I mean … about … about … my body.

(I wished Nuru was able to name whatever it was about her body that was so hard to articulate. Yet again, this triggered a strong feeling of shame within me, as I waited for her response that was accompanied by long pauses.)

C: Umm … and … my … my … p-pr-pry …
(The words could not come out, and it felt like a road that was too difficult to travel.)
T: I wonder if you were trying to say "my privates".
C: [sustained silence]
T: I am sitting here with a deep sense of shame and perhaps there are things about your body that might be too difficult or painful to talk about and just to assure you that it is alright to talk about those things when you are ready.
C: [silent with face down]
T: [silent but maintained gaze]

This was another perfect moment to assure Nuru of my capacity to hold that which was probably too much for her to bear.

> Holding and containment models a partnership that holds the emotional capacity to be with the other and facilitate conditions of change. (Stern, 1985, p. 160)

Nuru maintained a long silence, at the end of which she looked at me and said:

C: I just can't say it! It brings chills to my body just thinking about it … never mind!
T: I just felt chills in my body as you spoke, and I am really curious about it.
C: Umm … like girls go through a lot … [in a whisper while looking down]
T: I notice the whisper in your last statement, and I am wondering what is going on for you right now.
C: [sigh] Umm … I mean … I mean … Never mind! I hope we won't go! (Yet again, Nuru was dismissive and registered real worry about going to their country.)

T: Gosh, something seems really hard to say, and going back to your country seems quite scary?
C: It is!!! If only Mum would convince Dad to go with my brothers and leave us behind, but she doesn't seem to get it. I thought she cared but … umm … maybe not!
T: I do sense your anger and helplessness. If you could have a magic word right now, what would it be?
C: Can somebody please listen to me!

I recalled during our timeline exercise how Nuru consciously or unconsciously omitted the details for the period between her eighth and tenth years. On reflection, I realised her sister would be seven years in two months. If Nuru experienced FGM at eight years, time was ticking for her sister, hence the sense of danger and a cry for help, in order to protect her, before it was too late. Perhaps the desperation came from a place of knowing Mum was not able to protect her younger sister since she failed to protect Nuru.

T: I hear you and I hope you feel listened to in this moment.

Nuru looked straight into my face and nodded, which felt like a genuine response. However, she maintained a long silence whilst her face looked dejected. It was time to verbalise my concerns and signpost Nuru to relevant agencies for more help.

T: I feel your worry, concern, and desire to be heard. I am also worried and concerned over you and your sister's safety. I am aware there are some cultural practices like female genital mutilation that young girls are forced to undergo in some countries, and I do wonder if you might have experienced it while you were in your birth country.
C: [*prolonged silence, tearful and looking down*] … Umm, don't know what to … umm … what to say …
T: I know it is a difficult and sensitive subject and you might not be ready to talk about it right now … but I'm really concerned about you and your sister's safety.
C: [*silence*]

Whatever Nuru was resisting seemed too frightening to verbalise. By this time, I had a strong conviction that I was dealing with an FGM situation. There were too many red flags. I reflected on the evident pain and anger that Nuru was unable to express, the frustration that she expressed in "never mind", the unfairness and double standards for men and women, the scary and unsafe world, especially for girls, taking the character of a butterfly with its beauty but also fragility and vulnerability, the imaginary story of two sisters running away from danger and across the bridge to a place of safety, her body language when she coiled and put her hands over her lap, my accompanying bodily reaction of a sharp pain through my lower abdomen and the "my … my … p-pr-pry …", "I mean … I mean …", which Nuru laboured to name but could not, and the numerous occasions Nuru brought up the issue of her disapproval in regard to herself and baby sister travelling to their country. Perhaps this was a eureka moment pointing towards a traumatic experience in her country of birth, hence her protectiveness over her younger sister.

T: I notice your long silence. I'm aware we only meet once a week. I feel it would be good to give you some numbers that you can call for help at any time, any day, if you are afraid that something might happen to you or your sister.
C: [*nodded, made eye contact, and her demeanour changed*]
(At this point, I reiterated my concerns for Nuru's safety and informed her that I would like to discuss it further with her Mum or teacher, so that we can both support her. I reassured her that all this would be done in confidence.)
T: How do you feel about that?
C: Umm … I don't know … umm … maybe my teacher.
T: Okay, thanks Nuru.

Before Nuru left, I gave her the NSPCC and National FGM Centre helplines and the local NHS FGM clinic contact details. She gladly took the details and said she would save them in a protected folder on her phone. I also told her about specialist FGM National Health Service clinics that offer physical assessments, and that I would be happy to discuss this with both Nuru and her Mum, if she allowed me to.

As I watched her go out of the door, I vividly recalled young girls being taken away during the long holiday to "visit an aunt", only to return with an unusual walking style due to the raw wound, leaving the rest of the girls guessing what may have happened.

I later notified Nuru's parents that I would be contacting her teacher to find out how she was getting on in school. I had a good conversation with the teacher the next day. When I informed her about my concerns, she confirmed that she was not aware of any issues but would investigate. I did wonder, though, if Nuru was masking her feelings due to the shame that is associated with the subject of FGM, or feared getting her parents into trouble. Going forward, I recommended that the teacher and safeguarding officer monitor Nuru and her sister for any evidence of or intended harm. It was crucial that we maintained our strong rapport and working alliance. A week later when I met with my supervisor, we felt it was important for the school to consider escalating the matter further to involve social services so that the child protection practice could be activated, particularly for Nuru's younger sister, whom we felt was a potential FGM candidate.

> Good management of risks associated with FGM require coordination between child protection agencies, law enforcement officials, health practitioners and services and representatives of affected communities. In the UK, section 47 of the Children Act 1989 requires a strategy meeting with local authorities, children's social services, health professionals, police, referrer (often a school) as soon as practicable (within 2 days at most).
> (Costello, 2015, p. 231)

Work continued with Nuru leading the pace. Occasionally, I checked with her so that she felt heard, allowed time for feedback, acknowledged her vulnerability, and affirmed her courage when dealing with daunting material. Although she never named the elephant in the room, her body language and responses were clear indications. Furthermore, the pointers from her life story as well as the coincidence of the triggers, the age at which the behavioural and mental health challenges started, were telling.

Apart from providing the parallel support to Nuru, I incorporated psychoeducation for her parents, hoping this would give them a better understanding of mental health and equip them to develop strategies on how to support Nuru. I imagined Mum was possibly nursing her own physical/mental wounds and would, therefore, not have the capacity to attend to Nuru if she was not supported. This was a worrying scenario if no action was taken. During one of our meetings, I mentioned the FGM cultural practice and the effects on the girls' mental health, wondering if this was something that was practised in their community. Dad seemed dismissive, saying, "That's irrelevant." Instead, he blamed the "bad" influence of social media on mental health. He became quite defensive, saying, "Social media is the cause of many problems among the young people and Nuru is no exception; her siblings have no issues!" His reaction spoke volumes. I told them I only asked that question to ensure we were dealing with the root problem. I reminded them of Nuru's uniqueness as a person and that there was nothing like "a one-size-fits-all" approach, even in parenting. I suggested that Mum and Dad facilitate a one-to-one talk with Nuru in regard to their intended holiday before the end of the school term and to let me know how that goes. Dad said Mum would talk to Nuru.

Engaging with Dad was difficult to navigate. However, our engagement with Mum culminated in a trusting relationship within the triad and working alliance. Shortly afterwards, Nuru started talking about her conversations with Mum. I will never forget the excitement and contentment on Nuru's face during our twentieth session (of a total of twenty-four sessions) while exploring having a conversation with Dad, saying he seemed more open to discussions and accommodated different views. This was good progress, although it felt like we were just beginning. Meanwhile, Nuru and I explored alternative ways of expressing the unspeakable through journalling, symbols, creativity, drawing, or on the sand-tray. We thought together about self-resourcing, mindfulness, creating a safe space, talking, reflecting, and exploring feelings. In the ensuing sessions, Nuru seemed to develop a sustained sense of being in control.

In the following reflective parents meeting, Mum seemed more present and actively tried to contribute to discussions regarding Nuru's support. The domino effect as a result of this exchange was a real sense of attunement. Jernberg and Booth say parents provide a "reliable, supportive presence that guides and regulates the child's experience"

(2010, p. xi), while Novick and Novick refer to "restoration of the parent–child relationship leading to a lifelong positive resource for both" (2005, p. 17).

As we approached the endings, there was an ongoing conversation about Mum and the girls being left behind because Nuru was adamant she would not go with them. At fifteen years old, and being "Gillick competent" (Smaranda, 1985), I believe Nuru was becoming more aware of her rights and her place in the family. Although no concerns had been raised by the time our work ended, the school and children's department promised to remain vigilant to ensure the children's safety. I also recommended to the safeguarding officer that they familiarise themselves with The National FGM Centre UK document for schools in order to understand the FGM practice, risk indicators, and how to explore concerns and make referrals to relevant authorities where necessary. I felt it was important to give Mum contact details of specialist therapeutic and medical FGM clinics (Dahlia Project, Manor Gardens, NHS-University College London Hospital) with whom she could get in touch for support and physical assessment, even though there was no disclosure yet as to whether or not Nuru had experienced it. Obviously, she would liaise with Nuru before she took any steps, as discussed during our parenting meetings earlier.

Opponents of FGM as well as studies undertaken in the last decade by Benhrendt and Moritz (2005), Elnashar and Abdelhady (2007), Osinowo and Taiwo (2003), and Chibber and colleagues (2010) reveal the traumatic mental, psychological, and physical health consequences the victims suffer. Furthermore, the victims experience excruciating pain, severe blood loss, and shock (Wilson, 2021, p. 57). All this can leave them permanently disfigured and mentally wounded for life.

> Physiological and psychological trauma is likely to be most severe, if it is perpetrated by a caregiver, during childhood. (Allen, 1995, p. 14)

There is no doubt that the experiential trauma, due to the painful ordeal and observable permanent physical scarring, is devastating. Furthermore, the victims are exposed to infections such as HIV, hepatitis B, psychosexual problems (painful sex, incontinence, etc.)

They are re-traumatised through flashbacks and nightmares and often suffer depression, anxiety, PTSD, shame, and low self-esteem (Hearst & Molnar, 2013; Reisel and Creighton, 2015).

Besides, the girls go through it when they are underage and their bodies are still developing, after which some are married off to adult men back in their country of birth. Their husbands, who are usually mature men, expect the underage girls to honour their conjugal obligations. This further exacerbates the girls' ordeal during sex and subsequent birth processes. As a result, they are likely to experience accidental tears to their genitalia which would re-traumatise them or possibly cause death.

FGM is outlawed in most African countries, including my birth country Kenya, as well as here in the UK since 1985. Anyone aiding or performing FGM can be charged and jailed for up to fourteen years. The first person in the UK to be convicted of FGM was a mother of three and her partner (Summers & Ratcliffe, 2019).

Unfortunately, the battle against FGM is far from over, as evidenced by the extract below from a recent Kenyan Newspaper:

> Infant FGM is still rampant. The healthcare workers and parents are colluding to carry out the "cut" on baby girls during birth, as a new tactic of evading arrest for practising FGM. (Ngotho, 2022)

Due to the invasive and cruel nature of FGM, some of the girls may require long-term therapy, even in adulthood. The physical and mental scarring is a permanent reminder of the process. In this regard, it is important that the psychotherapist, parents, medical professionals, social workers, religious leaders, teachers, and government agencies work together to establish an effective all-inclusive intervention model and ensure there is no missing link. Besides, applying a combination of therapeutic and medical model would substantially complement the work with FGM victims.

Mwisho

Towards our ending, I became aware of a real change of trajectory with Mum, who was becoming much more collaborative, possibly appreciating the progress we were all making, as well as the positive change on Nuru. We thought together about healthy ways of accommodating Nuru's resistance and exhibited mannerisms, through dialogue and curiosity. The parents seemed to understand and appreciate that Nuru's stage of development (Erikson, 1963, pp. 234–235) and changing social environment could present some crisis as she develops a sense of self. As we prepared for the endings, I was confident of a good flow of communication and the relational fabric being repaired.

In the course of our work with Nuru, I became aware how important it is to give the young person a voice. Similarly, having parents on board was key, as they impact the work (positively or otherwise).

> Parental movement from the "closed" to the "open" system of self-regulation is the overarching criterion of change. (Novick & Novick, 2005, p. 168)

I recall, during my first two meetings with Nuru's Dad and Mum, how I picked up a real sense of pessimism around therapy. It was important to manage expectations right from the start as well as acknowledging how shameful, exposing, and unsettling it might be having to discuss some difficult issues with a stranger.

> Minority groups under-utilize counselling services due to their perceived mistrust, irrelevance and insensitivity to their cultural norms by the Western oriented counsellors. (Nelson-Jones, 2002, p. 291)

Mila na Desturi

It is crucial that the therapist is culturally competent, particularly when working with FGM victims, who are mostly from ethnic minority backgrounds. There is a need to be aware of stereotyping, prejudices, power imbalance, family dynamics, and contradictory world views to ensure objectivity, when the therapist's therapeutic vision is not blurred by life experiences (Lago, 1996). Coincidentally, both Nuru and I were born in the same geographical zone, and we shared some cultural similarities. This has benefits, but also brings some complexities. Often, the parents would ask leading questions or my opinion.

It was a tricky balance how I responded, while constantly ensuring professional boundaries were maintained. I wondered how they would have handled it if the therapist was of a different ethnicity. I endeavoured to maintain an open-minded curiosity, whilst being aware of my own perspective.

> Helpful factors when working therapeutically with survivors of FGM includes having cultural respect, knowledge and understanding, being non-judgemental/accepting and listening to the client. The most unhelpful factor is having "a general lack, or assumption of, awareness or understanding." (Jackson, 2017, p. 4)

My work with Nuru was a reminder of how trauma, re-traumatising, and secondary and vicarious trauma can linger long after a senseless action like FGM has been experienced. Emphatically feeling Nuru's pain was terrifying enough to flood me with vicarious trauma which I believe mirrored her experience. Obviously, this was evidence of my unprocessed material from the past in relation to FGM, which I was not aware of prior to working with Nuru. I often sat with anger and a sense of helplessness recalling my peers narrating their harrowing ordeals with FGM. I was able to work through and process my difficult feelings in my personal therapy. Perhaps Ifrah's true-life story in the film *A Girl from Mogadishu* (McGuckian, McGuckian, King, Abdi, & Antonio, 2020) gives a good summary of the mental and physical agony caused by FGM. Born in a refugee camp in Somalia, Ifrah was subjected to FGM at an early age and later trafficked to Ireland as a teenager, where she was eventually given political asylum.

My work with Nuru gave me a better understanding of the long-term mental and physiological health implications experienced by victims of FGM and how to intervene integratively. My knowledge of the legal issues was broadened, as was understanding the need to work in alliance with other agencies. Likewise, I hope this chapter offers the reader an insight into the negative effects of FGM practice and highlights the dilemmas and the need for the therapists' cultural competency.

In the past, research has generally focused on the physiological effects of FGM and how to intervene medically and not much on mental and psychological consequences and therapeutic support. Searching for relevant articles that specifically look at the therapeutic model for children and young people was difficult. An article written by the co-founder of Daughters of Eve, Leyla Hussein, states:

> The UK primary health services, GPs and hospitals primarily focus on the physical effects of FGM, such as chronic urinary tract infections, painful periods and acute and chronic pelvic infections that can lead to infertility. The emotional and psychological effects are ignored. Therapy is a chance to heal, a start of self-acceptance. (BACP, 2013, p. 25)

This calls for more work and an open dialogue. There is hope, as more organisations are working together to tackle FGM from different angles, creating awareness and developing a holistic intervention in liaison with affected communities. Here in the UK, the NSPCC and police provide an untraceable telephone number that victims can call if they are worried about being forced to undergo FGM. In addition, specialist National FGM support clinics have been opened in different parts of the UK to treat girls/women who have undergone FGM or are at risk. These can be accessed via this National Health Service link.[1] They are able to offer free support or direct the victims accordingly. The NHS has produced leaflets in different languages (Welsh, Amharic, Arabic, Farsi, French, Indonesian, Kurdish, Somali, Swahili, Tigrinya, Urdu) in order to reach out to many in practising communities. More details are available via the links provided at the end of this chapter.

It is ironic that most of the charities working with FGM victims are domiciled in the West even though many FGM cases are typically found in developing countries. This makes me wonder what therapeutic support is available at the grassroots, where the act is happening. Are there enough trained professionals to deal with the issue? Food for thought.

---

[1] https://www.nhs.uk/conditions/female-genital-mutilation-fgm/national-fgm-support-clinics

Special Swahili terminology

Mila na Desturi	Traditions and customs
Mwanzo	Beginnings
Mwisho	Endings
Nuru	Light
Tohara (Kukeketa)	Act of female genital mutilation

References

Abusharaf, R. M. (2006). Editor's introduction: The custom in question. In: *Female Circumcision* (pp. 1–26). Philadelphia: University of Pennsylvania Press.

Ahmadu, F. (2001). 14 rites and wrongs: an insider/outsider reflects on power and excision. In: B. Shell-Duncan & Y. Hernlund (Eds.), *Female "Circumcision" in Africa: Culture, Controversy, and Change* (pp. 283–312). Boulder, CA: Lynne Rienner. doi:10.1515/9781685850036-015 (last accessed 4 January 2023).

Allen, J. G. (1995). *Coping with Trauma: A Guide to Self-Understanding*. Washington, DC: American Psychiatric Press.

Amman, R. (1991). *Healing and Transformation in Sandplay*. USA: Open Court Publishing Company.

BACP (2013). Log in—BACP—British Association for Counselling & Psychotherapy. [online] www.bacp.co.uk. Available at: https://www.bacp.co.uk/bacp-journals/therapy-today/2013/december-2013/articles/talking-point (last accessed 14 January 2023).

Banks, E., Meirik, O., Farley, T., Akande, O., Bathija, H., & Ali, M. (2006). Female genital mutilation and obstetric outcome: WHO collaborative prospective study in six African countries. *The Lancet, 367*(9525): 1835–1841. doi:10.1016/s0140-6736(06)68805-3 (last accessed 13 January 2023).

BBC (2016). FGM is child abuse, says UN Population Fund chief. *BBC News*. [online] 15 July. Available at: https://www.bbc.co.uk/news/health-36805117 (last accessed 14 January 2023).

Behrendt, A., & Moritz, S. (2005). Posttraumatic stress disorder and memory problems after female genital mutilation. *American Journal of Psychiatry, 162*(5): 1000–1002. doi:10.1176/appi.ajp.162.5.1000 (last accessed 5 January 2023).

Berg, R. C., & Denison, E. (2013). A tradition in transition: Factors perpetuating and hindering the continuance of female genital mutilation/cutting (FGM/C) summarized in a systematic review. *Health Care for Women International*, [online] 34(10): 837–859. doi:10.1080/07399332.2012.721417 (last accessed 5 January 2023).

Berg, R. C., Denison, E., & Fretheim, A. (2010). Systematic review (continued). [online] Available at: https://www.fhi.no/globalassets/dokumenterfiler/rapporter/2010/rapport_2010_23_factors_genital_mutilation.pdf (last accessed 5 January 2023).

Bradway, K., & McCoard, B. (1997). *Sandplay: Silent Workshop of the Psyche*. London: Routledge.

Chibber, R., El-saleh, E., & El harmi, J. (2010). Female circumcision: obstetrical and psychological sequelae continues unabated in the 21st century. *The Journal of Maternal-Fetal & Neonatal Medicine*, 24(6): 833–836. doi:10.3109/14767058.2010.531318 (last accessed 5 January 2023).

Costello, S. (2015). Female genital mutilation/cutting: risk management and strategies for social workers and health care professionals. *Risk Management and Healthcare Policy*, 8: 225. doi:10.2147/rmhp.s62091 (last accessed 9 January 2023).

DeDomenico, G. (1995). *Sand Tray-World Play: A Comprehensive Guide to the Use of the Sand Tray in Psychotherapeutic and Transformational Settings*. Oakland, CA: Vision Quest Images. Available at http://visionquest.us/VQISR/SandtrayWorldplay_The%20Tool_.pdf (last accessed 9 January 2023).

Dellenborg, L. (2004). A reflection on the cultural meanings of female circumcision: Experiences from fieldwork in Casamance, Southern Senegal. In: S. Arnfred (Ed.), *Re-thinking Sexualities in Africa*. Uppsala: Nordic Africa Institute.

Elnashar, A., & Abdelhady, R. (2007). The impact of female genital cutting on health of newly married women. *International Journal of Gynecology & Obstetrics*, 97(3): 238–244. doi:10.1016/j.ijgo.2007.03.008 (last accessed 11 January 2023).

Erikson, E. H. (1963). *Childhood and Society*. London: Grafton.

Erlich, M. (1986). *The Injured Woman. Essay on Female Genital Mutilation*: Paris: L'Harmattan.

Europe (2019). FGM in Europe. [online] End FGM. Available at: https://www.endfgm.eu/female-genital-mutilation/fgm-in-europe/ (last accessed 14 January 2023).

Gruenbaum, E. (2006). Sexuality issues in the movement to abolish female genital cutting in Sudan. *Medical Anthropology Quarterly, 20*(1): 121–138. doi:10.1525/maq.2006.20.1.121 (last accessed 11 January 2023)

Hadi, A. A. (2006). A community of women empowered: the story of Deir el Barsha. In: R. M. Abusharaf (Ed.), *Female Circumcision* (pp. 104–124). Philadelphia: University of Pennsylvania Press.

Hearst, A. A., & Molnar, A. M. (2013). Female genital cutting: An evidence-based approach to clinical management for the primary care physician. *Mayo Clinic Proceedings, 88*(6): 618–629. doi:10.1016/j.mayocp.2013.04.004 (last accessed 11 January 2023).

Hosken, F. P. (1979). The Hosken Report: Genital and sexual mutilation of females. [online] Google Books. Women's International Network News. Available at: https://books.google.co.za/books?id=mPyxAAAAIAAJ (last accessed 11 January 2023).

Jackson, C. (2017). Counselling professionals' awareness and understanding of female genital mutilation/cutting: Training needs for working therapeutically with survivors. *Counselling and Psychotherapy Research, 17*(4): 309–319. doi:10.1002/capr.12136 (last accessed December 2022).

Jernberg, A. M., & Booth, P. B. (2010). *Theraplay: Helping Parents and Children Build Better Relationships Through Attachment-Based Play*. San Francisco: Jossey-Bass.

Johnson, A. G. (2005). *The Gender Knot: Unravelling Our Patriarchal Legacy (revised edition)*. Philadelphia: Temple University Press.

Lago, C. (1996). *Race, Culture and Counselling*. Maidenhead, Berks: Open University Press.

McGuckian, M., King, A. N., Abdi, B., & Antonio, M. C. (2020). *A Girl from Mogadishu*. [online] IMDb. Available at: https://www.imdb.com/title/tt7552790/ (last accessed 13 January 2023).

Nelson-Jones, R. (2002). *Essential Counselling and Therapy Skills: The Skilled Client Model*. London. Thousand Oaks, Calif.: Sage Publications.

Ngotho, S. (2022). Loitoktok: Alarm over infants being subjected to FGM at birth. [online] Nation. Available at: https://nation.africa/kenya/news/gender/loitoktok-alarm-over-infants-being-subjected-to-fgm-at-birth-4057430 (last accessed 13 January 2023).

Novick, K. K., & Novick, J. (2005). *Working with Parents Makes Therapy Work*. Lanham, MD: Jason Aronson.

Osinowo, H. O., & Taiwo, A. O. (2003). Impact of female genital mutilation on sexual functioning, self-esteem and marital instability of women in Ajegunle. *IFE PsychologIA*, *11*(1). doi:10.4314/ifep.v11i1.23446 (last accessed 11 January 2023).

Reisel, D., & Creighton, S. M. (2015). Long term health consequences of Female Genital Mutilation (FGM). *Maturitas*, [online] *80*(1): 48–51. doi:10.1016/j.maturitas.2014.10.009 (last accessed 11 January 2023).

Shell-Duncan, B., & Hernlund, Y. (2001). *Female "Circumcision" in Africa: Culture, Controversy, and Change*. Boulder, CO: Lynne Rienner.

Siegel, D. J. (2012). *The Developing Mind: How Relationships and the Brain Interact to Shape Who We Are*. New York. The Guilford Press.

Smaranda, E. (1985). *Gillick v West Norfolk and Wisbech AHA: The Right of Adolescents to Make Medical Decisions and the Many Shades of Grey*. [online] Available at: https://core.ac.uk/download/pdf/234650818.pdf (last accessed 13 January 2023).

Stern, D. N. (1985). *The Interpersonal World of the Infant: A view from Psychoanalysis and Developmental Psychology*. New York: Basic Books.

Summers, H., & Ratcliffe, R. (2019). Mother of three-year-old is first person convicted of FGM in UK. *The Guardian*. [online] 1 February. Available at: https://www.theguardian.com/society/2019/feb/01/fgm-mother-of-three-year-old-first-person-convicted-in-uk (last accessed 13 December 2023).

Weber, A. M., & Haen, C. (2005). *Clinical Applications of Drama Therapy in Child and Adolescent Treatment*. New York. Routledge.

Wilson, A-M. (2021). *Overcoming: My Fight Against FGM*. Oxford: Lion Hudson.

World Health Organization (1998). Female genital mutilation. [online] Available at: https://apps.who.int/iris/bitstream/handle/10665/42042/9241561912_eng.pdf (last accessed 13 January 2023).

World Health Organization (2008). Eliminating Female genital mutilation. An interagency statement. [online] Available at: https://apps.who.int/iris/bitstream/handle/10665/43839/9789241596442_eng.pdf?sequence=1&isAllowed=y (last accessed 13 January 2023).

World Health Organization guidelines on the management of health complications from female genital mutilation, (2016). [online] Available at: https://apps.who.int/iris/bitstream/handle/10665/206437/9789241549646_eng.pdf (last accessed 13 January 2023).

Important links

https://www.28toomany.org
https://www.endfgm.eu (a European network)
https://www.forwarduk.org.uk
https://www.integrateuk.org
https://manorgardenscentre.org/dahlia-project
https://nationalfgmcentre.org.uk
https://www.nhs.uk/fgm
https://www.nspcc.org.uk
https://www.orchidproject.org
https://www.uclh.nhs.uk/our-services/find-service/children-and-young-peoples-services/childrens-female-genital-mutilation-fgm-service

CHAPTER 7

Working with children and young people in the Orthodox Jewish community

Zisi Schleider

Introduction

Working therapeutically within the Orthodox Jewish community without adequate knowledge of this vastly rich population is akin to trying to read a book starting on the middle page. The Orthodox Jewish community is structured so that many of it needs are met from within, thereby creating a more insular environment. Interactions beyond the community tend to be more limited. When it comes to mental health, this is an area from which the community will reach out for further help (Bilu & Witztum, 1993, p. 199). Within the community, Rabbis, parents, and teachers are becoming more aware of their children's increasing mental health needs (Schnall et al., 2014, p. 167). In many sectors of the community, Jewish fiction and non-fiction magazine articles openly discuss mental health issues, bringing awareness to the importance placed on therapy (Friedman, 2021, p. 28–29). Orthodox Jewish families prefer to use therapists from within their own or neighbouring Jewish communities. However, there is a significant shortage of Orthodox Jewish child and adolescent psychotherapists. Rabbis are "overwhelmed with pastoral and counselling work and would welcome more professional support for their flock" (Loewenthal, 2006, p. 130). Although there are currently more Orthodox Jews training in psychotherapy, which will offer the community more culturally appropriate support, there is still a clear and urgent need, and opportunity, for qualified psychotherapists to reach this community.

Witztum and Buchbinder state, "The therapeutic challenge posted by the Ultra-Orthodox patients far exceeds that posed by the typical cross-cultural therapy situation" (2001, p. 119).

Being that I am in a unique position, as a member of the Orthodox Jewish community and as a child and adolescent psychotherapist, I personally have experienced a lack in understanding of my cultural and religious requirements, making them seem shrouded in secrecy. Winnicott states, "There is no such thing as a baby" (1960, p. 39). When working with children, we are also working with parents, the extended family, and the child's community. To cross the invisible borders and to reach my community (perhaps similarly to other minority groups, too), bridges of compassion and understanding need to be built; bridges built in personal therapy with my non-Jewish therapist. Although I do not claim to be an "expert in religion" (Plante, 2007, p. 10), I endeavour to contribute, in this chapter, to guide those who wish to work within this community, to be a reference to turn to.

The Orthodox Jewish community

In wider literature, the Orthodox community is interchangeable with the term ultra-Orthodox. For simplicity, the term Orthodox Jew is used throughout this chapter for both groups. The Orthodox Jewish community is complex and diverse and a subgroup with distinctive values (Zuk, 1978, pp. 103–109), yet it is a population generally found to be under-researched (Sharman & Jinks, 2019, p. 3). One of the reasons suggested for this is that Orthodox Jews are often not regarded as a separate ethnic minority and, instead, have been largely attributed an invisible status (Arredondo & D'Andrea, 1999). Weinrach urges that those "committed to multicultural counselling must embrace the notion that Jews are a culturally distinct group" (2002, p. 312).

Orthodox Jews follow a traditional form of Judaism involving strict compliance to the Torah, the teachings found in the Old Testament that govern a person's relationship with G-d and with fellow humans. G-d's name is written with a dash as it is considered holy. Deuteronomy 12:4 forbids erasing, destroying, or desecrating the name of G-d, so it is not written fully and therefore cannot be obliterated.

The family is the central social unit (Margolese, 1998, pp. 38–44), and so Jews tend to live in communities close to each other, accessing the infrastructure of Jewish schools, synagogues, and kosher food (Loewenthal & Rogers, 2004, p. 4). Whether within the family or business, everything is guided by the Torah (Schnall, 2006, p. 277). Rituals and traditions, such as daily prayers, Sabbath, and holiday observances, and the finer details of dress, diet, and speech, play a fundamental role in Orthodox Jewish life (Wikler, 2001, p. 80). Whilst easily misunderstood by the outside, Orthodox Jews usually find these instructions inspiring, containing, comforting, and meaning-making.

The Jewish community's insularity is due to the maintenance of the culture and also to anti-Semitism (Holliman & Wagner, 2015, p. 59). The predominance of anti-Semitism can mean that Orthodox Jews are reluctant to seek support outside the community (Sharman & Jinks, 2019, p. 3), in an attempt to be as self-sufficient as possible—except in the area of mental health care, where there is acknowledgement of the necessity for "experts from the 'other side'" (Witztum & Buchbinder, 2001, p. 118). Despite recognition for this support, Orthodox Jews have been shown to underuse mental health services provided by the dominant culture (Margolese, 1998, pp. 37–38).

The Rabbi's role and suspicion of therapy

Historically, there has been Rabbinical opposition towards psychoanalysis, which led Orthodox Jews to reject 'outside' therapists, viewing them as "sinners and heretics" (Bilu & Witztum, 1993, p. 206). Rabbis are considered the link in an unbroken chain in the receiving of the Torah, so, unsurprisingly, families feared their religious laws becoming violated in psychotherapy. The Jewish community operates in a hierarchical system, and the Rabbi interprets the Torah's teachings and offers guidance in a world which holds differing hostile values to the community. The community's reliance on and connection to their Rabbi is paramount. The Rabbi provides guidance on matters relating to spiritual, business, and family matters. Psychotherapists' engagement with Rabbis and community leaders is therefore crucial if children and young people within the community are to be referred and supported in accessing therapeutic services (Sharman & Jinks, 2019, p. 8).

Orthodox Jews are wary of the 'outside' therapist who may unknowingly breach social and sexual mores, or, for example, "prohibitions against speaking badly of others" (Loewenthal, 2006, pp. 130–131). A command in the Torah, "Honour thy father and mother" (Exodus, 20:12), directs the Orthodox Jew in how to treat and speak about parents. From an early age, children are instructed against improper speech and are taught the need to respect elders, and negative expressions of anger are actively discouraged. This may lead children to feel conflicted and unsure of what is allowed to be felt and spoken in therapy. This is likely to create a tension in building trust with a therapist. Specific adaptations are therefore required of the therapist in their ability to accommodate the child's religious laws, and it would be helpful for the child to experience the therapist's curiosity and openness to learning these laws.

Speech is significant, and the therapist is advised to be cautious around the use of everyday colloquial language that may be offensive or laden with innuendo for the child. The child's mother-tongue may not be English and/or may be heavily imbued with Hebrew or Yiddish, and trust can be built in the therapeutic relationship where the therapist understands some key phrases from the child's first language. Consultation with Rabbis and community leaders endorses encouragement and support in the therapeutic process and guards against the therapist introducing ideas or activities that conflict with the child's religious views. Whether the 'outside' therapist practises independently or within an agency such as Child and Adolescent Mental Health Services, it would be wise to factor into any treatment plan additional time for a working alliance with the community and/or wider system to counter any suspicions that may be raised (Bloch, Gabbay, Knowlton, & Fins, 2018, p. 1704).

Many Orthodox children and young people may lack previous experience and understanding of the purpose of therapy and arrive with "unhelpful preconceptions" (Schnall, 2006, p. 279), especially if they attend therapy at the recommendation of their Rabbi. Simple attendance may be viewed as meeting their obligation; however, engagement in the therapeutic process cannot be taken for granted. There may be an expectation that this relationship will replicate that of the Rabbi's position in the community, predicated on education and instruction. Particular attention and sensitivity to the transferential and countertransferential dynamic will help the therapist in better understanding the child's understanding of their relationship.

In some instances, Rabbis' own fears and suspicions inhibit them from supporting outside therapeutic agencies, so focusing on building peer relationships within the community, engaging with community leaders, and psychoeducation may be a more fruitful bridge (Schnall et al., 2014). The culturally sensitive outside psychotherapist, willing and open to listen, learn, and adapt to what may appear to be strange and different customs and behaviours, may lead to Rabbis, community leaders, and school leaders feeling less afraid and suspicious. Schnall et al. found a significant decline in the mistrust of outside therapists, and this has led to an increase in engagement with outside therapists in the Jewish community (2014). Trust from the Rabbi and wider Jewish community will support the child's trust in the therapist.

The impact of anti-Semitism on working therapeutically with children and young people

When reflecting on working with Orthodox Jewish children, the implications of persecution over thousands of years, the transgenerational impact, and anti-Semitism must be considered. According to Stein, "terrible as was the experience of the Nazi epoch, Jews do not see it as an unprecedented or isolated period in their history, but as a recurrent historic role" (1984, pp. 5–35). Hass (1999) says that anti-Semitism has been called the longest hatred, and Lerner (1992) describes anti-Semitism as permanent "Jew hating". Even in times of peace, anti-Semitism persists. Passages in the New Testament describe Jews in demeaning and derogatory ways, which seem to be used as a "justification to proselytize Jews, which is, in essence, a repudiation of the legitimacy of Judaism" (Weinrach, 2002, p. 307). Perhaps this gives some perspective on the Jewish experience; present reality is based on historical and current factors.

Anti-Semitism also requires attention and consideration due to endemic influence in literature and its subliminal inference. Shakespeare portrayed Shylock in *The Merchant of Venice* as a greedy, vengeful, and jealous Jew (Shakespeare & Mahood, 1987). This is read, watched, and included in many school curricula. Fagin is depicted as a menacing, evil figure referred to as 'The Jew' 257 times in the first thirty-eight chapters of Charles Dickens' *Oliver Twist*. Without Dickens ever having met a Jew, he bought into the [Jewish] myth that "has poisoned the psyche of the Western World" (The Independent, 2005, p. 4) and which continues to peddle these unconscious biases against Jews.

The risks involved in a young person stepping out of the safe insularity of their Jewish community for therapy can understandably incite fear in both parents and child, making this an unsafe option accessed only when desperately needed. According to Samuels, the "Modern Jews live in the shadow of centuries of anti-Semitism" (1992, pp. 127–148). The inbuilt experience of hatred, conversion attempts, and fear is real and cannot be underestimated. Beck (1991) equates the Jewish experience of subliminal fear of anti-Semitism to most women's subliminal fear of rape.

To define clearly whether anti-Semitism has occurred, Weinrach suggests substituting the word Jew with a member of another minority. The need to use this substitution made me question whether Weinrach doubted the reader's ability to be open-minded and neutral to the assertions he is making in considering anti-Semitism is not racism. Weinrach relays the words of Martin Gerstein, former treasurer of the American Counselling Association: "You're surprised that there is anti-Semitism in the counselling profession? The whole world is anti-Semitic. Why should the counselling profession be any different?" (Weinrach, 2002, p. 303). Saper (1991) regards anti-Semitism today as mostly subtle, silent, and covert. Sadly, many of the issues Weinrach presented seem as pertinent today as then. This necessitates raising the subject of anti-Semitism, whether conscious or otherwise, that might surface when working with Orthodox Jewish young people. It is incumbent upon the psychotherapist to examine their reactions and feelings to Weinrach's article.

Freud was a secular Jew who viewed religion as a fallacy, "a universal obsessional neurosis" (Freud, 1927, p. 104). Whilst Freud's writings may be unfamiliar to the Orthodox Jew, his views on religion are considered "heretical" (Margolese, 1998, pp. 42–43) and serve to bring suspicion to therapy. For Orthodox Jewish adults and children, the therapeutic experience may be an "encounter fraught with danger", encouraging changes not welcomed by the child or the community, requiring interactions that are discouraged or forbidden (Heilman & Witztum, 1997, p. 523). The client may arrive concerned that the therapist has ulterior motives or is anti-Semitic (Schnall, 2006, p. 278). The child may be suspicious of the therapist who is a representative of the "unchaste, evil, impure and decadent secular world" (Bilu & Witztum, 1993, p. 201).

Transgenerational trauma

The Jewish worldview is profoundly affected by historical persecution, which looms large in the community's awareness (Gabbay, McCarthy, & Fins, 2017, p. 548). The Holocaust is a recent chapter in a long history of hatred and massacre of Jews, and this trauma, in differing and disparate ways, "has marked the psyche of every Jew the world over" (Beck, 1991).

A study carried out fifty years after the Holocaust found that 57 per cent of survivors still met post-traumatic stress disorder criteria, with 74 per cent exhibiting symptoms of PTSD (Trappler, Braunstein, Moskowitz, & Friedman, 2002, pp. 2–7). These studies correlate with the supposition of transgenerational trauma as a communally felt experience. As a grandchild of Holocaust survivors, I have witnessed and felt the transgenerational trauma within my community. This is revisited when aged Holocaust survivors share their wartime experiences and remains a current theme in community lectures and current literature for adults and children.

It could be hypothesised that Jewish children arrive in therapy today with similar felt experiences, both conscious and unconscious. The Holocaust is present and alive to many, and this may feature in the therapy work on an unconscious level (Schnall, 2006; Weinrach, 2002). These felt experiences, together with fears of the therapist's unconscious anti-Semitism, is likely to create a significant reluctance, mistrust, and ambivalence in Jewish clients. It is crucial the therapist is cognisant of the historical persecution, intergenerational trauma, and anti-Semitism, and understands that they themselves may be perceived as representatives of an evil non-religious world. This may also apply to people of different ethnicities and cultures.

Stigma and shame in the Orthodox Jewish community

Parents from the Orthodox Jewish community are reluctant to seek external mental health support for their children for fear of secular influence and because of the communal stigmatisation of mental health (Bloch, Gabbay, Knowlton, & Fins, 2018, p. 1704). Stigma is a key barrier to preventing Orthodox Jewish children and adolescents accessing mental health support (Wikler, 1986, p. 115). Margolese concurs: "When they present for treatment they do so with reluctance and shame." Asking for help with mental health can cause the child to be shunned and lose social status, impacting the immediate family and beyond (1998, p. 40). There is "societal stigma and fear of the influence of secular ideas" (Bloch, Gabbay, Knowlton, & Fins, 2018, p. 1702) and "suspicion, anxiety, and defensiveness" (Wikler, 1986, p. 114). Loewenthal found that stigma and non-attendance were caused by conflict between "values inherent in psychotherapy and Jewish values" (2006, p. 128). Fear of lack of confidentiality and privacy also impacted therapy attendance. Clients' concern for confidentiality could be seen as "paranoid" (Wikler, 1986, p. 118). Primary school parents were shown to be concerned about future school acceptance (Sharman & Jinks, 2019, pp. 7–8).

Schnall et al. conducted a follow-up study on barriers to mental health twenty-five years after the original study and found that 90 per cent of the community's mental health needs were still inadequately met, with no significant change in clients seeking treatment from a mental health professional. Many clinicians cited stigma associated with mental health needs as the reason for this (2014, pp. 163–169) and this continues to impede access to outside professionals still today (Sharman & Jinks, 2019, pp. 7–8).

According to Cinnirella and Loewenthal (1999), and Hawthorne, Rahman, and Pill (2003), Muslims, people of colour, Christians, and other ethnic-religious groups also find accessing mental health services particularly discrediting/stigmatising. Mojtabai found stigma to be one of the most prominent impediments to treatment in minority communities (2007). Stigma is raised repeatedly in the literature of the Orthodox Jewish community, who may associate accessing help with extreme mental and physical health problems and the fear that this could severely jeopardise any matrimonial prospects (Gabbay et al., 2017, p. 546). Any therapist working with children and young people from an ethnic-religious minority needs humility regarding what they know and an inquisitiveness to learn what they do not. Further cultural research may deliver similarities that can be used for other minority communities.

Culturally specific countertransference

Countertransference is the therapist's feelings "that are caused by the actions on us of the child's unconscious communication" (Klein & French, 2012, p. 15). Clarkson defines countertransference as the psychotherapist's response to the therapeutic relationship (1992, p. 154). According to Strean, therapists have a general responsibility to always monitor their countertransference, especially with religious clients or their material, as both positive and negative countertransferential reactions are found (1994). Sandler explains how "exploring the countertransference can be useful in refining therapists' reflexive thinking" (cited in Toledano, 1996, p. 296). Weinrach notes how Jews evoke strong emotions in others (2002, p. 302), and Witztum and Buchbinder define some of the diverse countertransference reactions that the therapist may experience in this cross-culture relationship, which include disgust, surprise, "even attraction to the fierce religious commitments of ultra-orthodox patients ... either clear idealizations of religious values and life-style or overt hostility" (2001, p. 120).

Envy can evolve within the countertransference with religious clients; "a non-religious therapist may envy the kind of maternal warmth generated by the patient's lifestyle" (Margolese, 1998, p. 44). Melanie Klein defines envy as "the angry feeling that another person possesses and enjoys something desirable" and the "envious impulse to take it away or spoil it" (Klein, 1977, p. 181). Comas-Diaz and Jacobson similarly found therapists "were extremely biased, ranging from a total idealization of (the other's) value system to, more frequently, manifesting hostility and rejection" (cited in Bilu & Witztum, 1993, p. 206).

Bilu and Witztum consider it a requisite for mental health professionals working with Orthodox Jews to recognise and examine the religious component in countertransference (1993, p. 207). A sense of exclusion from the community felt by the therapist could lead to an unintended attack on the client and derailment of the therapeutic relationship. Witztum and Buchbinder warn of the danger in leaving feelings unattended; "strong countertransferenial feelings cause biased themes and attitudes and diagnostic and treatment mistakes" (2001, p. 120) and can leave the therapist feeling deskilled and fearful of wrongdoing.

Self-exploration by the therapist

Arredondo et al. encourage the therapist, working with a distinct cultural group, to examine their own cultural self-awareness (1996, p. 57), necessitating reflection of their own biases, beliefs, and lifestyle, in order to allow space to engage with the Orthodox Jewish child's practices and traditions. Working successfully in any minority community requires openness, curiosity, and acceptance of the whole client, with their "attributions and taboos", to allow growth to happen. "Culturally skilled counsellors should attend to, as well as work to eliminate biases, prejudices, and discriminatory contexts … develop sensitivity to issues of oppression, sexism, heterosexism, elitism and racism" (Arredondo et al., 1996, pp. 67–73).

The Dimension of Personal Identity Model (PIM) is an educational tool encouraging self-exploration, appreciating the full complexity of the individual (Arredondo et al., 1996). The PIM considers the multicultural perspective of an individual's affiliations, memberships, and subcultures. Using questions and discussion points, the therapist can influence interactions with clients, recognise their limits of expertise, understand how their communication style can clash with their clients', and raise awareness around stereotyping (Arredondo et al., 1996). The authors identify skill learning, research about mental health particular to the ethnic group, urge respect of beliefs and values with recognition of cultural-linguistic characteristics, knowledge of the family structure and hierarchy, and an understanding of cultural verbal and nonverbal cues (1996, pp. 47–73). The PIM gives therapists the opportunity to address their own biases, thus viewing with a clearer lens the Orthodox Jew without the centuries of subliminal stereotyping. Interestingly, this paper, which is so relevant, does not specifically reference the Jewish Community once.

In his RRICC model, Plante brings an in-depth understanding of respect, responsibility, integrity, competence, and concern. He considers these elements necessary in cross-cultural therapeutic relationships, explaining the "compelling ethical principles and issues to consider in spirituality and psychology" (2007, p. 2). One could argue that all therapists should be aware of their processes, and this is the reason personal therapy and supervision are an integral part of the training and ongoing practice of the psychotherapist.

Respecting clients' beliefs

Due to the insularity of the Orthodox Jewish community, children can be confused when exposed to external ideas from the therapist that the community does not allow—even something as seemingly innocuous as suggesting specific sports to manage aggression (Schnall, 2006, p. 279). The backlash from the family and community is perhaps the most challenging aspect of the therapy's survival. Other minority groups, such as Mormons, who also have guidelines governing their behaviour, are likely to experience this too.

Parents may fear that the outside therapist may influence an adolescent if presenting doubts or questions about their religious beliefs. When complex issues arise, the client's involvement of the Rabbi can be beneficial (Margolese, 1998, p. 49). The therapist could communicate with Rabbis or community leaders/members where appropriate and with respect to general data protection regulation (GDPR), giving no identifying details about the child or specific environment. In this way, they could explain/discuss the relevant issues in therapy. They could also have connections with respected Orthodox Jewish therapists and supervisors, who understand the particular community the child comes from.

Ogden (2004, p. 1356) defines Bion's container–contained as "not a thing but a process" wherein the child's thoughts and feelings can be digested, thus developing a new capacity to make sense of themselves (Klein, 2012, p. 36). Rogers' client-centred approach is a "conscious renunciation and avoidance by the therapist of all control over or decision-making for the client". Perhaps this is a good model to begin with Orthodox adolescents and children, as it protects the client's beliefs, avoids interpretations, suggestions, or challenging the client, with the therapist "experiencing a positive, acceptant attitude toward whatever the client" is at the moment (Rogers, 1980, pp. 115–116).

Some children do abandon Orthodox Jewish practices, and discussions with advisors, Rabbis, and teachers can be useful in exploring these issues. Loewenthal and Roger's study (2004) of twenty-one charitable organisations shows how they function with ongoing liaison and the Rabbi's approval, which is implicitly understood and trusted within the community. Organisations will often manage safeguarding issues and manage disclosures. Witztum and Buchbinder describe the "thousands of small aid organisations" supporting communities to be self-sufficient (2001, p. 118). The therapist needs some communal knowledge of who to approach in some of these delicate situations, how far to work with a client, or when to refer the client to a religious therapist (Heilman & Witztum, 1997).

Diversity training, whilst difficult to access, can be helpful (Schnall, 2006). When working with young, vulnerable children, the parent entrusts the therapist to uphold their values and show respect to the protected and insular world the child inhabits. The position of "not knowing" and being curious and open to learning can help explore the "personal meaning of cultural or religious issues" (Toledano, 1996, p. 293) and evaluate the role Judaism plays in the child's life (Holliman & Wagner, 2015). Asking questions of community members or staff is possibly the most accessible way of gaining insight and knowledge into a child's mannerisms, behaviours, or actions. The Israeli television drama *Shtisel* (2013) depicts a fictional Orthodox Jewish family living in a small area in Jerusalem. The characters are played by secular unaffiliated Jews, who learnt how to walk, talk, and act like Orthodox Jews and to speak Yiddish. It demonstrates how it is possible to learn the etiquette of engaging with the Orthodox Jewish Community.

This popular Netflix series represents a snapshot of life in one branch of Hassidic Orthodox Jewish community living. This exact lifestyle is not replicated throughout all Orthodox Jewish communities. However, it could be instrumentally useful as part of the induction of a therapist coming from the outside into the Orthodox community. When a therapist understands the culture, it greatly benefits the building of a positive therapeutic alliance.

Secular views can be experienced as existentially threatening and can overwhelm the Orthodox child, adolescent, or their parents, particularly at the start of therapy. Religion is the fabric of Orthodox Jewish identity, and the therapist has a responsibility to protect the child's culture. It is essential the therapist use their power in the relationship wisely.

Bilu and Witztum explore the creation of a "meaningful therapeutic discourse, a persuasive rhetoric of healing, tailored to the patient's cosmology and all-embracing value system" (1993, p. 201). Witztum and Buchbinder consider developing knowledge and respect about a child's customs as "a standard pre-requisite" in cross-cultural dyadic relationships (2001, p. 123).

Diversity and LGBTQ+

The integrative child and adolescent psychotherapist's role is to work with, in an age-appropriate way, all parts of their client's worlds, including their sexuality and individual identity. Part of the tension of working as an 'outside' with the Orthodox community will engender additional complexities, as exploration of the young person's relationship with the LGBTQ+ community might conflict with Torah values. However, it is still possible for the 'outside' therapist who is "respectful, knowledgeable, and skilled to work within various value parameters" (Stolovy, Levy, Doron, & Melamed, 2012) to support the client through this journey, and this work can be enlightening and beneficial for the young person. Whilst therapy is a place for a child to explore their experiences, it is important for the therapist to have understanding, maintain sensitivity, and not influence or lead this exploration.

Conclusion

This chapter shows some of the specificity and complexity of the Orthodox Jewish family's lifestyle. It evidences four main cultural themes—stigma, transgenerational trauma, anti-Semitic concerns, and suspicion or fear of therapy from a religious perspective.

The main themes developed here are found to apply to all different communities within the Orthodox Jewish community. In the same way as commonality appears in different sects of the Orthodox Jewry, the same may apply to other minority groups. More diversity research is needed to assist the therapist in building relationships with different minority/ethnic cultures or communities and in advocating for improved cross-cultural therapeutic work, and more development is required in providing ethical training methods and incorporating accountability. Further research into ethical issues in therapy warrant attention in and of themselves, as indicated with Arredondo et al's or Plant's suggestions, as they rely on the integrity of the individual therapist.

There is an assumption that spending many years training and attending personal therapy and supervision qualifies one to work in any field of choice. Much of the therapist's personal process is dependent on their awareness, self-growth, and focus on continuously refining themselves, in much the same way as the skilled craftsman whittles, sands, and perfects his artwork. Working with minorities, such as the Orthodox Jewish community, may require re-evaluating oneself and revisiting personal therapy. There are, at present, no specific therapeutic models related to working with Orthodox Jewish families but, as this chapter demonstrates, there are many additional needs to be considered.

Therein lies the dichotomy: the person is a representative and part of a community, yet at the same time is a unique individual with past and present experiences woven into their current presentation that demands to be seen as such.

Ivey and Ivey address this dichotomy with this cautionary quote.

> Never make an assumption about an individual based solely on cultural understandings. Treat each other first and foremost as an individual. But, never consider an individual out of social contexts. (1997, p. 40)

References

Arredondo, P., & D'Andrea, M. (1999). How do Jews fit into the multicultural counseling movement? *Counseling Today, 14*: 36.

Arredondo, P., Toporek, R., Pack Brown, S., Jones, J., Locke, D. C. Sanchez, J., & Stadler, H. (1996). Operationalization of the multicultural counseling competencies. *Journal of Multicultural Counseling and Development, 24*: 42–78. https://doi.org/10.1002/j.2161-1912.1996.tb00288.x (last accessed February 2022).

Beck, E. T. (1991). Therapy's double dilemma: Anti-Semitism and misogyny. *Women & therapy, 10*(4): 19–30. https://doi.org/10.1300/j015v10n04_04 (last accessed November 2022).

Bilu, Y., & Witztum, E. (1993). Working with Jewish ultra-Orthodox patients: Guidelines for a culturally sensitive therapy. *Culture, Medicine and Psychiatry, 17*: 197–233. https://doi.org/10.1007/bf01379326 (last accessed March 2021).

Bloch, A. M., Gabbay, E., Knowlton, S. F., Fins, J. J. (2018). Psychiatry, cultural competency, and the care of ultra-Orthodox Jews: Achieving secular and theocentric convergence through introspection. *Journal of Religious Health*, *57*(5): 1702–1716.

Cinnirella, M., & Loewenthal, K. M. (1999). Religious and ethnic group influences on beliefs about mental illness: A qualitative interview study. *British Journal of Medical Psychology*, *72*(4): 505–524. https://doi.org/10.1348/000711299160202 (last accessed March 2021).

Clarkson, P. (1992). *Transactional Analysis Psychotherapy: An Integrated Approach*. London: Routledge.

Freud, S. (1927c). *The Future of an Illusion. S. E., 21*. London: Hogarth.

Friedman, A. (2021). Short-changed. *Ami-Living Magazine*, 27 January 2021.

Gabbay, E., McCarthy, M. W., & Fins, J. J. (2017). The care of the ultra-Orthodox Jewish patient. *Journal of Religion and Health*, *56*: 545–560. https://doi.org/10.1007/s10943-017-0356-6 (last accessed January 2021).

Hass, P. G. (1999). Science and the determination of the good. In J. K. Roth (Ed.), *Ethics After the Holocaust: Perspectives, Critiques, and Responses* (49–89). St Paul, MN: Paragon House. https://doi.org/10.1057/9780230513105_12 (last accessed December 2022).

Hawthorne, K., Rahman, J., & Pill, R. (2003). Working with Bangladeshi patients in Britain: Perspectives from primary health care. *Family Practice*, *20*(2): 185–191. https://doi.org/10.1093/fampra/20.2.185 (last accessed March 2022).

Heilman, S. C., & Witztum, E. (1997). Value-sensitive therapy: Learning from ultra-Orthodox patients. *American Journal of Psychotherapy*, *51*(4): 522–541. https://doi.org/10.1176/appi.psychotherapy.1997.51.4.522 (last accessed January 2022).

Holliman, R. P., & Wagner, A. A. (2015). Responsive counseling in Jewish Orthodox communities. *Journal of Counselor Practice*, *6*(2): 56–75. https://doi.org/10.22229/joc038712 (last accessed January 2021).

The Independent (2005). Dicken's greatest villain: The faces of Fagin. *The Independent*, 7 October. https://www.independent.co.uk/arts-entertainment/films/features/dickens-greatest-villain-the-faces-of-fagin-317786.html (last accessed December 2021).

Ivey, M. B., & Ivey, A. E. (1997). And now we begin: Multicultural competencies gaining approval. *Counselling Today*, April, p. 40.

Klein, M. (1977). *Envy and Gratitude*. London: Vintage.

Klein, R., & French, L. (2012). *Therapeutic Practice In Schools: Working With The Child Within*. London: Routledge.

Lerner, M. (1992). *The Socialism of Fools: Anti-Semitism on the Left*. Oakland, CA: Tikkun Books.

Loewenthal, K. M. (2006). Strictly Orthodox Jews and their relations with psychotherapy and psychiatry. *World Association of Cultural Psychiatry*, 128–132.

Loewenthal, K. M., & Rogers, M. B. (2004). Culture-sensitive counselling, psychotherapy and support groups in the Orthodox-Jewish community: How they work and how they are experienced. *International Journal of Social Psychiatry*, 50: 227–270. https://doi.org/10.1177/0020764004043137 (last accessed March 2021).

Margolese, H. C. (1998). Engaging in psychotherapy with the Orthodox Jew. *American Journal of Psychotherapy*, 52(1): 37–53. https://doi.org/10.1176/appi.psychotherapy.1998.52.1.37 (last accessed March 2021).

Mojtabai, R. (2007). Americans' attitudes toward mental health treatment seeking: 1990–2003. *Psychiatric Services*, 58(5): 642–651. https://doi.org/10.1176/ps.2007.58.5.642 (last accessed November 2021).

Ogden, T. H. (2004). On holding and containing, being and dreaming. *International Journal of Psychoanalysis*, 85(134): 1349–1364. https://doi.org/10.1516/t41h-dgux-9jy4-gqc7 (last accessed November 2021).

Plante, T. G. (2007). Integrating spirituality and psychotherapy: Ethical issues and principles to consider. *Journal of Clinical Psychology*, 63: 891–902. https://doi.org/10.1002/jclp.20383 (last aaccessed January 2021).

Rogers, C. (1980). *A Way of Being*. Boston, MA: Houghton Mifflin.

Samuels, A. (1992). National psychology, national socialism, and analytical psychology: Reflections on Jung and anti-Semitism Part II. *Journal of Analytical Psychology*, 37(2): 127–148. https://doi.org/10.1111/j.1465-5922.1992.00127.x (last accessed December 2021).

Saper, B. (1991). A cognitive behavioral formulation of the relation between the Jewish joke and anti-Semitism. *International Journal of Humour Research*, 4: 41–59. https://doi.org/10.1515/humr.1991.4.1.41 (last accessed December 2021).

Schnall, E. (2006). Multicultural counseling and the Orthodox Jew. *Journal of Counseling and Development*, 84: 276–281. https://doi.org/10.1002/j.1556-6678.2006.tb00406.x (last aaccessed October 2020).

Schnall, E., Kalkstein, S., Gottesman, A., Feinberg, K., Schaeffer, C. B., & Feinberg, S. S. (2014). Barriers to mental health care: A 25-year follow-up study of the Orthodox Jewish community. *Journal of Multicultural counseling and development*, 4: 161–173. https://doi.org/10.1002/j.2161-1912.2014.00052.x (last accessed October 2021).

Shakespeare, W., & Mahood, M. (1987). *The Merchant of Venice*. Cambridge: Cambridge University Press.

Sharman, S., & Jinks, G. H. (2019). How are counseling and therapeutic services experienced by Orthodox Jewish primary schools in North-West London? What are the cultural sensitivities, attitudes and beliefs of senior staff members in these schools? *Mental Health, Religion and Culture*, 22(4). https://doi.org/10.1080/13674676.2019.1571027 (last accessed October 2020).

Shtisel (2013). Film directed by Alon Zingman. Netflix.

Stein, H. F. (1984). The Holocaust, the uncanny, and the Jewish sense of history. *International Society of Political Psychology*, 5: 5–35. https://doi.org/10.2307/3790829 (last accessed November 2022).

Strean, H. (1994). *Psychotherapy with the Orthodox Jew*. Northvale, NJ: Jason Aronson.

Stolovy, T., Levy, Y. M., Doron, A., & Melamed, Y. (2012). Culturally sensitive mental health care: A study of contemporary psychiatric treatment for ultra-Orthodox Jews in Israel. *International Journal of Social Psychiatry*, 59(8): 819–823. Doi.org/10.1177/002076400004600205 (last accessed December 2022).

Toledano, A. (1996). Issues arising from intra-cultural family therapy. *Journals of Family Therapy*, 18: 289–301. https://doi.org/10.1111/j.1467-6427.1996.tb00052.x (last accessed May 2021).

Trappler, B., Braunstein, J. W., Moskowitz, G., & Friedman, S. (2002). *Holocaust Survivors in a Primary Care Setting: Fifty Years Later*. http://www.research-consultation.com/InformationArticlesonMentalHealthProblems_11.asp https://doi.org/10.2466/pr0.2002.91.2.545 (last accessed 20 February 2022).

Weinrach, S. G., (2002). The counseling profession's relationship to Jews and the issues that concern them: More than a case of selective awareness. *Journal of Counseling and Development*, 80: 300–314. https://doi.org/10.1002/j.1556-6678.2002.tb00195.x (last accessed January 2023).

Wikler, M. (1986). Pathways to treatment: How Orthodox Jews enter therapy. *The Journal of Contemporary Social Work*, 113–118. https://doi.org/10.1177/104438948606700207 (last accessed March 2021).

Wikler, M. (2001). Sustaining ourselves: An interdisciplinary peer supervision group for Orthodox Jewish therapists treating Orthodox Jewish patients. *Journal of Psychotherapy in Independent Practice*, *2*(1): 79–86. https://doi.org/10.1300/j288v02n01_07 (last accessed September 2021).

Winnicott, D. W. (1960). The theory of the parent–infant relationship. In: *The Maturational Processes and the Facilitating Environment*. New York: International Universities Press.

Witztum, E., & Buchbinder, J. T. (2001). Strategic culture sensitive therapy with religious Jews. *International Review of Psychiatry*, *13*: 117–124. https://doi.org/10.1080/09540260124954 (last accessed March 2021).

Zuk, G. H. (1978). A therapist's perspective on Jewish family values. *Journal of Marriage and Family Counselling*, *4*: 103–109. https://doi.org/10.1111/j.1752-0606.1978.tb00501.x (last accessed December 2022).

CHAPTER 8

Go well: bearing witness to the grief of young clients in therapy

Tasha Bailey

Too often children are left out of the conversation when a family or community experience grief, loss, or change. Not having the language or understanding of grief can also leave children vulnerable to carrying their mourning without it having the opportunity to breathe and be witnessed.

In the following chapter, I will discuss the ways that grief can arise in the therapy room with children and young people and how this can be explored through metaphor and play. I will also demonstrate my role as a witness and co-facilitator along their journey through clinical examples. This includes how grief can show up in the closure of therapy and how this can be an opportunity for past experiences of loss and abandonment to be connected with.

Children and grief

Grief is a natural reaction to the loss of a relationship. Whether this loss comes from the permanent death of a lost one, separation, disruption, or change, it has the potential to cause emotional pain and to disrupt our thoughts, feelings, and path of development (Fiorini & Mullen, 2006a).

Grief is as an individual process with its own momentum, which encapsulates coping with fear, pain, and the new version of ourselves without our loved one (Samuel, 2018).

When we experience grief, we go through a push and pull of holding on and moving forward, between the past and future. This is described within Stroebe and Schut's dual process model, where we hold onto two reins during grief (Stroebe & Schuts, 1999). In one hand, we experience loss-orientated pressures. These are thoughts, feelings, and memories which connect us to our pain and mourning. In the other hand, we hold onto a restoration-orientated rein. This connects us to thoughts, feelings, and events about the needs of our daily life and the hopes of our present and future. We oscillate between these two modes as a normal way of coping. The loss-orientated rein brings up strong and difficult emotions, whilst the restoration-orientated rein brings us hope and forward motion.

For children and young people, grief could involve losing a parent or family member, moving school or house, or even having to change teacher at the end of the school year. Whether it is a bereavement, transitional change, or the end of therapy, children come up against goodbyes all of the time. However, children are often left out of the conversation when it comes to loss. Fiorini and Mullen describe how Western society has a "death-phobic culture" since it avoids open conversation around grief and loss with children and young people (Fiorini & Mullen, 2006b, p. 31).

As suggested by Kübler-Ross, we live in a society where "death is viewed as taboo, discussion of it is regarded as morbid, and children are excluded with the presumption that it would be 'too much' for them" (Kübler-Ross, 1969, p. 6). This causes a fundamental problem for children with unprocessed grief, leaving many of them with emotional and behavioural difficulties as a result. Furthermore, it is believed that children grieve "in spurts" (Himebauch, Arnold, & May, 2008, p. 242). As they move through various developmental stages, their understanding of grief and death changes, which leaves them to re-grieve at each developmental age. This suggests that children need more opportunities to grieve throughout their lives than they are often given.

Bearing witness to grief

When grief enters the therapy room, I take the approach of self-directed therapy, actively participating in the experience of growth and learning for the child (Axline, 1947). I am careful to not introduce anything outside of what the child is bringing themselves. Instead, I follow their lead and make gentle, play-focused invitations to deepen the material they share. This also involves maintaining restraint of any impulse "to take over the client's responsibility" which imposes our own stories onto the play (Axline, 1947, p. 16). Therefore, this involves me listening out for the child's limits, yet stepping "out of the way quickly so as not to interfere with the forces of play" (McCarthy, 2007, p. 22).

According to Kessler, grief needs to be witnessed by someone who is fully present with the magnitude of that loss and without trying to change or fix it (Kessler, 2019). As a therapist working with children who have lived through grief, my role is to bear witness to their pain without needing to reframe it or rescue them from it. I will demonstrate this through my work with Jasmine, a nine-year-old girl who had experienced various forms of grief in her life, especially centring around her mother.

Jasmine is of white British and Black Caribbean heritage and was referred due to displaying withdrawn behaviour and peer difficulties. The school were aware of how much loss she had experienced over the past few years and were concerned about her being in year five and the loss of primary school as her only constant. Jasmine had been in foster care for two years after being a young carer and separated from her siblings, who had been adopted or fostered outside of the borough. Her mother had various physical conditions as a result of her ongoing substance and alcohol dependency. During our therapy together, her mother died due to heart failure, and Jasmine was given little autonomy over the funeral plans. This was unfortunate, since not being involved in discussions around the death of loved ones and the rituals honouring their life can be a detriment to a child's grieving process (Fiorini & Mullen, 2006a).

Often when I made invitations to think about the loss of her mother, Jasmine looked at the floor and changed the subject. This indicated that talking about the death of her mother was too intense, and this was a form of self-protection. I wondered whether any invitations I made to reflect on her loss needed to begin within the safety of metaphor. As suggested by McCarthy, when "the child is protected by the symbol, [the work] can go straight to the heart of the matter" (McCarthy, 2007, p. 41).

I noticed that Jasmine had a fascination with historical figures, stories, and events, which made it difficult for her peers to connect with her. In the therapy space, I began to invite her to share these interests more with me, which included Buddy Holly and Elvis Presley. I noticed that she came to life when she spoke about their music, but especially their deaths and legacies. As she became more comfortable, she began to bring in books, song lyrics, and internet clippings that meant a lot to her. Developmentally, preadolescent children who are aged eight to twelve years old have an understanding that death is final and irreversible (Himebauch, 2008). Children in this age group are more likely to intellectualise death, which can lead to a morbid curiosity and interest, as Jasmine presented in her own interests.

What was uncovered was that these historical events and people were also symbols of her relationship with her mother and maternal family. Not only did these represent her mother's interests, but each held their own themes of death, mourning, and longing. For example, her favourite book, *The Highway Man*, told the poetic narrative of separated lovers who were waiting to be reunited but tragically died before this could happen. At the end of the poem, the two lovers are reunited only by death. I was reminded of Jasmine being separated from her own mother several years before, as she was moved into care, and her hopes that, one day, she could live with her again—but death interfered.

Each of her fascinations were actually clues that brought her closer to her mother and to her own grief. Bowlby and Parkes describe yearning and searching as fundamental parts of grief and mourning (Bowlby & Parkes, 1970). During this time, the grieving person holds onto reminders of their loved one so as to fill the relational void that has been left behind. This is characterised by a deep longing, sadness, and anger. For Jasmine, I noticed how she was projecting those emotions into the stories that she was bringing.

One way that this took shape was during a session where she was energetically sharing her recent research on World War I, another favourite interest of hers. I asked Jasmine if she wanted to recreate it in the room. Her face immediately lit up as she stood up and began directing us in how to transform the therapy room into a World War I battleground. When the room was set up, she invited us to dress up as soldiers on opposing sides. We wore hard hats and used paintbrushes as weapons and blankets to set up our bunkers. We found a large, unused piece of wood and used this as our shelter. Before battle, Jasmine told us that we needed to write letters to our loved ones, which took up most of the time and space of our play. We narrated our letters to each other, and also voiced our thoughts as soldiers at war missing our families back home. Will we ever see them again? It felt as though together we were naming the questions that Jasmine herself had been left with over the last few years in foster care and again at the death of her mother. We then laid our heads to rest before going into battle, where neither of us won. Through projection and role play, we had begun to hold the energy of loss together. Despite being on different sides of the battle, I was witnessing her character's grief and she was witnessing mine.

Before the end of the session, I carved out considered time for us to tidy the room and de-role. I asked Jasmine what she was left with from the experience of our play. She was calm and engaged as she told me how much she had enjoyed the role. We had been in the trenches of yearning and searching, as our characters had sat in fear and longing. Somehow, we had managed to touch a deep place within the visceral feeling of grief, despite it being a place that Jasmine had shut down from when I had invited us to go there verbally. It displayed how "when we are with others, we cannot be broken" (Estes, 2008, p. 117).

The following week, Jasmine wanted to recreate the same play again. But as we began to set up our war zone, we discovered that the wooden board which had become our shelter was now somehow broken. Jasmine gasped and I observed how frantically she wanted to rescue it. She immersed back into play, as the wooden board turned into a person in need of help who she named Destiny.

Shifting us from soldiers in the trenches to a heroic surgeon and nurse, Jasmine's desperate attempt to piece Destiny back together filled me up with sadness and panic. Jasmine's demeanour became controlling as she ordered me to get materials, with little eye contact for anything but Destiny. She drew big, alert eyes on her with a nose and no mouth, eager to bring life back to her. It appeared unbearable for things to be broken and irreparable, and my mind went to her broken family and all that she had already lost. Her protest behaviour was willing Destiny to be alive and a communication of distress in the face of separation and loss (Bowlby & Robertson, 1952).

In reality, I could see Destiny could never be repaired, but supported Jasmine whilst she used glue, tape, and paint. Making my voice as gentle as I could, I said, "I don't think she's going to make it, Doctor." However, Jasmine became even more wishful, promising to throw a celebratory party for Destiny if she survived. Jasmine's bargaining and magical thinking appeared to be her response to grief, with the belief that she could reverse the loss (Nielson, 2012). In a powerful way, Jasmine was trying to control her "Destiny", and reverse the presence of loss in her life.

Jasmine was satisfied with the operation, but as soon as we lifted Destiny up, she fell apart again. I paused, observing Jasmine and experiencing a sensation of sadness and loss within my own body. Jasmine's voice softened when she eventually broke the silence. "She needs to have a funeral," she said. Jasmine's head was bent down and her energy appeared solemn. I detected her need for control had dropped, and now she seemed lost and fragile. I noticed this with Jasmine, and she told me she was really sad that Destiny was gone. Despair had arrived and Jasmine had reached a point where she had to accept that there was no going back and her Destiny had changed. This made space for hopelessness to exist. We were in mourning and the "unutterable misery" (Bowlby, 1980, p. 9). There was a long pause in the play, allowing space for us to observe and digest these feelings.

We moved into a funeral scene, standing by Destiny's departed body. I invited Jasmine to say any parting words. Instead, she improvised a song of mourning. She sang the following:

> "You were our shelter, you were our saviour, but the war took you in the end, we are going to miss you, we will always remember you, as long as you remember us too."

As she sang, I thought about the loss of her relationship with her mother, and even the loss of parts of herself. Our shelter had gone, but our relationship had survived the emotional turbulence of the unconscious material. Samuel names how "death steals the future we anticipated and hoped for, but it can't take away the relationship we had" (Samuel, 2018).

As shown in these sessions with Jasmine, the power of creative expression and play in therapy is multifaceted, impacting on her process and the therapeutic bond. Each step of the play brought Jasmine and me closer in relationship as we played out her emotional experiences. With me as her companion, she was able to travel through her experiences of vulnerability through metaphor. As further described by Malchiodi, "the arts provide a safe transitional space that allows the child to experiment until attaining integrity and control (Malchiodi, 2015, p. 122.)

This opened space for Jasmine to use metaphor to explore the multiple parts of her grief. In the power of metaphor and play, there had been despair, hope, fight, and acceptance embodied by the characters and their narratives. We had played out the unspeakable.

Bearing witness to collective grief and social injustice

Collective grief can be described as the effect of an extreme change or loss on a group, community, or nation. Events such as the death of Her Majesty the Queen, the Grenfell Tower fire, and the 9/11 terrorist attacks all led to grieving communities. This shared loss is heightened by the exposure of these events on the news and on social media, as well as how these stories of loss can trigger other experiences of trauma and grief we might have already been through. Collective grief can be particularly difficult when it centres around the loss of a public figure or person we do not know directly.

Children can be aware of the collective grief surrounding them, without the words to voice or make sense of it. In this case, this can instead show up in therapeutic play, which is what happened with my five-year-old client, Dylan. I met Dylan whilst working in a behavioural support setting for primary school children. He was of Black British Caribbean heritage, with a diagnosis of global developmental delay. Despite his physically and cognitively young age, Dylan had been excluded from his mainstream primary school after several suspensions due to displaying violent behaviour in the classroom. Dylan had family support around him, but his father was within the criminal justice system. He had some difficulties with his speech, finding it hard to express what he meant, and therefore play was an important part of his communication.

I worked with Dylan for nine months before he was transitioned back into mainstream school. During that time, there was a political incident in the global news. George Floyd, an African American man in Minneapolis, had been brutally killed by the police during a trip to the grocery store (Hill et al., 2020). This news of anti-Black racism and social injustice was widespread and spoken about in many communities around me, including at the setting where I worked with Dylan. I noticed teachers talking about it in the staffroom with rage, grief, and fear.

As a Black British woman, I had felt an ancestral heaviness from this collective grief. A wave of racial trauma responses had journeyed through me, from fight and flight to freeze and dissociation. Seeing the footage of an innocent Black man being murdered had not only wired my fears for myself and Black people in my life, but they also wired my intergenerational racial trauma. I was reminded of being Dylan's age and being aware of Stephen Lawrence, a young, innocent Black man in London killed for his racial identity. Though I was only young and couldn't make sense of the narrative, I believe this was my first realisation that being Black did not equate to being safe. According to racial identity development theory, Black and Brown children are mostly oblivious to their difference from dominant society due to having to conform to White norms, values, and behaviours (Helms, 1990). It is only through being confronted with critical incidents of racism, directly or indirectly, that there is an awakening to realising the inequalities in terms of race (Singh, 2019). As a child witnessing the injustice of Stephen Lawrence's murder, a dissonance occurred in my young mind as I became subconsciously aware that safety and privilege was not granted to me or people who looked like me. The loss of my right to safety as a person of colour is something I have had to re-grieve throughout my life.

During this time, Dylan's play changed in the therapy room. Usually, we would move from corner to corner of the room, playing with different materials. But this particular week, he moved straight to a costume box dedicated to police attire. He looked through the plastic handcuffs, police badge, and police hat, before handing it over to me.

"You be police, you have to catch me," he smiled.

"Oh, I have to catch you? Okay. What happened?" I asked.

"Ummm, I'm a robber." Dylan directed the story. He was going to steal a toy and my role as the police was to tell him to stop and put his hands up and then I would have to shoot him. When he instructed this, I felt a lump in my throat. Knowing the context of what was so loud in the news that week, the storyline of this play had a different heaviness with it. Knowing the full reality of what was happening, I found myself wanting to resist the role of identifying with the aggressor (Klein, 1946, p. 102). I allowed myself to bear this, whilst quietly wondering what might be going on for Dylan.

The story played out, and Dylan dramatically dropped onto the floor in the most theatrical death. But just a second later, he sat up and said, "Not really, I'm not dead. Your turn!" He didn't allow us to sit with his character's death, and I wondered if this felt uncomfortably vulnerable for him or whether his young mind was unable to grasp the permanence of death. For pre-school children aged two to six years old, death is seen as reversible, temporary, and within their egocentric sense of control (Himebauch, 2008).

As he requested, we switched roles, and he became the police and I became the robber. My unease did not shift, but I felt myself being guided by the play. Surprisingly, when I died, Dylan announced that I was dead and fell into hysterical laughter. His laughter went on and on as he bent double, holding his stomach. The sound of his laugh felt uncomfortable and unfamiliar, and I wondered whether this was his false self in action, masking something more vulnerable and anxious (Winnicott, 1960, p. 144).

Dylan then demanded that we repeat this story again and again in these roles, and so we repeated it in a loop. For the first few times when I was killed, Dylan would continue to laugh. But eventually, his response shifted. He picked up the toy medical kit and brought it over to me as I lay on the ground. Compassionately, he began to use the stethoscope to listen to my pulse and looked through the ear scope. He gave me medicine and bandages. He then patted my shoulder and told me that I'm okay now. He had found a position in the story which felt most accessible for him to witness and help make sense of the narrative. I was curious as to whether he was projecting the themes of what was happening globally into the safe space of our therapy room for him to piece together his thoughts and questions. As his role changed and developed from an authority figure to a caretaker, I found myself thinking about the care that was needed in the community around him in their collective grief.

Being a child who found communication difficult, Dylan was able to use role play and me as a co-actor to tell the story of something he didn't have words for. He didn't return to that play again; however, my work on the collective grief around him continued. As Dylan had showed me, there needed to be more space to heal and grow systemically. I began to work with the teachers in the school to provide them a space to reflect and grieve. This felt important, especially within a school with a high proportion of primary-aged Black boys who had already been rejected by society in being suspended from mainstream schooling. The school staff were deeply affected by the social injustice which had occurred, and held great fears for the young boys they taught, who would grow up to eventually be Black men like George Floyd and Stephen Lawrence. We opened space for them to grieve, so that they could open space for their pupils to do the same in an appropriate way.

Bearing witness to the end of therapy

> *"When you need me, but do not want me, then I must stay. When you want me, but no longer need me, then I have to go."*
> —Nanny McPhee

One of the most important moments in therapy with children and young people is the ending of therapy. After creating a trusting and safe relationship between therapist and child where powerful and unique material has had the opportunity to breathe, it can be difficult to begin the work of saying goodbye. For many children who have experienced loss and grief, endings in therapy have their roots within these losses and can resurface feelings which the therapist must be aware of. For this reason, I believe the therapist has an ethical responsibility to prepare and collaboratively work through the ending with the client. Goodbyes in therapy can be a final source of nurture for the client to take with them into the next stage of their life and can repair some of the processes left behind from abrupt and messy endings. And providing the child with a good enough ending now will support the possibility for them to seek therapy again later on in their lives.

Endings in therapy are most articulated within psychoanalytical thought, comparing the process to separation in early childhood. Margot Waddell explores how the first experience of separation is birth, where the infant is cut off from the warmth, nourishment, and company of the womb (Waddell, 1998). When he is left alone and away from the womb the first time, the infant is consumed with the fear of dying. These feelings of terror and panic are replicated later on in child development. Melanie Klein describes how the infant loses his attachment to the mother's breast during weaning and begins to mourn the feelings of love, goodness, and safety that came with it (Klein, 1940). Known as the depressive position, the infant is consumed with guilt and sorrow, believing he may lose the goodness of the mother forever (Klein, 1935, p. 145).

Bringing this back to the therapeutic bond, these pre-verbal memories of the difficulties of separation are replayed in the ending of therapy. As stated:

> The central emotional tasks are those of weaning and separation, ones which will be forever internally worked and re-worked, whether in life generally or, for some, in the particular setting of the consulting room. (Waddell, 1998, pp. 61–62)

Thus, the therapeutic bond becomes a vessel for past experiences of grief. Since endings are positioned between past and future, it brings with it ambivalent feelings of hope, regret, accomplishment, disappointment, loss, and gain (Holmes, 1997). Adding on to this, endings are paradoxical, whereby the client has to be held in mind by the therapist whilst also being appropriately let go (Lanyado, 2004).

To support the child for the afterlife of therapy, it is important to support them in making sense and meaning of the presence and absence of the therapeutic bond. For Klein's guilt-stricken infant, he gains the impulse to repair his relationship with the mother, turning inwards to create a version of the mother within him. This process of internalisation is defined by Klein as:

> The baby, having incorporated his parents, feels them to be live people inside his body in the concrete way in which deep unconscious phantasies are experienced—they are, in his mind, "internal" or "inner" objects. (Klein, 1940, p. 127)

What Klein describes here is an internal representation of the parent, which they can return to when needing an internal source of love, warmth, and company. Such ideas are supported by the concept of the capacity to be alone, where, through internalising a good relationship even after it ceases to exist, maturity and sufficiency of living can be reached (Winnicott, 1958, p. 417). As a result, these internal good objects are within the individual's inner world and are available for projection at suitable times. These same processes occur in therapy as it draws to a close and the child takes with them the experiences that came from the psychological safety and therapeutic bond with the therapist. With a considered process of ending, the client will be left with "a remembered voice of compassionate understanding and as an internal presence backing her up" (DeYoung, 2015, p. 165).

In preparing my client for closing our therapeutic bond, my role is to first bring awareness and clarity about our ending. As we do this, we explore and make sense of the accompanying emotions that are brought into the room, observing conflicts which may concur. Next, I invite the client to gain some control over the process of ending by inviting them to reflect on the therapeutic process. By reflecting on "the experience of therapy and to contemplate how it feels to lose the relationship with the therapist", the therapist is able to avoid the client's reactive behavioural patterns towards separation (Lanyado, 2004, p. 127). Having a space to reflect and think about ending will give the client a new meaning to ending. Lastly, ending therapy with children and young people can be uniquely difficult due to the nature of the therapy and its longevity being determined by external factors, leaving the child and therapist with less control over when the sessions end. Therefore, I must be aware of my own feelings in ending with the client to avoid colluding with the client's own resistances to closing. In all of this, I am weaning the client by encouraging a gentle separation, clarifying our individual identities through reflections on the therapy and the ending. In demonstrating these priorities, I will discuss my work with fourteen-year-old Lucia.

Lucia was of Spanish heritage, and her maternal grandmother had been her primary carer until she suddenly died when Lucia was four years old. Since then, Lucia and her family had moved from country to country every couple of years due to her father's job. This was a difficult pattern for Lucia, who had difficulty in maintaining relationships with her peers, as she was always fearful of how long she would get to stay in one place. However, her parents reassured me that they would not be moving again, at least until Lucia finished secondary school. This would be the longest period that she would stay in one school.

Her referral came as a result of her low mood, anxiety, and difficulty maintaining friendships. We were contracted to work with each other for just a year, which was spoken about in our therapy agreement. Because of this, from the beginning of our therapeutic bond, Lucia viewed our ending as a threat. This arose within her her biggest dilemma: how much can she trust and share with me if I'm going to leave her eventually? Such a dilemma was understandable with the amount of disruption she had experienced. Additionally, her transitions had impacted on her sense of cultural identity, as she was forced to adapt to new cultures and language with each move.

Assessing Lucia's preoccupied fears of abandonment, a way of supporting her was to embrace thinking about the ending from the start (Holmes, 1997). To prepare her, I named our ending several times throughout our time together, and school breaks became our dress rehearsals, an opportunity to explore the absence of our sessions. During these moments, I would ask Lucia about our comings and goings in the therapeutic relationship, and what goodbyes had been like for her when she was younger. She began to talk about some of her early experiences of bereavement, such as the friends she had made. Though she and her family had left those places and people, she described it as being that her friends had abandoned her. I was curious about this, leading her to share how she wrote letters to her friends, but they never replied back. She felt forgotten. Tears streamed down her face as she voiced her early experience of loss, now having the words and safety to explore it. Seeing loneliness as the biggest threat in her life, Lucia believed having her grandmother present and available would have changed everything. Just as Klein explored in her idea of the depressive position, Lucia was in a place of guilt and sorrow in losing a maternal figure and source of goodness forever (Klein, 1935, p. 145).

As she shared this with me, I found myself feeling remorseful, picking up on the blame she was projecting onto her friends. Furthermore, I felt culpable for being another person who was transiently present in her life, before leaving her alone again. Her continuous disappointment in relationships made me feel like I was a disappointing object, and I wondered whether this was how she felt about herself as someone who was always left behind. Within early years of development, the emotional availability and presence of the caregiver is crucial for the baby's emotional security (Emde, 1988). My thoughts took me to the loss of Lucia's maternal grandmother as a primary object, and the impact this may have had on Lucia's own mother, and whether she was a disappointing object for Lucia in toddlerhood. With loss in the environment of her infancy, she would have grown up knowing that things were not as good as they might be (Murdin, 2015). By encouraging Lucia to reflect on what life "could have been", she was able to reflect on some of this disappointment. Moreover, a new experience of ending was forming for her, where the ending and experience of endings could be thought about and verbalised, varying from past experiences (Lanyado, 2004). Furthermore, I thought of my role as the "passing stranger" who "pushes us through the channel to the step", validating how I could support her in the ending (Estes, 2008, p. 184).

To support Lucia's separation from therapy, we prepared a calendar together detailing a twelve-week countdown until our last session. Lucia had chosen to do this though drawing twelve circles, each titled with the date of our remaining sessions. Then each week, she would draw a picture within that dated circle, bringing the future of the ending into the present moment. This is a practice which has followed me into all of my therapeutic endings, as it provides the client with a physical representation that can be seen and thought of. By facilitating an arena for experiencing the ending and its processes, therapists are allowing their clients to progress through the conscious and unconscious levels of mourning (French, 2012).

In the third session before the ending, Lucia drew an angry dragon on our calendar. Remaining in the metaphor, I tenderly asked Lucia about the dragon and its anger. Anger is "a natural reaction to the unfairness of loss" (Kessler & Kübler-Ross, 2005, p. 16), and I wanted to facilitate Lucia's connection with it without judging or forcing meaning out of it. She described how the dragon was angry at someone he liked and so was felt unable to show his anger. When I asked how the dragon would show his anger if he could, she told me "he wants to turn his back, slam the door, and never come back again." She voiced that he felt out of control and paralysed. I verbally empathised with the dragon's overwhelming and stuck feelings, which gave Lucia an invitation to slip out of the metaphor. Adolescent children, who have a more adult concept of death (Himebauch, 2008), are more able to think abstractly and existentially than younger children. With this in mind, Lucia and I were able to dip into the metaphor and dip out for deeper reflection together. In talking about life after therapy, she communicated her experience of lonely nights, numbness, and fears about her impulses to self-harm. And though she explained her inability to cry, in the here and now her eyes were becoming glossy.

As she spilled out her feelings of despair and fear, I felt moved. Within my own body, I felt growing warmth of compassion and tenderness building up within me, and my own eyes grew wet. She saw this, and tears began to fall from her cheeks, as though they now had consent.

By engaging the shadow of the angry dragon that week, it was given permission to be embodied for the penultimate session, which Lucia had forgotten to attend. As previously agreed in our contract, if she ever forgot, I went to her class to find her. She came when she saw me, but Lucia walked in silence as we walked down the corridor together. As we walked to the therapy room, she ignored me to walk with friends with her back turned to me. I felt rejected and lost, sheepishly following her. I was reminded of the dragon, who so angrily wanted to turn its back on the person he liked. Murdin describes how lateness is the client's way of attacking the therapist's parental authority on time (Murdin, 2015).

In the room, Lucia sat down, and the room went silent. After a moment, she let out a loud sigh. "I don't want to talk today, but it's too quiet in here, so you have to do the talking," she said. Lucia voiced how she did not want to talk today, yet when silence fell, she requested that I fill it. We explored Lucia's resistance: she didn't want to come today and she didn't want to come for the ending. Her self-protection against the goodbye was to avoid it, yet despite this, she had come into the room with me. Though her words and responses to me communicated her frustration and anger, her presence and attendance showed her longing to break an unconscious pattern.

In the final session, we reflected on the experiences of coming into the therapy and saying goodbye: the safety, humour, and validation but also the awkward, fearful, and lonely parts too. Articulating my own gratitude to Lucia in all that she had shared of herself in our process together, I told her I would always remember her. She received this with watering eyes, before declaring, "I'm not going to cry today." Instead, she moved over to the doll's house, which she had never done before and previously rejected as "childish". After restructuring the furniture, she picked out two small figures: a small baby and an elderly woman. Silently and carefully, she placed them in the living room of the dollhouse. First, she placed the elderly woman on a sofa, and then the small baby on her lap. Lucia then closed the doll's house, ready for us to say our goodbye.

This closing image of Lucia's doll's house reflected so much on her journey towards ending. I thought of the grandmother that she had grown up with and lost, and the child within her that was left behind. She had left a part of her loneliness and despair there to be held within the safe and structured innocence of the doll's house. It was a space for me to continue to take care of the lost and vulnerable baby. Additionally, as Lucia would move further into adolescence in the afterlife of our sessions, I wondered if she had left behind a part of her childhood which she had been mourning. Lucia's fears had shifted in the final weeks as she felt more able to be tender to her solitude. Noticing this reminded me of how we are more able to tolerate aloneness once we feel truly understood (Holmes, 1997).

Conclusion

Whilst finding the words to explore and make sense of their emotions can be difficult, play and metaphor have proven to be helpful tools in supporting children and young people with grief. At each developmental age, creative projection and role play can be accessed to reach material which is otherwise not verbalised. We have seen this in the way that

Jasmine was able to give a funeral to Destiny in the way that she wasn't able to plan a funeral or say goodbye to her mother. We also journeyed through as Dylan repetitively played out a narrative of injustice and fear, which I held in the room for him and outside the room for the community around him. And finally, we observed this as Lucia transitioned out of therapy with me, whilst also re-grieving the loss of her grandmother and previous chapters in her life.

Each narrative of loss has been unique. Yet at the heart of it is the need to have that grief worked through alongside a compassionate and reflective witness who can hold what might be beneath the surface of play.

References

Axline, V. M. (1947). *Play Therapy: The Inner Dynamics of Childhood.* New York: Houghton Mifflin.

Bowlby, J. (1980). *Attachment and Loss, Vol. 3: Loss, Sadness and Depression.* New York: Basic Books.

Bowlby, J., & Parkes, C. (1970). Separation and loss within the family. In: E. J. Anthony (Ed.), *The Child in His Family* (pp. 197–216). New York: Wiley.

Bowlby, J., & Robertson, J. (1952). A two-year-old goes to hospital. *Proceedings of the Royal Society of Medicine, 46*: 425–427.

De Young, P. A. (2015). *Relational Psychotherapy: A Primer.* Hove, UK: Routledge.

Emde, R. N. (1988). Introduction: Reflections on mothering and on re-experiencing the early relationship experience. *Infant Mental Health Journal, 9*: 4–9. https://doi.org/10.1002/1097-0355(198821)9:1<4::AID-IMHJ2280090103>3.0.CO;2-J (last accessed 17 December 2022).

Estes, C. P. (2008). *Women Who Run with the Wolves.* London: Rider.

Fiorini, J. J., & Mullen, J. A. (2006a). *Counseling Children and Adolescents Through Grief and Loss.* Champaign, IL: Research Press.

Fiorini, J. J., & Mullen, J. A. (2006b). Understanding grief and loss in children. *Vista.* Retrieved 25 November 2022, from https://www.counseling.org/docs/default-source/vistas/understanding-grief-and-loss-in-children.pdf?sfvrsn=9dd7e2c_10 (last accessed 19 December 2022).

French, L. (2012). *Therapeutic Practice in Schools.* Hove, UK: Routledge.

Helms, J. (1990). *Black and White Racial Identity: Theory, Research, and Practice*. New York: Greenwood Press.

Hill, E., Tiefenthäler, A., Triebert, C., Jordan, D., Willis, H., & Stein, R. (31 May 2020). How George Floyd was killed in police custody. *New York Times*. https://www.nytimes.com/2020/05/31/us/george-floyd-investigation.html (last accessed 16 December 2022).

Himebauch, A., Arnold, R. M., & May, C. (2008). Grief in children and developmental concepts of death. *Journal of Palliative Medicine*, 11(2): 242–243.

Holmes, J. (1997). Too early, too late: Endings in psychotherapy. *British Journal of Psychotherapy*, 14: 159–171. https://doi.org/10.1111/j.1752-0118.1997.tb00367.x (last accessed 22 May 2022).

Kessler, D. (2019). *Finding Meaning: The Sixth Stage of Grief*. London: Ebury.

Kessler, D., & Kübler-Ross, E. (2005). *On Grief and Grieving*. London: Simon & Schuster.

Klein, M. (1935). A contribution to the psychogenesis of manic-depressive states. *International Journal of Psychoanalysis*, 16: 145–174. https://www.sas.upenn.edu/~cavitch/pdf-library/Klein_Contribution.pdf (last accessed 1 June 2022).

Klein, M. (1940). Mourning and its relation to manic-depressive states. *International Journal of Psychoanalysis* 21: 125–153.

Klein, M. (1946). Notes on some schizoid mechanisms. *International Journal of Psychoanalysis*, 27: 99–110.

Kübler-Ross, E. (1969). *On Death and Dying*. London: Routledge.

Lanyado, M. (2004). *The Presence of the Therapist*. Hove, UK: Routledge.

Malchiodi, C. (2015). *Creative Interventions with Traumatised Children*. New York: New York Press.

McCarthy, D. (2007). *If You Turned into a Monster: Transformation Through Play: A Body-centred approach to Play Therapy*. London: Jessica Kingsley.

Murdin, L. (2015). *Managing Difficult Endings in Psychotherapy: It's Time*. London: Karnac.

Nanny McPhee. (2005). Film directed by Kirk Jones. Universal Pictures.

Nielson, D. (2012). Discussing death with paediatric patients: Implications for nurses. *Journal of Paediatric Nursing*, 27(5): 59–64.

Samuel, J. (2018). *Grief Works: Stories of Life, Death and Surviving*. London: Penguin.

Singh, A. A. (2019). *The Racial Healing Workbook*. Oakland, CA: New Harbinger.

Stroebe, M., & Schut, H. (1999). The dual process model of coping with bereavement: Rationale and description. *Death Studies*, *23*(3): 197–224. https://doi.org/10.1080/074811899201046 (last accessed 1 June 2022).

Waddell, M. (1998). *Inside Lives: Psychoanalysis and the Growth of the Personality*. London: Karnac.

Winnicott, D. W. (1958). The capacity to be alone. *International Journal of Psychoanalysis*, *39*(5): 416–420.

Winnicott, D. W. (1960). Ego distortion in terms of true and false self. In: *The Maturational Process and the Facilitating Environment: Studies in the Theory of Emotional Development* (pp. 140–57). New York: International Universities Press.

Part III

Neurodivergence and differently wired brains

CHAPTER 9

Working therapeutically with uniquely wired children

Sasha Morphitis

Ryan was a warrior
Fighting was his game
He had no words till he was 5
And hated things to change
But change they did, again and yet again,
He moved house and city, changed his school
They even changed his name.

Ryan was frustrated
Being "taught" he could not bear
"Do this", "do that" the people said
But rules just were not fair
Not one rule made sense to him
As no one said the reason
He might as well use his fists
He knew he'd never please them.

Ryan had a temper,
It sparked from a demand

> *"Look at me" "go there", "stop that", "no more"*
> *He must be in command*
> *Inside he felt so anxious, scared and so confused*
> *"Does PDA even exist?" The adults were bemused.*
>
> Sasha Morphitis

I have always found myself drawn to working with children with challenging (or atypical) behaviour, children who struggle in the mainstream education system, who find it hard to cope with relationships, who seem hard to reach and easily dysregulated. These children are often misunderstood. The way they behave, present, and exist in the world is often perceived as problematic. I have had the fortune of getting to know many neurodiverse children (and adults). They are all unique but have collectively taught me that if afforded a supportive environment to thrive and understand themselves, they shine as bright as stars.

A past student attending a workshop I led on working therapeutically with autistic clients questioned the whole purpose of the workshop. "Just because someone is autistic doesn't mean they need therapy necessarily." A true statement indeed, and I would like to be clear about the distinction surrounding my work and interest. I do not share the skills or intentions of a behaviour therapist seeking to change the external presentation or turn the differences into seemingly more socially acceptable versions of their neurodivergent selves. In that regard, my approach with autism spectrum disorder (ASD), attention deficit hyperactivity disorder (ADHD), or other presenting neuro-differences can seem, in some ways, no different to therapy with neurotypical counterparts.

The therapeutic stance I take encompasses acceptance and understanding (and helping others to understand) the individual child's ways of being in the world. For me, the therapy is not about correcting the autism but about being curious about the internal emotional landscape and individual sensory and communication differences. Helping the child to find the "self" as well as celebrating strengths within the child's differences, therapy can also include supporting challenges such as emotional/sensory dysregulation, gaps in development, and difficulties relating to and communicating with others.

I have gone on to further my training in DIR Floortime—"Developmental, individual-difference, relationship-based (DIR) model ... referred to as the 'Floortime' approach" (Greenspan & Wieder,

2006, p. x)—so that I can support children with neurodevelopmental conditions more effectively as a psychotherapist. DIR is a model created specifically as a treatment for children who are not developing along a typical trajectory, that is, children with speech or developmental delays and social communication challenges, such as autism spectrum condition. The goal of this model is to support children:

> To master critical abilities missed or derailed along their developmental path, namely, the ability to relate to others with warmth and pleasure, communicate purposefully and meaningfully…and to varying degrees, think logically and creatively. (Greenspan & Wieder, 2006, p. xi)

I will focus on a few common themes in my lived work experience by sharing two case studies. The first highlights aspects of a therapeutic journey of an autistic adolescent. I will discuss what relational aspects support the therapy and share some theories informing my practice. The second case is an autistic, preschool child with developmental challenges. I share how I work dyadically with a parent and child, with the integration of a DIR approach.

Case study: Poppy, eighteen

An email arrives in my inbox from a concerned mother requesting "Therapy for my daughter". In the short message, I sense both desperation and ambivalence towards seeking help. "My daughter, Poppy, eighteen, has been suffering with her mental health for some time, has recently been diagnosed with ASD. She has finished school, has made no future plans, does not eat, barely leaves her room … I don't know what to do to help her. I think she may need a few sessions of therapy." After a quick phone call, we arrange to meet on Zoom for a parent assessment, which she agrees that both she and her husband will attend.

It is not uncommon that parents seek help for their child in adulthood or late adolescence, particularly when their child has a neurodevelopmental condition. This can be due, in part, to only seeking support once their child has reached crisis, which can become exacerbated and more apparent at transitional ages, such as leaving school. Often the individual's chronological age is mismatched to their developmental age, which has nothing to do with intelligence or academic ability. They can seem and behave younger in some capacities, such as social skills or self-care. Often, there is a sense that the individual themselves feels they cannot cope with adult responsibilities, and they need more help than their neurotypical (NT) peers to become independent, struggling to live up to the socially accepted norms and expectations of age. This is particularly true if they have not received any support until now, with executive functioning skills such as self-organisation and time management.

Sometimes this discrepancy can come from either the parent's desire for the child to reach independence before they are ready, or, conversely (and often due to parental anxiety), infantilising the child. It is hard for parents to get the balance right between supporting capacities and supporting self-agency. If parents are referring their child, who is chronologically no longer in childhood, I like to remain curious about this. Is there a discrepancy between chronological and developmental age? Which aspects of development are younger and why? Which have been missed or derailed? Where is this perspective coming from: the client or the parent? For example, is it a parental perspective, infantilising their neurodevelopmentally different child, or do parents yearn for their child to "act their age", functioning at higher capacities than the individual feels capable of, or are there genuine deficits viewed by both parent and adult child?

> On Zoom, the parents are on time, seated side by side at their dining room table with a bookshelf full of books behind them. They present as smart, tidy, academic, and a little ill-at-ease with the forewarned personal nature of this meeting.
>
> I attempt to put them at ease, thanking them both for attending and naming how strange it might feel to divulge personal information to a stranger, assuring them it is both common practice and will support the therapy. I also explain that the information they share will help me understand more, I am not here to judge, and they are perfectly within their right not to answer any question that feels uncomfortable.

I often work with parents and certainly always meet with them. I always approach this work with compassion and acceptance, holding in mind that most parents do their best in their own given circumstances.

Approaching with curiosity and understanding is more effective support for the child than judgement and blame.

> On enquiring about their family cultural heritage, mum explains they are "British-Asian". They were both born in Jaipur, in Rajasthan, to observing Hindu families. Father's family moved to England in 1980, and he was entirely educated in England. Mother grew up speaking mostly English and Hindi; she moved to England to study at university. She is now an academic and lecturer. Father is in finance, and they had met through family connections shortly after university and were married within three months of meeting.

Given that my future client is a person of colour, racism is an important factor in a family member's life experiences. I do not wish to diminish the importance and therapeutic relevance of the complex issue of race and racism by not focusing on this aspect of the client's intersectionality. The way one is treated and perceived by others, and then how those perceptions are interjected, adds a context to self-understanding and self-identity that is always part of the therapeutic dialogue. However, this case study for this chapter focuses mostly on neuro-difference and how that affects the therapeutic relationship.

> Poppy has an older brother, gifted in technology, head boy at school, involved in many extra-curricular activities and a wide social group. The parents are bemused at how different their two children are and describe how Poppy seems like a child from a different family.

A diagnosis, such as ASD, ADHD, or pathological demand avoidance (PDA), should not define a child. They are terms that often instil confusion, stereotyping, and even stigma and shame in wider society, resulting in parents occasionally avoiding diagnosis and denying challenges until (and only if) their child reaches crisis point. Autism and other neurodivergence often run in families. "Well, I got by and there is nothing wrong with me," can be the defensive presentation of parents who had to survive without support. It can be too painful to witness your child struggle in similar ways.

Within my work, I am regularly confronted by the human struggle in the face of difference. Many clients I have worked with experience punishment, bullying, social anxiety, the idea they are "not normal", "weird", "lazy", "difficult", or just "badly behaved". In a neurotypical world, a one-size-fits-all approach within the education system confirms the negative bias towards difference. School behaviour policies, assessment processes, class sizes, and even what and how children are expected to learn within the mainstream education system do not support educators to provide an environment where all children can thrive. In my experience, many schools do not question their approach, which largely focuses on the management of children's behaviour with rewards or sanctions. Behaviour is something to be disciplined and controlled, rather than a communication of an internal experience.

> Children's (and our own) behaviours are an outward reflection of the complex workings of the brain-body connection, their platform. When we stop to consider what their behaviours are telling us about their platform, we have our first clue for building resilience. (Delahooke, 2022, p. 31)

Being on the autism spectrum (or having any other difference) should not equate to being less than, bad, wrong, or broken, and yet this is often the self-perception of many neurodivergent individuals. From the earliest age, children introject this negative valuing of themselves and it becomes their sense of self. Developing self-esteem is derailed, and psychological damage has been caused.

> Expectations of other people and how they will behave are inscribed in the brain, outside conscious awareness, in the period of infancy, and they underpin our behaviour in relationships throughout life. (Gerhardt, 2004, p. 24)

The parents describe Poppy's early years as quiet but troubled. She spoke late and only when necessary. She never settled in environments away from home, struggled to maintain friendships, and seemed compliant and aloof. Mum remembers that Poppy had a "transitional object" (Winnicott, 1953, pp. 89–97), a rag doll with a fixed-smile expression, which would go everywhere with her. It was not allowed to be washed, replaced, or taken off her. (If it was, she would become nonverbal, scream, cry, and hyperventilate until she struggled to breath; occasionally she passed out.) She carried it from the ages of three till eight, until it smelt, the smile had worn away, and Poppy became worried it was contaminated with germs. At eight, she discarded the doll and transferred her affections to a piece of rag, which she could hide in her pocket or bag. Dad chipped in with, "She did used to have friends, but it would only be one person at a time."

In my experience, it is common for an autistic child to continue a relationship with a transitional object for longer than their neurotypical peers. It can be an object that helps the child feel safer when outside the home: a form of self-regulation and comfort for an autistic child who continues to feel easily overwhelmed. It can also act as a social mediator with peers, something to "break the ice" with social interactions, having an object to talk about. It can even be due to relating more to the object, comforted by its predictability, unlike other children. Depending on the environment, the specific object, and the age of the child, it can also be a target of mockery.

At secondary school, things had gone downhill for Poppy. Parents describe how she had become socially isolated. They encouraged her to join drama, sports, and other groups, but gave up when leaving the house would end in screaming rows and panic attacks. By fifteen, Poppy was refusing to eat with the family and started losing weight, which caused much embarrassment to the parents and wider family. Poppy had become a problem. She cut her own hair very short, refusing to wear a sari or anything feminine. As the mother described this behaviour, she shifted uncomfortably in her seat and looked down, avoiding my gaze. She continued explaining that at sixteen, Poppy was diagnosed with an eating disorder and depression. CAMHS was suggested, but the mother explained in a tiny and matter-of-fact voice, that "it would have brought shame on their family". By eighteen, after a bout of ineffective anti-depressants, she was diagnosed with autism.

During this Zoom meeting, the father was quiet, saying little other than a few disapproving comments.

An additional external obstacle for the autistic individual is the fear of autism and difference within the family system, which is often difficult to navigate. Many cultures deem learning differences as a source of shame: something to hide, to not speak openly about in case of being ostracised by their community. The cost to the child, unless this perspective is compassionately challenged, is huge, and when autistic traits are misunderstood and left unsupported, the cost is increased by the serious mental health conditions that may result.

> Late-diagnosed autistic children often have high levels of mental health and social difficulties prior to their autism diagnosis and tend to develop even more severe problems as they enter adolescence. (Mandy et al., 2022)

The parents both admit that they have no understanding of ASD (nor depression or eating disorders) and have not talked openly with Poppy about any of these subjects. It becomes clear that their style of parenting has been to continue as if there are no challenges. They explain how, when Poppy is difficult, they get angry and sometimes punish her, by taking away her phone and sending her to her room. The father makes a comment about it having been easier when she was young, as she would just get a smack if she didn't listen. Hearing some of their own difficult experiences as children and how they were parented helps me to adopt a quiet, unspoken understanding of their defensive position.

I ask what they hope Poppy will get out of embarking on therapy. Dad says, "I would like for her to feel like a normal, happy girl." Mum says, "I would like her to work on her ASD, to join our family meals, and take part in life more." She then asks how long it will take.

After explaining that therapy is not a quick fix and it can take time to feel differently, I reassure them that seeking support for their daughter is the most courageous and helpful thing they could be doing right now. After a few more questions, they seem nervous of the future, but happy to finance a possibly long-term process.

The first time I meet Poppy, I am struck by the contrast of how little physical space and how much psychological space she takes up (energetically, she has a heavy presence). I greet her at the door, welcoming her into the room. She almost whispers hello as she enters, looking all around, as if checking for danger. She has the appearance of a younger child, closer to fourteen than eighteen, slim frame, long limbs, short hair. It would be hard to assume her gender on first impression. Her movements are small, awkward, and staccato. She wears glasses, which appear oversized and slide down her face, rarely pushing them back to the bridge of her nose, possibly using them as a shield to hide her searching eyes.

As she sits on the edge of the chair, her wide-eyed yet flat expression alerts me to her hypervigilant state, I feel a rush of fear and anxiety, "reactive countertransference" (Clarkson, 2003, p. 90), which I imagine is exactly what Poppy is experiencing now. I begin with warmth and curiosity, expressing both my pleasure in meeting her and my desire to get to know her. I ask a few questions about how she is feeling and her thoughts on why she thinks she is here. These are met with shrugs and "I'm not sure", which becomes a common response in the initial sessions. I am suddenly aware of myself, my naturally fast pace, passionate expressions, and affective empathy. I lower and slow my voice down, and name that I can see how difficult this is for her.

> Sometimes the fear that a client brings into therapy is an overall dread of interpersonal connection. Genuine connection is a powerful threat, for it makes him feel unbearably vulnerable. (DeYoung, 2015, p. 59)

For Poppy to experience relational safety, she initially needs to protect her identity from me. Getting to know her is an elusive experience. I am aware of the dance we are in: I move towards her with words or curiosity, she moves away. It is all too much. Poppy feeling seen is possibly such a foreign experience that it may overwhelm her if there is too much, too soon.

I attune to Poppy's physical expressions of dysregulation by noticing her movements, sensing in my body what I am feeling in response. "Attunement represents the sharing of affect intersubjectively, which leads to its co-regulation" (Hughes, 2011, p. 22). When her eye contact wanes and she looks down on the floor, or she starts to fiddle with her sleeves by rolling them up and down, I feel her shift into discomfort. I feel intrusive, so energetically step back. We are going to need to move at her slow pace instead of uncovering her defences too fast, too soon; by verbalising what I see in her, I aim to contain these feelings.

I recognise that to begin with, I am the threat, and no wonder, as relationships are possibly experienced by Poppy as dysregulating, critical, expectant, and/or confusing.

> If I can free him as completely as possible from external threat, then he can begin to experience and to deal with the internal feelings and conflicts which he finds threatening within himself. (Rogers, 1961, p. 54)

I attempt to adopt a quiet energy and gently mirror Poppy's physical position. "One person reflecting another's inner state" (Stern, 1998, p. 144). Silence seems equally threatening to Poppy. When it comes, she squirms in her seat, looks above my head, around the room, then searches my face as if looking expectantly to find the answers to what she should be doing or saying. I reassure by normalising her experience of discomfort empathically. "I think silence doesn't feel great to you. No wonder you feel uncomfortable, you don't know me yet." She nods and looks me straight in the eyes. I have seen her and now she wants to see me.

We play a game of questions; rolling a ball to each other, we take it in turns to ask and answer questions in order to get to know each other. We stick to facts about our likes and dislikes: "What is your favourite thing to do/eat/watch?", etc. I am happy to disclose these things about myself, as it helps us to build rapport and trust. We discover some differences and some similarities between us. We start each session with this game for a few weeks. I discover Poppy likes to talk about novels, cooking programmes, and recipes. Once on these subjects, her eyes sparkle, her speech quickens, and she is engaged. If I ask questions that may bring up emotions, for example "What makes you feel happy?", it is responded to with a small shrug and "I'm not sure." Facts are more comfortable than feelings.

When I ask her to choose two objects in the room that she likes and two she doesn't, she hesitates. When I suggest drawing, she asks me what colours she should use for her picture. I ask her what colours she would like to use: again, "I'm not sure." I sense she does not trust her own ideas and thoughts, seems frightened to voice opinions, possibly in case I judge her or disagree and abandon her. I respond with: "Sometimes, when I'm not sure, it's really that I'm worried I'm going to get it wrong." She looks at me with recognition and nods. I then ask her how she feels in her body when she is not sure. She freezes to the spot and her eyes glaze. "I think feelings can be scary sometimes, but I do a lot of asking about them, not to scare you, but because they help us understand ourselves better. They are useful messages."

Initially with clients on the spectrum, I aim to titrate (Heller & LaPierre, 2012, p. 205) naming their feelings, as often they are something they struggle to name and identify in themselves. With Poppy, I balance naming a few things I see in her with disclosing a few of my own feelings and intentions. My aim with self-disclosure relates to remaining congruent. Staying true to my own reality will encourage Poppy to accept her own reality (Rogers, 1961, p. 33). In addition, by modelling my own thoughts and intent, I am supporting Poppy to further develop her mentalizing capacity (Fonagy, Gergely, Jurist, & Target, 2004). Lastly, my self-disclosure meets her need for things to remain transparent and straightforward. I also attempt to empathically normalise a client's experience by hinting at the universality of it.

After a few weeks there is a shift. She seems physically more at ease. I can name things more directly and even name my own misattunements as a way of modelling that adults are not always right, can own mistakes, and that relationships can survive rupture. "I think my question was confusing for you, too fast, too many words. Can I start again?" We begin sessions in the same way each week (always discussing a recipe); the continuity and predictability are comforting. Poppy likes it if I disclose that I have watched the same cooking programmes. A few times she makes recommendations, which I diligently watch. I sense that the idea of being held in my mind outside of these sessions is a necessity for building rapport and trust. As well as the sense of agency she may develop, she has the feeling that "I can suggest something and Sasha will watch it; perhaps I am important enough to have opinions and things to recommend." I feel huge warmth and tenderness towards her. Not just when she is chatting, but also when frozen. I sense she can feel this, as I begin to receive more eye contact and willingness to share ideas. With this warmth, perhaps her shame is waning.

Acceptance of each fluctuating aspect of this person makes it for him a relationship of warmth and safety, and the safety of being liked and prized as a person seems a highly important element in a helping relationship. (Rogers, 1961, p. 34)

I suggest a sand-tray of Poppy's experience at school. Choosing objects to represent her peers, teachers, and herself is a useful vehicle in exploring feelings through projecting them onto something outside of herself and our relationship, a "third-space" (Lee, 2004) between us. It becomes clear that her experience of school, where she was bullied "for being weird and a tomboy", and of racial discrimination was traumatic. She can now bear my empathy. "Naming an experience brings sensations and emotions into consciousness" (Heller & La Pierre, 2012, p. 242).

She begins to recognise how her body reacts to overwhelming social situations and how, in the moment, she is almost outside of herself, dissociated, numb, an autonomic shutdown. She describes it as "being behind a thick sheet of cracked ice". Poppy recognises how from very early on, even as a young child, she spent much of her time in a "sympathetic nervous state". Another sand-tray uncovers a mobilised state she would automatically adopt when at home, sitting at the family dinner table, with all the noise and expectations to eat. It leads to a "meltdown" (rocking, crying, biting her fingers), or she runs to her room and crawls under her bed. Feeling full of food, or emotions, or even sensations, overwhelms her, and then she is behind the ice again.

There is a high prevalence of eating disorders within neurodivergent individuals (Nickel et al., 2019, p. 708). This can be related to the sensory system becoming overwhelmed by textures, smells, or tastes, and often is a coping mechanism, which, like self-harm, attempts to regulate the emotional overwhelm. With Poppy, there was the added ritualistic routine behaviour of weighing food and counting calories that helped her feel in charge of herself, creating a distraction from negative, intrusive thoughts about herself.

People can learn to control and change their behaviour, but only if they feel safe enough to experiment with new solutions … our priority is to help people move out of fight-flight states, reorganise their perception of danger, and manage relationships. (Van der Kolk, 2014, p. 349)

During one session, after asking Poppy how something her teacher said made her feel, I noticed she glazed over. I suggested we do a body scan, so she could tune into what was going on in her body in the present moment. Enough trust had built between us at this point for me to suggest it. By now, she would have refused if felt it too much. We drew around her body on a large, rolled-out piece of paper and put it to one side. I guided her through different parts of her body, inviting her to tune in to the sensations and, if possible, emotions. After the scan, I asked her to draw on her body on the piece of paper what she felt and where she felt it. Her body was full of expressive, colourful scribbles and her head just black clouds. She was not yet able to name emotions, but sensations were now available to be acknowledged.

In the coming months, after a year of therapy, Poppy becomes aware of her challenges with interoception, one of the less known senses (Kranowitz, 2005, p. 54). For example, her not feeling the glasses slipping on her nose, not noticing feeling hot or cold (wearing a jumper in summer even though she is sweating), and not recognising how she feels emotionally. She explores her senses through sensory play, allowing herself to revisit a stage of childhood where these opportunities had passed her by because she had stood on the sidelines watching others. She sinks herself into non-verbal play with materials she loves. She set her own challenge of creating a sensory box at home of objects to touch, smell, and sooth. We use a lot of body-work techniques, sensory play, breathing, meditation, self-holding, and helpful regulatory, self-stimming behaviour like rocking, tapping, and spinning. If we are talking for a while, I pause her and ask: "Can you tune in? What are you experiencing, where do you feel it?" She begins to build a clearer understanding of self, by first understanding her physical experiences and then by exploring some introjected trauma wounds.

> The more the child can be assisted to define herself, the stronger the self becomes and the more opportunity there is for healthful growth. (Oaklander, 2007, p. 28)

She begins to understand that she has introjected the sense that she is aloof, unfriendly, and unsociable, and masculine, non-feminine, even alien.

Her anxiety at being around others and her low self-worth are deeply rooted in her psyche, a reaction to previous relational experiences, at home, at school, and in the wider community of her family. She believes she is unable to socialise, but begins to understand more about her sensitive sensory and autonomic nervous systems and even possible unintended relational trauma.

Poppy's therapeutic journey lasted eighteen months. In some ways, it felt there were still so many areas to explore. However, she had courageously explored her vulnerabilities and ended up more aware of herself and with a raised self-esteem. She joined a cookery course and a book club and began to make some social connections through these passions. She started her own food blog and began to enjoy using different textured food to create original sensory dishes. She began to realise she had strengths which she was in control of utilising.

Floortime therapy

At the heart of much of my therapeutic work, particularly when working with younger children, is supporting the bond between parent and child. Part of the developmental individual-difference relationship-based (DIR) philosophy is that parents are the "play partners", the best therapeutic intervention a child can have. The "R" in DIR highlights the importance of relationships and how the child is related to. A parent's capacity to connect with their child in a non-invasive, supportive, and empathic way is deemed to be a cornerstone of the child's development. The idea that the main caregiver's "good-enough" (Winnicott, 1965, p. 146) attunement (Stern, 1998, p. 139) to their infant's needs, their containment and co-regulation (Gerhardt, 2004, p. 197) of discomfort, the provision of a safe, secure loving bond (Bowlby, 1988), is well-established in the world of child psychotherapy and therefore creates a happy integration with Floortime Practice.

DIR encourages the parents, through the support of the therapist, to not only look at the more systemic and relational issues at play but to have deeper curiosity into what is happening for the child in terms of their senses, their development, and their ways of thinking and communicating. It creates a framework for the practitioner to support the people in the child's external world to be observers of the child's internal world and therefore help to build on areas of development that have been missed or derailed; to see the "whole child", not just a generic list of deficits.

> Almost all human learning occurs in relationships … To bring about this learning, relationships must foster warmth, intimacy, and pleasure. The regulatory aspects of relationships (for example, protection of the child from over or under stimulation) help the child maintain pleasure in intimacy and a secure, alert, attentive state that permits new learning and development to occur. (Greenspan & Weider, 2006, p. 257)

Case study: Sara, three-and-a-half

Speaking to Sara's mother (Penny) on the phone for the first time felt like a familiar experience. All families bring different circumstances, but this conversation, like so many others before, gave a strong impression of a parental internal conflict: on one hand, huge love for their child and desperation to seek help that offers support and some answers; on the other, the grief experienced from having confirmation that their child is different and not what they had fantasised prior to conception. Another familiar theme in this conversation was a child parented by two individuals who in so many ways are not on the same page. Many families I meet have this struggle, but sometimes it can seem heightened when they are parenting a child that is wired uniquely.

I already know at this stage that the work going forward will be predominantly supporting the parents; helping them to understand that Floortime therapy is not about fixing their child and making the autism go away and that their child is a process that has nothing to do with a label or diagnosis. It has everything to do with discovering who the child truly is and encouraging them into relationships, through playful, meaningful, joyful, and reciprocal interactions. Floortime is no miracle cure, but with commitment and hard work from the parents, the rewards for them (connected, loving relationships with their child) are far-reaching. Sometimes, this means coaching the parents to parent in a completely different way to previously. This cannot be done without compassion and understanding of the parents' own journey and the recognition that they are often beginning from the position of feeling they are getting it all wrong and they are to blame.

My experience with many families is that when children are highly sensitive and/or have developmental trauma, parenting with authority and discipline is frustratingly ineffective. Working with foster parents confirmed to me that adopting a therapeutic parenting approach (Naish, 2018) avoiding conflict and focusing on co-regulation is most effective. It is also helpful to approach behaviour with "connection before correction" (Golding, 2015), which encourages positive relating as the backdrop to setting boundaries. Feeling valued, loved, and understood is essential for self-esteem to remain intact with emotionally dysregulated children.

Parents who seek a diagnosis are generally wanting to understand and find the right support for their child. However, unfortunately, the diagnosis does not translate into understanding their child or their specific individual differences. Therefore, much of my work focuses on supporting the environment (the external relationships) to support the child. As a therapist, I offer modelling and coaching and deep emotional holding, containment, and co-regulation; I am an observer and witness to the internal states of the child; and a translator, deciphering what the behaviour might be communicating about the individual differences and the functional emotional developmental capacities (FEDCs) (Greenspan & Wieder, 2006) and therefore the internal experiences. The child's thoughts, feelings, and sensations (psychological and physiological states) can then be understood, by the child themselves and by others. Interactions with others become emotionally meaningful to the child and therefore a source of joy and connection.

> Sara's father, Phillip, does not attend the parent consultation. According to Penny, he didn't believe there was anything "wrong" with Sara, and since the recent ASD diagnosis he has spent less time with the family and more time at work. I sense this is an area of conflict and possibly great sadness. I explain that Phillip can join the process at any point he feels open to it,

knowing that trying to entice him will possibly destabilise his strong defence of denial and may also mean that the work becomes more like couples therapy than Floortime practice. We agree to move forward with Penny alone receiving my support. The information I glean from this consultation is useful to understand some of Penny's main concerns: Sara does not speak, and Penny does not understand her behaviour. She has tried many things, from time-outs to sticker charts, but nothing works. Sara does not interact with other children, so Penny has stopped arranging play dates, as it causes too much shame. Sara has no bedtime routine, has big meltdowns at home, and when distressed has started to scratch her skin and hit or bang her head. She has a dummy, is not yet potty-trained, wants to be on the iPad as much as possible, and eats only five different foods.

Nursery observation

Sara has attended nursery three days a week since she was one-and-a-half, when her mother returned to work. The staff have known Sara for two years. Inside the classroom, she does not engage with others and flits from place to place picking up toys or objects with seemingly no intent to play nor any understanding of how to play with each object. She does not answer to her name and turns away if someone attempts to speak to her.

I notice Sara prefers to be outside. She runs up and down the outside space, her legs seem uncoordinated, running fast and out of control; she trips over a few children and crashes into the fence. She does this several times. It becomes apparent that this is a regular activity—one that Sara loves and the staff do not. A teacher comes out, with a stern voice says, "No Sara", takes her by the hand, and sits her on the time-out chair with a sand timer. Sara sits and stares off into the distance. A few children approach and stare. Sara responds by roaring at the children and tensing her fingertips towards them (as if she is a lion). When the sand runs out, Sara gets up and begins running towards the fence. The crash is big and shakes the fence, she turns, smiles, and runs back to begin again. The whistle blows and it is inside time again.

The children sit on the carpet; it is noisy. Sara hides under the teacher's table, flapping her hands, rocking, and looking out of the window. She seems distressed. "Rocking behaviours in autistic individuals may reflect a naturally occurring biobehavioural strategy to stimulate and to regulate a vagal system that is not efficiently functioning" (Porges, 2011, p. 223) The teacher puts on music and Sara emerges from under the table, jumps up and down and flicks her fingers. She seems to like the song.

Young autistic children do not develop typically. They struggle to understand what the behaviour, expressions, intentions, or actions of others mean. They also lack self-awareness/understanding. Williams explains that being autistic is less about being caught in a bubble of self and more about having no concrete perspective on what self is at all. The intense focus on sensations is due to feeling them as "foreign" (Williams, 1996, p. 14): therefore, they struggle to make emotional meaning from the world around them (Janert, 2000, p. 2). There is too much competing and confusing information, and this can lead to a turning away from relationship. Their focus is on gaining regulation, usually through sensory input, which often presents as self-stimulatory behaviours. Sara crashing against the fence is meeting a high need of proprioceptive input; the crash helps her feel where her body is in space, giving her regulatory feedback. To the outside eye, this behaviour can seem purposeless and/or destructive, but it is serving a need.

DIR Floortime practice asks us to look for clues about what the behaviour is communicating. What is difficult and needs regulating? Which senses are overwhelmed or underwhelmed? Until we understand the internal experience, the child will remain stuck in patterns of behaviour that serve as coping mechanisms, managing dysregulated psychological and physiological states.

Greenspan and Wieder talk of "individual differences" and "functional emotional developmental capacities", the former being individual ways of processing the world through the senses and the latter being where the child is developmentally: their capacity to engage, relate, join in, problem-solve, make links, think, and communicate.

The Floortime therapy

Before the first session, I explain that Floortime works best if parents are the play partners, meaning that part of my work will be coaching Penny on her interactions with Sara. Penny expresses mild disappointment that

I am not going to "do all the therapy". When we unpack this, we find that this need for me to magically fix her child without her involvement comes from a deep-rooted anxiety that she is a bad mother. I feel warmth and compassion for her; she has a harsh inner critic. We look deeper into these fears and this self-judgement of being inadequate. She is reflective and able to see from where these fears stem in her childhood and present life. She is reassured that we are going to be a partnership where we bring compassion and reflection rather than judgement and perfectionism. We will film parts of our sessions so that we can reflect after the therapy in a parent consultation on Zoom.

Parental grief around diagnosis or recognising developmental differences is often exacerbated by feeling unneeded, as the social cues of reciprocity are not returned from their infant.

> It appears that autism is associated with autonomic states that remove the individual from direct social contact by supporting the adaptive defensive strategies of mobilization (i.e., fight-or flight behaviours) or immobilization (i.e., shutdown). (Porges, 2011, p. 221)

The more the child is seen to be self-absorbed and not needing the parent, the more the parent can cut off, withdrawing from the child. If this is left unsupported and unnamed, it can feed into psychological defence mechanisms, which a child will subconsciously adopt in order to survive. It can lead to attachment difficulties. Helping parents to understand the internal states of their child can release them from self-blame. Understanding that reciprocity simply cannot be the chosen priority for their child, due to dealing with confusing and dysregulated internal states much of the time, is reassuring for parents who feel unwanted or superfluous.

> If a child avoids us, do we take it as a personal rejection and either shut down and stop trying or get too intrusive and try to force her to pay attention to us? Asking those difficult questions, we can then fine-tune our strategies to meet the child's special sensitivities and needs. (Greenspan & Weider, 2006)

The child does not necessarily enjoy or yearn for a life of solitude. Children with social communication challenges are not "anti-social"; many, as they grow, yearn for connection. In fact, particularly in infancy and early years, they need more social interaction than typical children, set at their pace in order to help gently entice them out of self-absorption and into reciprocal exchange. Using high affect, co-regulation, and non-verbal playfulness is a helpful place to start, encouraging the parent to not take it as rejection, but a message something is not right.

I see it as an important part of the triad between parent, therapist, and child that the parents' own internal world, sensory system, nervous system, and psychological defences need to be explored. It is a recommended assessment phase in DIR that not only the child's individual differences but the parent's and therapist's capacities be analysed in order to create a best-fit programme, considering all who are involved in the interactions. We cannot pour from an empty cup. We also cannot support a child to return to a regulated state if we, as adults, are dysregulated. This needs some sensitive exploring too and is always approached from a strengths-based perspective.

> I glean a lot of information about Sara's sensory profile during our first session. When Penny comes near her, Sara moves her head away. I notice Penny is wearing a strong perfume and make a mental note to discuss a possible smell sensitivity later. When there is a car horn outside, Sara freezes with a wince, and when there is a small sound (like the fridge humming), Sara notices it and looks towards the sound, moving only her eyes rather than her head, side-glancing. I sense there is overwhelm with sights, sounds, and smells.
>
> Sara changes activities from running into the soft furniture, crashing two objects together (cars or animal objects), and lying on the carpet staring out of the window, while stamping her feet on the floor. She does these alone, and repeats them all, as if I and her mother are not there. It gives the impression of needing to frequent her own personal universe, where no one else exists, except when she has a need to be met, which occurs rarely. She needs to remain autonomous and has an ability to self-regulate by dissociative, sensory play.

Penny attempts to interact—firstly, to check the nappy; she is ignored. Then to suggest a puzzle, a book, some Play-Doh; all invitations go unacknowledged. I whisper to Penny, "try to join in with what Sara is doing." When Sara is bashing two cars together, Penny says "Cars … vroom vroom. Blue car, red car." Sara changes activity to banging her feet on the ground; "Bang, bang," echoes Penny with words. Interaction is still frustratingly out of reach. I notice a flush of red on Penny's cheek and a dejected expression. I name what I see. "You are trying so hard to be part of what Sara is doing and feeling pushed away; doesn't feel great, must make you just want to give up." Mum smiles and nods, tears prick. I explain that what I also see is Sara working very hard to attain a level of homeostasis and that often doesn't involve someone else. I explain that we will talk more on Zoom about this and offer to take a turn at being the "play partner" for a while, which Penny gratefully accepts.

I initially use no words, just my body to join in, copying Sara's activity and moving with the changes. She notices me next to her also bashing my feet on the floor; she then gets up and goes back to crashing animals this time. I crash animals too, firstly just my own, then singing a made-up little song with only the words "crash" and "bash" in it. Sara stops and listens, then takes one of my animals and continues, so I take another and start crashing it onto different parts of her body (gently) just saying "crash … leg" … "crash … head" etc. Sara giggles, I have found a way in. As I extend the game, I am careful to use a soft voice with huge animation in my facial expressions, attempting high affect without matching it with volume. As I am choosing a body-part to crash on, I extend the anticipation with a long "Ahhhhhh" before it lands. After waiting for where it will land, she begins to offer me her foot, then hand, then knee etc. The game is playful, silly, and fun, without the bombardment of language or expectation of how it should be played. It also seems to meet the sensory needs, adding stimulation for what is underwhelmed, taking out what overwhelms.

On the Zoom consultation, I firstly explore Penny's rejection and reframe it through a sensory lens of Sara's need. I ask "Have you noticed the games of crashing she does? Sara is proprioceptive seeking, she likes to get feedback in her body and muscles, it possibly helps her know she is here, a kind of body-feedback sense of self. It is also possibly cause and effect … 'when I do this, something happens'." Then I attempt to help Penny question her way of joining in. "Why did you name the colours, and make the car noise?" We discuss how as adults, we often unlearn how to play. We get stuck in our own thinking and lose the natural curiosity of childhood. Animals makes sounds, we learn colours, numbers, houses are painted like this, flowers like that. Penny immediately sees how irrelevant her comments were to what Sara was interested in. "So actually, she was focused on the movement, not what the objects were or sounds they make." "Yes, bingo! You've understood already," I encourage. Next, I explain some Floortime goals, to give what we are doing some reasoning, and explain what I was doing in the play. The first goal is to "follow the child's lead or harness their natural interests"; the second is "to bring the child into a shared world" (Greenspan & Wieder, 2006, pp. 178–179).

We discuss Sara's sensory profile and how we are going to adapt: soft voices, big expressions, no perfumes, lots of physical play, low lighting. I share the intention of "being the most interesting thing in the game" in order to make the interaction as relational as possible. We also discuss regulation, which is the first developmental capacity. I explain that Sara is often able to self-regulate, but usually by doing something self-stimulatory and alone. It will not help Sara reach the next stages of development, nor encourage two-way communication, if our interactions are intrusive, controlling, or misattuned; this would only dysregulate her. Therefore, Penny and I must join Sara, follow specifically what she is interested in with curiosity and playfulness. We need to be careful not to obstruct her ideas by injecting our own too soon. We must assume that her ideas are purposeful and join her with acceptance.

We plan how Penny is going to join, mirror, and attune to the specifics of what Sara is doing. If she is crashing, Penny will crash with her; if she is jumping, Penny will jump too. If Penny is not sure yet, she will wait, watch, and wonder, until she has understood. Sara has a good sense of humour it seems, so Penny is going to re-engage the playful silliness from childhood she feels she has since lost.

Over the next few sessions, there is connection, attunement, and, I can see, attachment beginning to build. Sara is running into the sofa; Penny, without a word, (just playful sounds of "weee … crash"), runs and lands on the sofa. Sara smiles; a game ensues of taking it in turns to run and crash on the sofa. There are giggles, warm looks, eye contact, and cuddles. Hardly any words were spoken, but a lot of relating was done. The biggest shift in the early sessions was Sara looking into her mother's face to gauge a reaction to something, no longer self-absorbed. They are now play partners. "The precursor to the mirror is the mother's face" (Winnicott, 1971, p. 149). Penny had to be brave; some of the ideas did not work at first, so I would tell her, "It's ok, just chuck that idea out the window, wait, and observe and try something else."

Over the coming months, our sessions' focus shifts and grows. Sara enjoys the same set of games during my visits, and we revisit them each time. One game is hiding objects in Play-Doh and pretending we cannot find them; when Sara finds them, we sing a song (again made-up), which says hello to all the objects. There are quite a few physical games, one being Penny and I turn Sara into a sandwich by piling cushions on her body—"here is the tomato, here is the cheese …" Then the final cushion is the bread, which gets squished down, adding a little pressure, which Sara loves, and she giggles and says, "again!" Another version is making her into a wrap by using a blanket. Penny and I playfully discuss what filling she is going to be. Then the wrap falls apart as we unroll the blanket, and the filling (Sara) falls out.

We practise language in a meaningful, relational context. Penny's initial technique of attempting to entice words from Sara by withholding objects was frustrating Sara and causing a rupture between them. If Sara wanted a yogurt, Penny would hold it away and repeat the word—"Yogurt? Say Yogurt"—until Sara moaned and cried. Instead, we practised assuming purposeful meaning from all interactions and physical gestures. So, if Sara was pointing and moaning, Penny would say, "Oh, you really want a yogurt, yes, I understand." The same with play; Penny practised naming Sara's thoughts and emotions, so that Sara's internal experiences could be matched to what was going on relationally and then matched to language that fit the experience. "The caregiver's capacity to observe the moment-to-moment changes in the child's mental state is critical in the development of mentalizing capacity" (Fonagy et al., 2004, p. 54).

I helped Penny understand that by dismissing Sara's signs of distress (either by not acknowledging them, getting upset herself, or more overtly, denying them—"You're okay, it doesn't hurt"), Sara was denied feeling her emotions and sensations and acknowledging them as her real experience. I modelled the co-regulation of Sara's distress, by using acceptance and empathy, giving voice to the internal experience. During a skin-scratching episode, caused by the ending of a game she was enjoying, I sat close by and breathed myself calm. I spoke only empathic sounds to let her know I was here and witnessing the distress. Once she calmed, I said "Sara was *really* upset! It's so hard when a fun game ends."

We learn how to self-regulate by being in relationship with someone who understands what we are going through and takes responsibility for keeping us regulated. "The parent assists the infant in learning to regulate affect and any underlying emotions by matching the affect expression of these emotions and remaining regulated himself" (Hughes, 2011, p. 4).

On Zoom, Penny and I spoke about boundaries and her fear of saying "No" in case it caused a meltdown. She recognised that the meltdowns would cause a lot of anxiety and fear in herself and that she just wanted that feeling to go away. She understood that her own distressed state was exacerbating Sara's dysregulation. She came to understand how the "interbrain connection" (Shanker, 2017, p. 59) between her and Sara meant that if she shared the same anxiety and became overwhelmed by it, her own capacity to co-regulate was derailed. It was important to work with Penny on her own regulation for her to remain calm in the face of Sara's upset. Penny began to track her own emotional states throughout the day, bringing her own thoughts and feelings into awareness. Instead of avoiding her and Sara's emotions, she practised containment, empathy, and regulating herself first; if Penny could bear Sara's feelings of distress, then Sara was more likely to bear them too. Surviving the meltdowns together helped them lessen in frequency and intensity.

During the year we worked together, we returned to the themes mentioned above many times and, of course, this was merely a snapshot of the therapeutic work in its entirety. It is never plain sailing, and there were many bumps in the road along the way. In some ways, the client is the attachment relationship between parent and child, and I had only been able to work with half of that dynamic. There was a period after the first few months where Penny almost disengaged from the work. Phillip was parenting Sara in the only way he knew how, with authority and discipline. Penny had found a new way of relating to Sara, and Phillip, not being on the same journey, was being left behind. This was causing more conflict in their marriage. I, and the therapy, were seen by both at times as a threat to their connection. It would have been optimal if I had found a way to engage Phillip. In this capacity, a big part of what could have been worked on was not available.

Sara now has ear defenders for certain activities, and a trampoline and swing to support her proprioceptive and vestibular needs. Sara loves any kind of messy play, so Penny and Sara started gardening together … and making mud pies. Penny discovered many of Sara's strengths: she can sing and dance, loves animals, and through song Sara now has many words, which is helping her manage life at nursery better. She has made friends with a little boy whose favourite activity is also crashing into things. The nursery have provided soft obstacles and mats that they can crash into together and giggle.

Conclusion

My therapeutic work with neurodivergent children has two main areas of focus: supporting developmental capacities and supporting self-esteem and self-understanding. It is paramount that both these areas be thought about in relationship with a safe, warm, compassionate other.

The first developmental capacity is regulation. Without regulation, all other developmental capacities are frustratingly out of reach. Younger children benefit from their parents and teachers learning how to support the development of this capacity through co-regulation. Older children and adults benefit from having a self-understanding, exploring what dysregulates them and how to self-regulate.

Individuals who are neurodivergent struggle to see and understand themselves, and the more that person exists in a neurotypical world, without an understanding environment, the more their self-esteem suffers. Therefore, the therapeutic work encompasses a relearning of who they are and a processing of traumatic, negative introjections.

References

Bowlby, J. (1988). *A Secure Base: Parent–Child Attachment and Healthy Human Development*. Abingdon, UK: Routledge.
Clarkson, P. (2003). *The Therapeutic Relationship*. London: Wiley.

Delahooke, M. (2022). *Brain-Body Parenting: How to Stop Managing Behaviour and Start Raising Joyful, Resilient Kids*. London: Sheldon Press.

DeYoung, P. (2015). *Relational Psychotherapy: A Primer* (second edition). Hove, UK: Routledge.

Fonagy, P., Gergely, G., Jurist, E., & Target, M. (2004). *Affect Regulation, Mentalization, and the Development of the Self*. London: Karnac.

Gerhardt, S. (2004). *Why Love Matters*. Hove, UK: Routledge.

Golding, K. (2015). Connection before correction: Supporting parents to meet the challenges of parenting children who have been traumatised within their early parenting environments. *Children Australia*, 40(2): 152–159. https://kimsgolding.co.uk/publication/journal-papers/connection-before-correction (last accessed 10 May 2022).

Greenspan, S., & Wieder, S. (2006). *Engaging Autism: Using the Floortime Approach to Help Children Relate, Communicate and Think*. Boston, MA: Da Capo Press.

Heller, L., & La Pierre, A. (2012). *Healing Developmental Trauma: How Early Trauma Affects Self-Regulation, Self-Image, and the Capacity for Relationship*. Berkeley, CA: North Atlantic Books.

Hughes, D. A. (2011). *Attachment-Focused Family Therapy Workbook*. London: W. W. Norton.

Janert, S. (2000). *Reaching the Young Autistic Child*. London: Free Association Books.

Kranowitz, C. S. (2005). *The Out-of-Sync Child: Recognizing and Coping with Sensory Processing Disorder*. New York: Skylight Press.

Lee, P. (2004). *Unexpected Gains Psychotherapy with Adults with Learning Disabilities*. London: Routledge.

Mandy, W. et al. (2022). Mental health and social difficulties of late-diagnosed autistic children, across childhood and adolescence. *The Journal of Child Psychology and Psychiatry*, 63(11): 1405–1414. https://acamh.onlinelibrary.wiley.com/doi/full/10.1111/jcpp.13587 (last accessed 10 May 2022).

Naish, S. (2018). *The A–Z of Therapeutic Parenting*. London: Jessica Kingsley Publishers.

Nickel, K., Maier, S., Endres, D., Joos, A., Maier, V., Tebartz van Elst, L., & Zeeck, A. (2019). Systemic review: Overlap between eating, autism spectrum and ADHD. *Frontiers in Psychiatry*, 10(708). https://www.ncbi.nlm.nih.gov/pmc/articles/PMC6796791 (last accessed 10 May 2022).

Oaklander, V. (2007). *Hidden Treasures: A Map to the Child's Inner Self*. London: Karnac.
Porges, S. (2011). *The Polyvagal Theory: Neurophysiological Foundations of Emotions, Attachment, Communication and Self-Regulation*. London: W. W. Norton.
Rogers, C. (1961). *On Becoming a Person*. London: Constable.
Shanker, S. (2017). *Self-Reg: How to Help Your Child (And You) Break the Stress Cycle and Successfully Engage with Life*. Toronto: Penguin Random House.
Stern, D. (1998). *The Interpersonal World of the Infant*. London: Karnac.
Van der Kolk, B. (2014). *The Body Keeps the Score: Mind, Brain and Body in the Transformation of Trauma*. London: Penguin Random House.
Williams, D. (1996). *Autism: An Inside-Out Approach*. London: Jessica Kingsley Publishers.
Winnicott, D. W. (1953). Transitional objects and transitional phenomena: A study of the first not-me possession. *International Journal of Psychoanalysis*, *34*: 89–97.
Winnicott, D. W. (1965). *The Maturational Processes and the Facilitating Environment: Studies in the Theory of Emotional Development*. London: Hogarth.
Winnicott, D. W. (1971). *Playing and Reality*. London: Tavistock.

CHAPTER 10

Is it too late? The contribution of the integrative child psychotherapist to those affected by fetal alcohol spectrum disorder

Anna Tuttle

Forty to fifty per cent of the children you meet in your therapy room are likely to have prenatal alcohol exposure (Department of Health and Social Care [DHSC], 2021). On first meeting, there will be no way to distinguish whether they have been exposed to alcohol in utero, and, if they have, to what extent this has affected them. Prenatal alcohol exposure (PAE) refers to a child being exposed to alcohol during pregnancy. As there is no safe level of alcohol consumption in pregnancy, causal links of impact cannot be drawn, and a myriad of maternal and fetal factors affect the breadth and depth of impact. For a child to have been given a diagnosis of fetal alcohol spectrum disorder (FASD), a multi-disciplinary team will have to have found evidence of severe impairment in three or more neurodevelopmental areas. This diagnosis is unlikely to be made, in the absence of physical markers, without confirmed PAE. This, along with other diagnostic challenges, means that FASD is under-diagnosed. For this reason, in this chapter, I will refer to prenatal alcohol exposure (PAE) more frequently than fetal alcohol spectrum disorder (FASD). Using indicators of PAE based on either parental disclosure or the constellation of difficulties a child presents with can, therefore, be more useful, as it can be assumed that PAE and FASD are much more prevalent than diagnostic rates suggest. A person with PAE will have typical features of exposure and will also present as uniquely as a fingerprint. PAE is complex, with co-occurring neurological, educational, physiological, psychological, contextual, and intergenerational factors that sustain their effect across the lifespan of the person affected. Research suggests that people with FASD will typically experience significant adversity. For example, increased risks of trauma, poorer physical and mental health, lowered life expectancy, use of toxic/addictive substances, and reduced earning potential all combine to perpetuate the intergenerational cycle of FASD (Gonzales et al., 2021). This neurodevelopmental disorder (NDD) caused by PAE is unyielding in its breadth and depth of impact. A meta-analysis of comorbidity of FASD outlined 428 conditions that co-occur in individuals with FASD spanning physiological and psychological domains (Popova et al., 2016). It is safe to assume that many more individuals with PAE may be affected in a similar way.

Until now, integrative psychotherapy for people with PAE has not been discussed. Even wider PAE-informed psychological interventions are limited in the literature base. The outcomes for those with diagnosed or undiagnosed FASD, where targeted support is not provided; the complex clinical picture caused by PAE; and high prevalence of alcohol use in pregnancy all contribute to the challenges on the individual, their family, and at a societal level. This highlights the need for contextual psychotherapeutic thinking. As integrative child psychotherapists, our interventions are often trauma- or attachment-focused, which may appear to be congruent with the needs of children with PAE. However, research has shown that the effects of prenatal alcohol exposure are not further deepened by subsequent postnatal neglect, leading to little change in neurodevelopmental outcomes (Mukherjee et al., 2019). This has significant implications for child integrative psychotherapists. How can postnatal neglect not have more impact? Even with my clinical experience in PAE, I was astounded, and began to assume that trauma might have more impact than neglect. Research had shown that children with FASD had higher levels of adverse childhood experiences (ACES) (except physical and sexual abuse domains) than the general population. Therefore, it was expected that children in the FASD sample would have more severe behavioural and cognitive difficulties. Yet despite higher ACE scores, with slightly higher behavioural difficulties, the research found that trauma did not lead to an increased impact on functioning when PAE is present.

Children with PAE usually have a higher number of ACEs, meaning that interventions are focused on trauma and attachment issues (Price, 2019). Yet trauma does not appear to make functioning any worse. So, whilst it is important that trauma is not overlooked, interventions that are formulated specifically for PAE are likely to be more effective than those designed for trauma. Within psychotherapy, and most other professions, there is limited understanding of PAE/FASD, with many myths and misconceptions. For instance, less than 10 per cent of children with PAE have the sort of facial features routinely assumed to suggest PAE. An integrative psychotherapy approach to working with children (and adults) with FASD has not, until now, been formulated, yet this evidence clearly indicates the importance of a shift from a routine approach informed by trauma and attachment to a psychotherapeutic way of thinking informed by PAE.

I have noticed how relieved I feel when children arrive with a FASD diagnosis rather than clear indicators of PAE and a best fit of multiple NDD diagnoses. This usually indicates to me that the parents who have arrived in my therapy space have had to navigate systems and fight for services for their child to even gain a diagnosis, and it is less likely they will have been offered support following FASD diagnosis compared to a diagnosis of other NDDs, which in itself is often limited. Chasnoff, Wells, and King (2015) highlighted the concern regarding diagnosis, finding that 86.5 per cent of adolescents with FASD had not been diagnosed or had been misdiagnosed. Many PAE features are developmentally expected in the pre-primary child; although differentiators are present, their subtlety, in combination with masking behaviours, provides identification challenges for non-specialists. Evidentially, recommended interventions to reduce the probability and severity of adverse outcomes include changes in the relational schema (Baldwin, 1997) between the adult and child. Using a PAE formulation, or preferably FASD diagnosis, enables this reframing, and the earlier this shift occurs, the greater the impact for the child (Malbin, 2017; Olson, Jirikowic, Kartin, & Astley, 2007). This, and the need for using a

PAE-informed approach (rather that one informed by attachment or trauma) led to Chasnoff, Wells, and King's (2015) stating:

> The great majority of children that are affected by alcohol are misdiagnosed and taking inappropriate medications or receiving ineffective therapy. FASD should be the differential diagnosis for any child who presents with behaviour problems.

This is particularly pertinent when considering the prevalence estimates. In the UK, prevalence estimates for FASD range from 3.24 to 17 per cent of the population (Lange et al., 2017). Diagnosis rates are much lower due to low professional awareness of FASD, lack of access to comprehensive MDT assessment, delays to the publication of a diagnostic criteria in the UK, and disorientation in professionals due to overlapping neurodevelopmental and physiological features. Challenges in diagnosis and data collection increase difficulties in obtaining reliable estimates of prevalence in the UK. It is known that alcohol use in pregnancy is not safe, and any exposure risks adverse effects from PAE. One approach to considering the scale of children with PAE in psychotherapy settings is to consider the level of PAE in the UK. The "Fetal alcohol spectrum disorder: Health needs assessment" (DHSC, 2021) outlined these rates using data from 2010 (McAndrew et al., 2010). The number of women who reported drinking in pregnancy was:

- 40 per cent across all groups
- 52 per cent of over thirty-fives
- 51 per cent in a managerial or professional occupations
- 46 per cent from a white ethnic background

A meta-analysis to establish global prevalence of alcohol use in pregnancy found the UK to be fourth in the world. Prevalence of FASD has been more widely studied in North America, with estimates of FASD in the US ranging between 3.1 and 9.9 per cent. The scale of potential challenge of PAE in the UK is heightened when considering the prevalence of alcohol use in pregnancy for the UK is 40 per cent compared to 10 per cent in the United States. This highlights the importance of a PAE-informed approach across education, psychotherapy, and children's services in the UK.

A family case study

Alice

At the age of four, Alice was placed with Diane and Stephen for adoption. She had remained with her birth parents, both dependent drinkers, until she was two-and-a-half years old. Alice's early life lacked stimulation, and while some language delays were evident, she had no global developmental delay (GDD). In foster care, the language delays improved, and when placed with her adoptive parents, reports concluded that she was meeting her developmental milestones.

In early-middle childhood, Alice struggled with concentration, and would move rapidly between unfinished activities, reacting impulsively to her wants and not waiting for them to be fulfilled. Sleep initiation (more than three hours) and disrupted sleep cycles were particularly challenging. As Alice approached middle childhood, the gap with her peers widened; dysmaturity and younger play preferences along with social communication difficulties became more visible. The transition to secondary school exacerbated these challenges, particularly when generalising learnt social skills to new contexts: for example, texting and emailing. This resulted in Alice becoming more withdrawn, avoiding social contact with groups, and seeking more relationships with adults, leading to her parents becoming concerned about her vulnerability to exploitation.

Alice always found it difficult to follow instructions and became anxious when she was unable to understand information. She had significant difficulties when comprehending a future event without concrete previous examples to support her understanding. This would lead to her becoming, as her parents saw it, "explosive" and "dissolving into tears". They said it was hard to support her or communicate with her during these episodes. Alice told me: "I am bad, I get things wrong all the time, I'm just thick, I'm not good at anything." Despite clear strengths and talents, she had significant difficulties with self-concept and self-esteem.

Alice found secondary school more difficult than primary school. Diane felt this was due to the increased sensory load, the transitions between different physical environments and different teaching styles, and the impact of "relational juggling" due to multiple teacher relationships. Diane and Stephen had concerns for Alice's ability to reach her potential and for her later independence in adulthood.

Alice was diagnosed with autism and attention deficit hyperactivity disorder (ADHD) aged seven. Diane and Stephen reported feeling relieved that she had been given a diagnosis, although they had felt confused as standard interventions for NDDs were ineffective and they had felt like "something else was going on". They reported that one ADHD medication had negative impacts and they decided not to pursue other options. Melatonin had been helpful for sleep initiation, with challenges remaining with sleep-cycle disruption and early waking. Their new neurodevelopmental paediatrician had previous experience with FASD and discussed the possibility with them. After genetic testing (to rule out a chromosomal abnormality that may have been impacting on her needs), Alice was diagnosed with FASD, aged eleven.

Her parents, teachers, and previous therapists had used therapeutic interventions more commonly used for autism and trauma. These had little impact. Social stories had not reduced her anxiety with unpredictable experiences, and feelings thermometers did not support communication of emotional regulation. Trauma-informed CBT (which Alice found especially dysregulating) and non-directive play therapy had not led to any sustained changes. The introduction of a sensory diet had been moderately successful (swinging on a hammock, kinetic sand, feeling the wind from a fan on her face, and body brushing). Educational provision within a smaller nurture unit at secondary school had also decreased her anxiety and reduced educational demands. However, Alice missed her friends, and this had become a source of rumination.

Freddie

Freddie was placed with Diane and Stephen at the same time as Alice, when she was four years old and he was one month old. His birth weight and length were on the bottom of the percentiles, with improvements when oesophageal reflux and milk intolerance were managed. Freddie met his developmental milestones. As a pre-schooler, his parents found his needs were increasing, beyond what they felt was developmentally typical. Diane shared:

> "He was three. He stopped going to sleep—bedtimes took forever, and he would hit us and throw things. He wouldn't

do anything we asked, he would break everything and fight us. He didn't seem to follow instructions, couldn't play, and was destructive. He would sometimes hit other children and show no remorse. We didn't understand, he came home to us as a baby, we felt like it must be our fault and began to blame each other."

When Freddie started school (aged five), child-to-parent violence (CPV) increased in frequency and severity. He became unsafe in the car, posing a risk to the driver. Following an ADHD diagnosis (at age six), an education, health, and care plan (EHCP) was implemented with regulation breaks, targeted educational intervention, provision of a low-stimulus environment, and a sensory diet.

Freddie's needs continued to grow in multiple contexts, particularly in areas of hyperactivity, impulsivity, inattention, cognitive processing deficits, and emotional dysregulation. The impact of fatigue and overwhelm from attending school had led to episodes of emotionally based school avoidance (EBSA) lasting a few days. When Freddie had a sustained break from school (for example, school holidays of more than a week), his parents reported a reduction in fatigue, displays of anger, violence, and oppositional behaviour.

To manage Freddie's needs, the school chose to teach him separately from his peers (aged seven), and when recalling this, Freddie said, "I missed my friends". Freddie had three school exclusions during Year Three and asked, "Am I still bad? 'Cos I got kicked out." I was surprised that his strengths had not been identified. What was supporting the development of his self-esteem?

Following Alice's medication experiences, Diane and Stephen had felt resistant to ADHD medication for Freddie. When recalling Freddie at age seven, Diane said:

> "I just couldn't cope with being hurt anymore. I felt like a battered wife—except I couldn't just leave. No one was coming if I rang the police. I wanted him gone. I knew we were at adoption breakdown. Stephen couldn't cope with him, so I could never leave them alone together. I was so exhausted. The only thing left to try was medication."

As Stephen's reflective capacity increased through parental reflective work, I asked him to recall this time. He said:

> "I feel ashamed to say it now, but I felt like he was evil. He was the devil child. He was abusing my wife, and I had to let him? Any man that did that I would have knocked him out—and I'm not that kind of bloke. It was hard enough dealing with Alice, but we couldn't cope with Freddie too. He was the bigger problem. He had to go. Diane convinced me that it was worth trying medication. That was the turning point. It took the psychiatrist a while to get the medication right, and I'm still not sure if it is, but life isn't as bad. Especially now I know it's his brain, not him causing this. It must be really hard living inside himself."

Once he started taking the medication, Freddie was able to be supported in the class environment more often, and shortly afterwards, he was diagnosed with FASD (aged eight). Despite scaffolding and accommodations, the increasingly complex language-based interactions with his peers, the demands of the curriculum, and the greater requirement to understand abstract concepts made the cognitive demands of school challenging. In my assessment, I became aware of indicators of loss and shame that he was experiencing. I wondered if this was connected to difficulties in sustaining peer relationships, scapegoating from other children at school, and a perceived low level of educational success. Challenging behaviours had increased at home owing to masking and the psychological impact of his primary disabilities, leading to these secondary effects.

Stephen said to me: "It's him causing this, maybe it's something genetic he has got from his birth dad, maybe he will be bad like him. Do you think he might be a psychopath?" I assessed that Freddie's parents were the interventional priority to support a shift in their relational schema; however, I also felt that Freddie was coming towards the end of his time in mainstream provision. I was also wondering if seeking an appropriate suitable educational provision may be of benefit to Freddie. Diane added: "Everyone keeps saying it's our parenting … but we've tried everything. All the traditional stuff, like sticker charts and consequences, just don't work."

Early diagnosis acts as an intervention to reduce adverse outcomes. Alice and Freddie were diagnosed at eleven and eight years old respectively.

Alex and Feldmann (2012) found that children who received a diagnosis at age eight years or younger had fewer behavioural difficulties longer term. Yet Streissguth, Bookstein, Barr, Sampson, and O'Malley (2004) found that diagnosis before the age of six offered the greater protection against secondary effects and tertiary impacts.

A new approach

I use a PAE-informed approach when a child presents with a combination of behavioural and cognitive challenges, until further assessment indicates this is not required. Before this change in my practice, I would have made sense of Alice and Freddie's presentation (Figure 10.1 and Figure 10.2) using an attachment and trauma lens. From a PAE-informed approach, I view these behavioural and cognitive challenges as secondary effects of primary disabilities caused by PAE. These secondary effects, or defensive behaviours (mapped in Figure 10.2), are normal reactions to distress caused by a poor fit between the person and their environment. Integrative child psychotherapists can have the greatest impact in this area of the intervention plan. Our expertise enables us to adapt our psychotherapy approach to provide individual psychotherapy with parental and contextual interventions to reduce both the severity and recurrence of secondary effects and tertiary impacts.

Facilitating a psychological shift in the adult carer's perspective of the behaviours of their child with PAE, from "won't" to "can't" and "bad" to "disabled", is the single most effective intervention that we can offer as psychotherapists (aside from referral for assessment and diagnosis that may further facilitate this). The earlier this reframing occurs in the individual's life, the greater the impact on the child's future (Malbin, 2017). A more positive relational schema in parents, educators, and extended family leads to increased contextual accommodations to improve the fit between the environment and the child. This shift also has the potential to lead to increased attachment security owing to improvements in the parent–child relationship through more appropriate parenting strategies and expectations.

The delivery of a combination of brain-based PAE psychoeducation and parental and educator reflective sessions is the most effective intervention. Catterick and Curran (2014), Malbin (2017), and Geddes (2022) have written useful texts for parents, educators, and other professionals to read.

	Primary disabilities (Many of these primary disabilities will be caused by PAE, and there are likely to be a range of other contributory factors that intersect)	Interdisciplinary interventions to reduce and/or prevent secondary effects
Apply to Alice and Freddie	- Inattention - Hyperactivity - Impulsivity - Cognitive flexibility problems - Receptive language - Working memory - Abstraction - Sensory avoidance/seeking - Emotional dysregulation - Dysmaturity - Slower processing pace - Generalising, forming links, and making associations - Sleep initiation/disrupted sleep cycles - Dental vulnerabilities - Blunted pain response	- Implement accommodations to reduce triggers with graded reintroduction when regulated and supported - Education health care plan (EHCP) including specialised classroom support and early intervention - Educational and/or clinical psychology providing baseline cognitive/psychometric testing and re-testing at key transitional points - Early intervention educational strategies (Olson & Montague, 2011) focusing on increasing adaptive executive functioning and child's neurodevelopmental profile (Figure 10.3). Research shows a correlation between executive functioning impairment and increased anxiety - Visual supports to support processing and retention difficulties - Regulation breaks in all settings when unable to choose own activity/stimulus level and/or when arousal levels are high - Emotional regulation intervention in early years. Adapt for FASD with higher adult ratio, increased structure for play and concrete play materials

		• Neurodevelopmental paediatrician to consider pharmacological-based interventions for sleep • Assessment for ADHD symptoms to provide access to ADHD medications, preferably prescribed using FASD research (for example, CANFAS medication algorithm) • Increased dental monitoring/intervention: fissure sealants, fluoride supplementation due to dental vulnerabilities • Individualised sensory diet • Auditory processing assessment • Occupational therapy: including sensory integration-based treatments or FASD–ALERT (Chasnoff, Wells, & King, 2015)
Specific to Alice	• Poor planning • Understanding money • Concept of time • Fine motor skill delay • Language acquisition delay • Aversion to food textures	• Developing strength areas, increasing protective self-esteem • Speech and language assessment and therapy (SALT) formulated for FASD, not wider NDDs, with a focus on integrative language • Social skills training to bridging existing one-to-one interpersonal skills to groups
Specific to Freddie	• Sugar-seeking to mediate cortisol • Poor social understanding/ superficial interactions • Tics • Physiological comorbidities	• Focus on developing strength areas to provide protective self-esteem • Dietary interventions: working with natural feeding pattern; use of food as medicine to regulate; dietetics monitoring • Medical monitoring

Figure 10.1 Primary difficulties: intervention plan

	Secondary effects	Interdisciplinary interventions	Psychotherapy-led interventions
		All interventions to be targeted to individualised domain on child's neurodevelopmental profile (Figure 10.3), using a PAE-informed approach rather than an attachment and trauma lens	
Apply to Alice and Freddie	- Socially isolated, unstable friendships, socially inappropriate, difficulties with navigating social relationships through technology - Shame-based responses/behaviour - Disproportionate emotional responses - Micro, macro, and relational transitional difficulties - Oppositional behaviours/non-compliant to instructions - Limited interventional impact	- Individualised social stories/comic strip stories (Gray, 1994) to interpret abstract social concepts - Anticipatory parental guidance to plan future interventions/support - FASD individualised parental support: families moving forward programme (Olson, Jirikowic, Kartin, & Astley, 2007) or emerging new models - MDT approach to identify strengths and challenges - Regulation and rest breaks, pacing of activities and supportive sensory interventions - Assessment and implementation of PAE and attachment-informed respite package	- Reflective parental session to process parental experiences - Reflective sessions with parents and wider contexts (individual and combined) to advocate for the child and implement reframing; brain-based approach; identification/implementation of accommodations; planning for long-term interventions - Repetitive interventions to increase causation linkages and generalisability - Psychoeducation supporting child's understanding of PAE (strengths and challenges) and co-creation of useful strategies using concrete explanations, repetition, and generalisations to a range of situations/contexts - Supportive psychotherapy: play-based and dialogic

Specific to Alice		• Desensitised, flat affect, depression • Fatigue • Social anxiety • Poor self-concept, feelings of failure, low self-esteem • Episodic self-harm	• Plan low arousal environmental breaks in busy/crowded or challenging environments • Reduce environmental risks and increase parental monitoring	• Life story work—repeated at different developmental stages using concrete adaptations and increased repetitions • Identify relational trauma, support reparative opportunities, implement relationship-focused parenting • Increase understanding of context of child on how to reduce impact of shame and identify shame-based responses
Specific to Freddie		• Regular lying (possible confabulation due to working memory and information-processing challenges)	• When more emotionally regulated, introduce adapted individually delivered social skills training e.g. incredible years child training programme	• Collaborative safety planning and risk assessments • Autism/ADHD mindfulness techniques adapted for FASD: slower concept introduction, visual integrations, concrete concepts, repetition, increased sensory/fidget objects • Increase understanding of context of child on how to reduce impact of shame and identify shame-based responses

(Continued)

- Child to Parent Violence, episodes of aggression within a range of contexts
- Exclusion from school

- (IY-CT) with adaptations for PAE: increase number/variety of vignettes; increase role play and coaching—outcomes suggest reduction in disruptive behaviour (Webster-Stratton, Reid, & Hammond, 2004) and peer relationship improvements
- Parallel planning of settings/interventions to reduce educational disruption

- Introduce therapeutically informed approaches that can be generalised to a wider context e.g. break-it-down boards
- Support context to understand challenges with boundaries with PAE exposure and ways to provide safety, boundaries, and containment
- Family-based safety planning for managing violence
- PAE-adapted non-violent resistance strategies using collaborative approach
- PAE-adapted dyadic interventions dependent on cognitive capacity

Figure 10.2 Secondary effects: indicative intervention plan

Once basic reframing and awareness has been possible, a co-creation can emerge that enables the development of accommodations, interventions, and strategies that are brain-based, individualised, and geared to the child's developmental age in each specific domain (Figure 10.3).

This psychotherapy-led, reflective work focuses on implementing relationship-focused parenting and caring approaches. It is important to eliminate inappropriate strategies: for example, learning-based approaches that focus on consequences and positive reward systems. These are inherently based on forming causal links and reasoning to manage behaviour; therefore, they are unsuccessful in brains that have impairments in executive functioning. Research shows that children with PAE are usually relationally engaging with high social motivation and a desire to please, which when present tend to counterbalance negative developmental outcomes (Olson, Jirikowic, Kartin, & Astley, 2007). Failing to succeed at a sticker chart with these personality traits and social motivators is likely to activate strong shame-based responses.

My core intervention (at times, this may be the sole intervention), in all cases of PAE, is parental reflective work. It is therefore important that I retain my core value of "curiosity not pathology". This is my commitment to avoid pathologising the child, the family (birth and current), and supporting others (the wider network and professionals). Each brings their own personal experiences, challenges, and strengths that will be important to this journey.

Diane: "I am so angry that we have to live this life because of the damage to their brains. I feel like I am grieving for the child they could have been."

The combination of grief and anger overlaid with hopelessness and helplessness in PAE is painful to hold. PAE/FASD is the most common preventable NDD. In 1973, a birth defects disorder attributable to PAE was recognised in France and the United States, leading to women in the United States being advised not to drink alcohol when pregnant in 1981, with explicit labelling placed on alcohol for sale in 1988. However, guidance was not changed in the UK until 2016 (DHSC, 2021).

The cost of this delay, in terms of the quality of life in those affected by PAE, is unquantifiable. Financially, the British Medical Association has estimated the annual cost of FASD in the UK is £2 billion. To implement a service to reduce the occurrence of secondary effects of FASD would need to be 28 per cent effective to be cost neutral (cited in DHSC, 2021). The positive impact of intervention would be wide-reaching across public sector services and beyond.

Those affected by PAE are not only children, their families, and those that support them. The burden of blame often lies with the child's birth mother, who may also be raising her biological child. In this case, Diane is an adoptive parent, and due to the challenges presented by PAE for her and her children's lives, I can understand why she feels angry towards their birth mother. However, PAE, in my opinion, is a feminist issue. PAE is another example of how cultural blame is magnetised towards women, often leaving men less accountable. A man may encourage or facilitate, implicitly or explicitly, alcohol consumption in pregnancy. Domestic violence, trauma, illicit drug use, exploitation, mental health difficulties, lack of educational opportunities, and lack of accurate or visible government guidance may all be contributory factors in a woman's apparent choice to drink during pregnancy. There are also women who are not trying to conceive or are unaware they are pregnant who drink alcohol. Maintaining a woman's freedom over her own body is essential.

The ever-present cultural and systemic view of "where is/was the mother" directly impacts self-concept, leading to shame-based parenting responses. A fundamental cultural shift is required to bring about change across the generations. I believe that mothering, in this cultural context, may be one of the hardest, most impossible jobs. Parenting a child who has PAE makes what may be an impossible job so much harder for Diane and Stephen.

It is important that I avoid any pull into confluence to blame the children's birth mother to shift the pathology away from the children. In my opinion, blaming the children's birth mother can be experienced (potentially unconsciously) by the adopted child as an attack on self. Providing Diane with a reflective space to explore (and witness) her sadness, desperation, anger, and fear whilst supporting an increase in her mentalizing capacity enabled a resolution of this process. On darker days, however, Diane still found she fell into this process of annihilation for a short time, each time with increasing awareness. Diane and

Stephen, like most adopters, entered the adoption process from a place of their own vulnerability, following loss and trauma; offering a space for processing of these experiences was also essential.

Stephen: "This isn't what I wanted having a family to be like."

Like many other families, Diane and Stephen knew that their children had PAE, and were told that this would not cause adverse effects because they did not have the supposedly characteristic facial features. The inaccuracies in the myths of PAE/FASD are staggering. In my clinical practice, I often work with a differential diagnosis, formulation, and intervention plan based on PAE/FASD when there is no confirmation of PAE. It was helpful for future intervention that Diane and Stephen were aware of the children's PAE, even though this did not change their expectations of what family life may be like. There are many reasons for unconfirmed PAE: for example, procedural/documentation issues, lack of engagement of birth parent, stigma attached to this diagnosis, and/or lack of diagnostic opportunities. Although the National Institute for Health and Care Excellence (NICE) guidance released in 2021 is expected to improve multi-disciplinary assessment, diagnosis, and support, this is not likely to have significant impact in the short–medium term.

There was a mismatch with Stephen's expectations of family life and reality that was unsurprising to me. Studies show that parents of children with FASD experience significantly higher levels of stress than children with other NDDs (Bobbitt et al., 2016), and prospective adopters are likely to have built their fantasy of parenting based on the prevailing models of family in their own culture. An important component of parental reflective work is to give space for parents to process the pain, loss, and grief they experience in raising their children compared to the children they imagined. Parents will often hold onto their fantasy of how family life should be, viewing the child as the problem, as a defence against depression (self-blame) or persecutory feelings (blaming others) to avoid the destabilisation of their own self-image of parenthood (Raphael-Leff, 2020). Increasing reflective capacity and reflexivity will only be possible once these experiences, fantasies, and defences have been processed through psychotherapy intervention.

A combination of parental reflective psychotherapy and increasing their opportunities to receive empathy through carer support groups was supportive for Diane and Stephen. They had often experienced criticism and judgement in the wider context due to people's perceptions of their brain-based parenting decisions. From my reflective work with the context of the family, a shared narrative emerged of their children's needs. This was especially positive in the dialogue between home and school. This increase in contextual support, empathy, and shared understanding reduced the degree of loneliness that they experienced, thereby increasing their resilience.

Stephen: "So it can't be fixed then?"

The effects of PAE are lifelong, although we currently have a clearer understanding of the impact and effectiveness of interventions during childhood rather than over the course of life. The primary disabilities caused by PAE are permanent and are likely to be lowered IQ or significant impairment in adaptive functioning; impaired abilities in maths and often in reading comprehension; significant compromise to executive function, specifically in problem-solving, impulse control, information processing, following through on directions, concept formation, and frustration tolerance (Arendt & Farkas, 2007).

Accepting the lifelong impact of PAE is challenging for children and parents. Stephen was focused on the possibilities of neuroplasticity. It was important that I carefully titrated evidence, communicated with empathy and containment, to hold his devastation when he began to realise this was not possible. At times, encouraging Stephen to put down his problem-solving talents and invite him to join my reality felt cruel. Yet shifting the focus from what was not possible to what was possible was essential. *Neurological repair is not possible* was a hard-hitting message that was crucial.

Exploring what was possible enabled Diane, Stephen, and me to co-create an intervention plan (similar to Figures 10.1 and 10.2) that offered opportunities to reduce secondary effects and subsequent tertiary impacts. Much of this plan was aspirational; services were not available to meet the needs of this family. By creating a shared reality of what was necessary, we were able to prioritise what we believed would be the most effective interventions for the children long term. This collaborative approach reduced Diane and Stephen's sense of helplessness, increased their agency and autonomy, motivated and sustained their engagement, and built trust in our therapeutic relationship to increase the likelihood of beneficial outcomes. Most importantly, their relational schema had been updated, reframing had occurred, and they were working together. This was the biggest indicator of the possibilities for Alice and Freddie's future.

As expected in a child with an FASD diagnosis, most of these primary disabilities are present for Alice and Freddie, and Stephen is right: these cannot be fixed, *and* interventions are possible.

Diane: "Where do we even start? We've tried so much, it's all too much. I'm exhausted."

A comprehensive holistic approach to assessment, formulation, and intervention planning is particularly important with a child with suspected PAE (or indicators that this may be an area to explore in more depth). My approach is to constellate the areas identified in the assessment to enable connections to be made. This can be a particularly helpful approach when working with PAE where the unwieldy depth and breadth of presentation and comorbidities can be overwhelming. PAE spans physical, psychological, social, and educational domains, and often specialist supervision is helpful to support this process.

One child with FASD, who had a stable postnatal experience, had over twenty common physical abnormalities along with significant neurodevelopment challenges. It would be remarkable for the number of these physical abnormalities to be coincidental and not linked to PAE. When viewed in combination with his cognitive profile, a fuller picture of the impacts of his PAE emerges. It can be useful to consider each feature of a child's neurodevelopmental, physiological, and attachment profile in conjunction with validated screening tools in the absence of diagnostic pathways. Through constellating this information, I am usually astounded by the cumulative challenge of these features, many individually below diagnostic thresholds, all combining to create secondary effects.

Figure 10.2 outlines the secondary effects experienced over the course of Alice's and Freddie's childhood that emerged at different developmental stages. Secondary effects are not unique to PAE; they occur for each of us when there is a gap between our abilities and environmental expectations.

The intersection of a child's primary disabilities can be a barrier to effective therapy interventions. It is important that all interventions (including psychotherapy) are adapted and prioritised based on the individual's primary disability profile (or, when unclear, to a general PAE primary disability profile) to increase the possibility of positive outcomes. Olson and Montague (2011) suggest that multi-interventions are more effective, and, speaking from my clinical experience, the ordering and phasing of these interventions should focus on the areas of greatest impact and likely effectiveness—working with the adults in the context of the child.

Alice: "Nothing makes me feel better."

Alice had a typical mixed neurodevelopmental profile. This is sometimes described as a spikey learning and developmental profile (Figure 10.3). In PAE, it is important to note that there will also be inconsistent performance across days. The targeting of interventions based on the specific developmental age of the domain (for example, social skills) that we were focusing on was essential.

Alice was experiencing high levels of shame, with challenges centred around self-concept and difficulties in managing peer relationships. I was also aware that the environmental adversity that Alice experienced

Domain	Age
Chronological age	13
Expressive language	18
Receptive language	6
Social maturity	7
Social skills	8
Living skills	9
Money and time concepts	7
Maths skills	6
Reading decoding	12
Reading comprehension	8

Figure 10.3 Example of a profile of a thirteen-year-old with PAE, using developmental ages for specific domains to illustrate functional impacts

in her early life may have exacerbated her brain-based vulnerability from PAE. Based on my mapping of the primary and secondary effects (Figures 10.1 and 10.2), I felt that Alice was likely to benefit from creative and play-based psychotherapy interventions, which would be in line with her social maturity and social skills. I hoped this could be a reparative relational experience through minimising demands and matching pace and interventions compatibly to her neurodevelopmental profile. Sentences longer than a "tweet" (Diane's phraseology) cause the child to lose the beginning of the intervention, so short, direct, concrete language is essential. I hoped that by working with play, we would have a way to communicate with each other that would not be as reliant on language, which had remained an area of challenge and shame for Alice.

I soon found that a non-directive approach was too overwhelming for Alice. Whilst this approach builds children's abilities in social responsiveness (Josefi & Ryan, 2004) and self-regulation, Alice was seeking more direction from me. Despite my view that the space was low-stimulus, Alice appeared overloaded with sensory input created by her own exploration of the play materials. To combat this, I reduced the availability of materials, and introduced play stations that would allow her unconscious process to unfold whilst reducing demands for her attention. I also discovered it was important to keep consistency of materials, processes, transitions, and timings (with visual cues) to adapt to her brain needs.

Over time, Alice was able to manage an increased flexibility of interventions in the therapy space. Working from an integrative perspective enables me to move through a blend of open-ended and structured therapeutic interventions. I also incorporated role play for social skills development, projective techniques so that Alice could act out some of her experiences, and mindfulness-based interventions that enabled an increase in regulatory capacity. Later in our work, I was able to introduce play-based yoga interventions with a co-therapist to integrate yoga, neuroscience, and play therapy, offering a multi-modal approach. It was essential that each individual therapy intervention was mapped to her unique intervention plan (Figures 10.1 and 10.2) so that her brain-based needs led the process.

Alice's brain-based needs took priority, and I consciously decided not to offer dyadic-based attachment interventions. This type of intervention was not appropriate for Alice, primarily owing to receptive and integrative language difficulties and prominent difficulties with cause-and-effect linking. However, this approach may be appropriate for other children with PAE. I felt attachment-strengthening activities would have more impact for Alice. Trialling, practising, and then generalising attachment-based activities from therapy to home increased attachment security. Another specific focus was on reducing attachment ruptures in relationships and creating opportunities for relational success. One intervention that facilitated this was the use of break-it-down boards (https://fasd.me) to understand precipitating, contextual, internal, and expectational factors, which enabled Alice to start to make cause-and-effect links (which may only ever be possible retrospectively) using a concrete approach. Alice was then able to make attempts to generalise these skills, and it is hoped that she will start to use this independently as she gets older or to identify other people to support her through interdependence (people with PAE are likely to need to "borrow" someone else's executive brain, even when in adulthood).

Stephen: "I am scared that Alice will do anything for love. I don't know what the future looks like for our children."

The combination of Alice's attachment experiences, her seeking relationships with adults owing to challenges in her peer relationships, her primary disability in impulse control, and her difficulties with abstraction and establishing cause-and-effect (Freunscht & Feldman, 2011) increased her risk of vulnerability to exploitation. Alice was beginning to seek access to technology independently and to seek more unmonitored time outside of the family home. This meant that safety was an important consideration as part of the therapeutic process. Concrete approaches to exploring risk were essential. Alice was able to engage with identifying risks through stacking building blocks, with the impact of one block too many causing the tower to crash as a helpful illustration. This collaborative, concrete, and visual approach is essential both to assess understanding and to improve potential retention, which, owing to difficulties with cause-and-effect and generalising between situations, will be challenging.

Risk profiles for the person with PAE are complex, and as the child gets older, the sphere of influence and the ability of parents (and the wider context) to accommodate needs and manage associated risks reduces. This can mean that the adolescent or adult with FASD may not have robust enough contextual support to accommodate their brain injury. The net effect of the chronic failure and frustration experienced by the individual (Malbin, 2017) when their disabilities have not been accommodated leads to secondary effects (immediate defensive responses). When these have also not been successfully mediated, the individual may experience tertiary impacts.

To the parent of a child with PAE/FASD, the prospect of possible tertiary impacts is devastating. As an integrative psychotherapist, I often feel hopeless. The odds *are* stacked against a child with PAE. Evidence of therapeutic impact with a child with PAE is subtle, and the positive impact of therapeutic work is focused on the absence of negative effects (secondary disabilities and tertiary impacts) rather than positive effects. To manage this, I hold both the hopelessness of these evidence-based statistics and the words that I share with parents:

> "Everything you do is for adulthood. Not for now. Any impact now is a bonus. Repeatedly switching interventions reduces our chance to make an impact. Consistency is key."

In my experience, therapy reduces the severity and number of secondary disabilities and also reduces the risk of tertiary impacts. I also believe that the shift in relational schema and an increase in parental support reduces the risk of relational trauma in the parent–child relationship, placement breakdown, and increased ACEs.

I remind myself of the possibilities of therapeutic intervention for PAE and to trust the process. Studies have shown that people with FASD:

- are five times more likely to attempt suicide than the general population (Huggins, Grant, O'Malley, & Streissguth, 2008)
- are more likely to be victims of violence. In Clark, Lutke, Minnes, and Ouellette-Kuntz (2004), 87 per cent of participants had been

victim to some form of violence; 77 per cent had experienced physical and/or sexual abuse; and 92 per cent of participants' caregivers felt their child was vulnerable to exploitation

Streissguth, Bookstein, Barr, Sampson, and O'Malley's 2004 study found, of all participants:

- 90 per cent had mental health problems
- 61 per cent had disrupted school experiences
- 60 per cent had contact with the criminal justice system
- 49 per cent had committed inappropriate sexual behaviours on multiple occasions
- 35 per cent had substance misuse problems
- 50 per cent had been confined (criminal justice or mental health)

To counteract these adverse life outcomes, it is significantly advantageous to diagnose FASD before the age of six, to have access to services for support, and to create a good and stable environment (Streissguth, Bookstein, Barr, Sampson, & O'Malley, 2004). The combination of their strengths, the commitment of their parents, support through psychotherapy and other provisions, with an accurate diagnosis, offered some protective factors for Alice and Freddie. It was not too late, and I wished they had started therapy sooner.

Diane: "I don't want Freddie to hurt the people he loves, I don't want him to be seen as a problem, I want people to see his talents."

My pull to work individually with Freddie was strong; he was similar to other children I had worked with. However, using Figures 10.1 and 10.2, I felt that the priorities for intervention were with the context. Freddie was often overstimulated by the environment or exhausted by the impact of being "a ten second kid in a one second world" (Malbin, 2004, p. 55), and his behaviours were a symptom of the poor fit between him and his environment.

I believe the primary disabilities relating to language are a large risk factor for secondary effects and tertiary impacts. Young children with PAE, like Freddie, are often described as very "chatty", charming, and engaging, and so their language difficulties are often missed, particularly due to their ability to mask and confabulate. Language skills are critical in the development and maintenance of peer relationships, and this gap widens between peers (generally age 7 to 10) when the narrative of play, stories, and social interactions tend to necessitate higher-level integrative language skills (Thorne, 2010). The more pervasive these difficulties, the greater the impact on peer relationships. The impact of increasing awareness of their disabilities, changes, and/or loss of peer relationships, and challenges with social interactions leads to further secondary effects, for example, low mood, anxiety, poor self-concept, and shame-based responses.

Diane and Stephen were offered parental reflective therapy as the core intervention, which focused on both their children. In addition to the support provided directly to them as carers, these sessions also focused on enabling them to make incremental changes in their parenting techniques to accommodate to Freddie's brain-based needs as they evolved. Gaining insight into Freddie's strengths and helping his parents build on these was fundamental to supporting his development of a healthy self-concept. Taking a strengths-based approach to preventing secondary disabilities is an area often overlooked in the psychological understanding of PAE, including in the research base.

My role as an advocate was fundamental in supporting Freddie and his parents effectively. Bringing psychotherapeutic insight to the advocacy for the family's needs was essential. This helped secure an appropriate support package to reduce the risk of adverse outcomes, and, critically, to prevent adoption breakdown. It made possible the introduction of a psychotherapeutically informed respite package before the family hit blocked care. This respite package offered Freddie opportunities to replicate relational successes, build relationships, and access wider opportunities, whilst strengthening the resilience of the parental relationship and providing much-needed self-care opportunities.

I am currently researching and developing a pre-adolescence integrated psychotherapy and speech and language intervention (SLT); in Freddie's case, this would have been a priority intervention to reduce secondary effects/tertiary impacts. As this is in its early stages of development, this was not available for Freddie; however, a psychotherapeutic PAE-informed SLT intervention was provided, enabling Freddie to communicate more effectively his needs in order to promote co-regulation. It can be useful to rehearse and experiment with social skills with older children and adults who are developmentally more able to accommodate the child with PAE needs. This increases the possibility of relational success and results in greater self-esteem impacts.

My final intervention was aimed at reducing Freddie's "relational juggling". Managing the PAE and attachment impact of multiple professionals was difficult for Freddie, whilst also being exhausting for his parents. Working with professionals to co-ordinate delivery of interventions was more effective. This meant each professional equipping either his parents, teaching assistant/teacher, or speech and language therapist with the skills necessary to deliver vital interventions. This innovative approach is challenging within traditional services, and ultimately is possible if each of us can relinquish some of our professional defensiveness to provide the most effective approach for the child with PAE.

Our voices

Alice and Freddie's journeys continue. I would like to finish this chapter with their words:

> "Listen to my struggle, find out about FASD, and then do something about it."

> "Don't just read the stuff my mum gives you and decide it's too difficult and keep doing what you do in the same way. 'Cos then I will feel like it's me that's failing. Ask me, I know what helps."

> "It's not my fault my brain does this stuff."

> "I'm not choosing to be wobbly."

> "Please stop using so many words."

> "You wouldn't make me try to see if I was blind."

> "You can't fix me, and I'm not broken."

References

Alex, K., & Feldmann, R. (2012). Children and adolescents with fetal alcohol syndrome (FAS): Better social and emotional integration after diagnosis. *Klinische Paediatrie*, *224*(2): 66–71. https://doi.org/10.1055/s-0031-1299682 (last accessed 28 November 2022).

Arendt, R. E., & Farkas, K. J. (2007). Maternal alcohol abuse and fetal alcohol spectrum disorder: A life-span perspective. *Alcoholism Treatment Quarterly*, *25*(3): 3–20. https://doi.org/10.1300/j020v25n03_02 (last accessed 13 November 2022).

Baldwin, M. W. (1997). Relational schemas as a source of if-then self-inference procedures. *Review of General Psychology*, *1*(4): 326–335. https://doi.org/10.1037/1089-2680.1.4.326 (last accessed 19 November 2022).

Bobbitt, P. S., Baugh, L. A., Andrew, G. H., Cook, J. L., Green, C. R., Pei, J. R., & Rasmussen, C. R. (2016). Caregiver needs and stress in caring for individuals with fetal alcohol spectrum disorder. *Research in Developmental Disabilities*, *55*: 100–113. https://doi.org/10.1016/j.ridd.2016.03.002 (last accessed 28 November 2022).

Catterick, M., & Curran, L. (2014). *Understanding Fetal Alcohol Spectrum Disorder: A Guide to FASD for Parents, Carers and Professionals.* London: Jessica Kingsley.

Chasnoff, I. J., Wells, A. M., & King, L. (2015). Misdiagnosis and missed diagnoses in foster and adopted children with prenatal alcohol exposure. *Paediatrics*, *135*(2): 264–270. https://doi.org/10.1542/peds.2014–2171 (last accessed 1 December 2022).

Clark, E., Lutke, J., Minnes, P., & Ouellette-Kuntz, H. (2004). Secondary disabilities among adults with fetal alcohol spectrum disorder in British Columbia. *Journal FASD International*, *2*(e13): 1–12. https://doi.org/10.1111/j.1468-3148.2007.00414.x (last accessed 17 November 2022).

Department of Health and Social Care (DHSC) (2021). Fetal alcohol spectrum disorder: Health needs assessment. https://gov.uk/government/publications/Fetal-alcohol-spectrum-disorder-health-needs-assessment/Fetal-alcohol-spectrum-disorder-health-needs-assessment#contents (last accessed 28 November 2022).

Freunscht, I., & Feldman, R. (2011). Young adults with fetal alcohol syndrome (FAS): Social, emotional and occupational development. *Klinische*

Padiatrie, *223*(1): 33–7. https://doi.org/10.1055/s-0030-1261927 (last accessed 28 November 2022).

Geddes, A. (2022). *A Complicated & Beautiful Brain*. Self-published.

Gonzales, K. L., Jacob, M. M., Merceir, A., Heater, H., Nall, L., Joseph, J., & Kuerschner, S. (2021). An indigenous framework of the cycle of fetal alcohol spectrum disorder risk and prevention across the generations: Historical trauma, harm and healing. *Ethnicity & Health*, *26*(2): 280–298. https://doi.org/10.1080/13557858.2018.1495320 (last accessed 1 December 2022).

Gray, C. (1994). *Comic Strip Conversations*. Arlington, TX: Future Horizons.

Huggins, J. E., Grant, T., O'Malley, K., & Streissguth, A. P. (2008). Suicide attempts among adults with fetal alcohol spectrum disorders: Clinical considerations. *Mental Health Aspects of Developmental Disabilities*, *11*(2): 33–41. https://doi.org/10.1177/07067437211053288 (last accessed 28 November 2022).

Josefi, O., & Ryan, V. (2004). Non-directive play therapy for young children with autism: A case study. *Clinical Child Psychology and Psychiatry*, *9*(4): 533–551. https://doi.org/10.1177/1359104504046158 (last accessed 17 November 2022).

Lange, S., Probst, C., Gmel, G., Rhem, J., Burd, L., & Popova, S. (2017). Global prevalence of fetal alcohol spectrum disorder among children and youth: A systematic review and meta-analysis. *JAMA Pediatrics*, *171*(10): 948–56. https://doi.org/10.1001/jamapediatrics.2017.1919 (last accessed 28 November 2022).

Malbin, D. (2004). Fetal alcohol spectrum disorder (FASD) and the role of family court judges in improving outcomes for children and families. *Juvenile and Family Court Journal*, *55*(2): 53–63. https://doi.org.10.1111/j.1755-6988.2004.tb00161.x (last accessed 28 November 2022).

Malbin, D. (2017). *Trying Differently Rather Than Trying Harder* (3rd ed.). Portland, OR: FASCETS.

McAndrew, F., Thompson, J., Fellows, L., Large, A., Speed, M., & Renfrew, M. J. (2010). *Infant Feeding Survey*. Health and Social Care Information Centre, Leeds, 2012.

Mukherjee, R., Penny, A., Cook, S. H., Norgate, A., & Price, A. D. (2019). Neurodevelopmental outcomes in individuals with fetal alcohol spectrum disorder (FASD) with and without exposure to neglect: Clinical cohort data from a national FASD diagnostic clinic. *Alcohol*, *76*: 23–28. https://doi.org/10.1016/j.alcohol.2018.06.002 (last accessed 10 December 2022).

Olson, H. C., & Montague, R. M. (2011). An innovative look at early interventions for children affected by prenatal exposure. In: S. Adubato, & D. Cohen (Eds.), *Prenatal Alcohol Use and FASD: A Model Standard of Diagnosis, Assessment and Multimodal Treatment* (pp. 64–107). Oak Park, IL: Bentham.

Olson, H. C., Jirikowic, T., Kartin, D., & Astley, S. (2007). Responding to the challenge of early intervention for fetal alcohol spectrum disorders. *Infants & Young Children*, 20: 172–189. https://doi.org/10.1097/01.iyc.0000264484.73688.4a (last accessed 28 November 2022).

Popova, S., Lange, S., Shield, K., Mihic, A., Chudley, A. E., Mukherjee, R., Bekmuradov, D., & Rehm, J. (2016). Comorbidity of fetal alcohol spectrum disorder: A systematic review and meta-analysis. *The Lancet*, 387: 978–987. https://doi.org/10.1016/s0140-6736(15)01345-8 (last accessed 10 November 2022).

Price, A. (2019). The impact of traumatic childhood experiences on cognitive and behavioural functioning in children with fetal alcohol spectrum disorders. (Unpublished doctoral thesis.) University of Salford, Salford, UK (last accessed 1 November 2022).

Raphael-Leff, J. (2020). Absolute hospitality and the imagined baby. *The Psychoanalytic Study of the Child*, 73(1): 230–239. https://doi.org/10.1080/00797308.2020.1690906 (last accessed 28 November 2022).

Streissguth, A. P., Bookstein, F. L., Barr, H. M., Sampson, P. D., & O'Malley, J. K. Y. (2004). Risk factors for adverse life outcomes in fetal alcohol syndrome and fetal alcohol effects. *Journal of Developmental & Behavioural Paediatrics*, 25(4): 228–238. https://doi.org/10.1097/00004703-200408000-00002 (last accessed 28 November 2022).

Thorne, J. C. (2010). Tallying reference errors in narratives: Integrative language function, impairment and fetal alcohol spectrum disorders (Unpublished doctoral thesis.) University of Washington, WA: US.

Webster-Stratton, C., Reid, M. J., & Hammond, M. (2004). Treating children with early-conduct problems: Intervention outcomes for parent, child and teacher training. *Journal of Clinical Child & Adolescent Psychology*, 33: 105–124. https://doi.org/10.1207/s15374424jccp3301_11 (last accessed 28 November 2022).

Part IV

Systemic issues and working within systems

CHAPTER 11

An ongoing conversation ... What (really) works in therapeutic residential care?

Kelly Brackett

> *Somehow, we've come to think of the children's home as full of bad children; that's where abuse starts.*
>
> (Lemn Sissay, 2017)

Introduction: a shocking reality

Let us start by facing the reality of health and social outcomes for our looked-after children and care leavers. The cost to them and society is unfathomable.

Looked-after children and care leavers experience significant mental deprivation (Engler, Sarpong, Van Horne, Greeley, & Keefe, 2022; Taylor, Di Folco, & Lou, 2018). This contributes to low academic achievement. The public finance cost of not being in education, employment, or training (NEET) is estimated to be around £56,000 over the working lifetime of each person who has been NEET (Gov.uk, 2012). In higher education, they are more likely to have lower entry qualifications, less likely to get a first- or upper-second-class degree, and less likely to be in full-time work (The National Network for the Education of Care Leavers, 2022).

Daw and Gill for Centrepoint (p. 15) found a quarter of homeless adults were in care, and adult self-harm is four to five times greater for those with a history of care than the general population (DfE, 2015, p. 6). Children leave care unprepared for independence and are vulnerable to exploitation; up to half of adult women engaged in sex work have at some point been in care as a child (Child Exploitation and Online Protection Centre, 2011).

The care-system-to-prison pipeline shows our abject failure towards looked-after children. A DfE review (MacAlister, 2022, p. 145) showed that care leavers make up a quarter of our prison population. Looked-after children are highly vulnerable to exploitation by criminal gangs as they search for a sense of belonging (Ribeiro-Addy, 2021). The operational dynamics of the justice systems disadvantage BAME children (Lammy, 2016, p. 17).

Looked-after children are also vulnerable to wider risk factors that impact on their substance use, such as self-harming behaviour, sexual exploitation, offending, or domestic abuse (Public Health England, 2021).

Looked-after children going missing from care are among those at highest risk. In 2020, some 3,033 looked-after children were identified by local authorities as being exploited. Of these children, 1,468 went missing—almost half (48%). The scale of exploited children going missing from local authority care is exceptionally high (Missing People & ECPAT UK, 2022).

Looked-after children are at a high risk of teenage pregnancy, which significantly increases intergenerational trauma (Fallon & Broadhurst, 2015).

Social care review

> *Our children's social care system is a 30-year-old tower of Jenga held together with Sellotape: simultaneously rigid and yet shaky.*
> (MacAlister, 2021)

Josh MacAlister's 2022 Social Care Review ("Review" hereafter) magnifies the fault lines in therapeutic residential care (Conway, 2009) and the state of the sector's political and social landscape. It captures a tidal wave of urgency, desperation, and the inequalities that children face. There is a call to wake up to the children's health and social care crisis (Lee-Izu & Perry, 2022, pp. 44–48).

MacAlister (2022) recommends "[i]mplementation governance and support" and recognises that "[s]ound policy too often falls down at implementation" (p. 238). He acknowledges that "[d]elivering this level of transformation within an already overwhelmed system will require excellent planning, long term investment in future models of care, and dedicated leadership" (p. 123). I agree with MacAlister that systemic responsibility lies in a society and culture change; leadership is a key aspect of moving the sector forward (p. 191), relational permanence is a crucial factor, and marketing requires some ethical reflection. However, I propose some caution.

(I refer to "looked-after children" as "children" hereafter.)

Direction

My MA research in 2020 focused on these key questions: What is "therapeutic" in, and of, therapeutic residential care (TRC)? What are the "active ingredients" and "glue" (Whittaker, del Valle, & Holmes, 2015, p. 332) that bind and underpin TRC, and how does it serve children and young people? (Brackett, 2020).

I discuss "organisational readiness" as an ethical responsibility for TRC to improve outcomes. There was a dearth of literature on leadership in TRC, yet leadership provides psychological safety and governance structure—the containment. Traditional leadership models that are visionary, transactional, and transformational limit the depth required to reach the complexity and pain of human behaviour in this field; they home in on "soft-skills". They do not break through to the "hate in the counter-transference" (Winnicott, 1949) that lives in re-enacting cultures which contain elevated levels of trauma and anxiety. A deeper layer of complexity is needed.

Dr Simon Western's "psychosocial influencing dynamic" model is, I propose, the ideal model of leadership, both in TRC and sociopolitically in the sector (2008, p. 36). The *psycho*dynamics of leadership and interrelational dynamics are within and between us, emotionally driven both consciously and unconsciously. *Social* dynamics influence how power and authority are socially constructed (material and symbolic resources, discourses, history, culture, and politics). *Influencing* leadership draws on vast resources to influence, from personality to coercive power. *Dynamic* leadership captures the movement of leadership in its fluidity that cannot be reduced to skills, competencies, or a way of being, but more rhythmic dynamic social processes.

The sector requires this sophistication of leadership that can embrace complexity to avoid *repetition of the same thinking* that exists in these spaces. Western's insight completes my research and provides hope in the face of desperation. Through his lens, I can look *through* my eyes, not *with* them, and observe the patterns of politics, education, and power (Bateson, n.d. 2019, 28:09–38:08). To avoid repetition, we must know our ontological patterning of what we have come to think we know.

The complexity of how we care requires new thought about thinking (Arendt, 1978) to build an effective road out of the chaos. Haraway (Haraway & Latour, 2020, 44:38) reminds us that care is closely wrapped up with control and *both* are needed; control is not a bad word. Care derives from the Latin root word *curare* meaning both poison and remedy. Our social care practices are not some kind of sentimentalised "being nice". To "live in caring" involves being in the thick of contradiction. Through Western's (2008; 2012; 2015) "five frames" of leadership and coaching, I propose questions that may challenge organisations.

Guided by a deep conviction, a longing for change, and hope, I draw my inspiration from the children who continuously teach us. They show us: "I AM HERE. I AM ALIVE!" albeit through despairing and pain-based behaviour. I see Winnicottian (1971, pp. 216–218) hope. The hopeless child, masked as compliant (Winnicott, 1960b), concerns me deeply. Like Havel (1991, pp. 181–182), my hope is not optimism but an "orientation of the spirit, an orientation of the heart".

I also see the child's uncelebrated creativity and heroism. Sissay (2012, 00:55) recognises why authors tell stories through the lens of children in, or raised in, care. Take Harry Potter; Pip from *Great Expectations*; Superman; Cinderella; Lisbeth Salander in *The Girl with the Dragon Tattoo*; Batman; Roald Dahl's *James and the Giant Peach*; and more. Do the haunting statistics mentioned cloud our ability to see children's uniquely patterned minds and extraordinary skills? Sissay (2017) reminds us to wake up to counteract the "bad" narrative (unconscious bias) that children's homes are full of bad children.

This abuse must end with us.

Therapeutic residential care (TRC)

The DfE (2019, pp. 4–6) describes a child looked after (under the age of eighteen) as accommodated or looked after by a local authority, which holds parental responsibility. Most of these children were looked after due to abuse or neglect. In 2022, the DfE reported that the number of children looked after by local authorities in England rose to 82,170, up 2 per cent on the previous year and continuing the rise seen in recent years. Figures were likely impacted by the pandemic (DfE, 2022).

There has been a steady increase in the provision of private sector TRC homes in the UK, which have taken varied forms, many employing (or buying in) clinical teams for a therapeutic provision. Most are eclectic in nature (Eclectic-TRC), and some evolved from a therapeutic community (TC) model (see https://therapeuticcommunities.org/ for more information on TCs including research, Haigh [2013] pp. 6–15 for examples of TCs' therapeutic environments, and Tomlinson [2021] for therapeutic model development).

Neglect and abuse inhibit the growth of a social and emotional developing mind, self, psyche, and hence, potentiality (Eluvathingal et al., 2006). Children arrive with fragmented developmental structures and depend upon the care from decision-makers and their carers to intervene and support healthy development. These early complex experiences include prenatal influences, early interpersonal trauma involving the primary caregiving relationships, disturbed and disrupted attachment relationships, and other significant losses. Adverse environmental experiences create a complex constellation of symptoms and a pervasive impact on development that is difficult to categorise. The DSM-5 inadequately captures the range and type of psychopathology seen in looked-after children in diagnoses such as quasi-autism, reactive attachment disorder, and complex trauma (DeJong, 2010).

Expectations

This work is not for the faint-hearted. Children view themselves, others, and their environments through insecure internal working models (Bowlby, 1988) and live in a state of survival. They rely on defences to avoid thinking, feeling, and remembering. Their trauma-bodies and nervous systems express ever-present memories (Porges, 2007; Van der Kolk, 2014). Their behaviours communicate "I'M HURTING", until they come to experience genuine safety and containment and develop relational "epistemic trust" (Csibra & Gergely, 2009, pp. 148–153). Survival behaviours include physical aggression, damage to property, absconding, extreme risk-taking, significant self-harm, dissociation, and/or suicidal ideation or intent. These require trauma-responsivity and emotional resiliency.

In my work, I became enmeshed and entangled in a complex system of mess, chaos, relational dynamics, culture, systems, policies, procedures, regulations, and external influences. I managed projections from desperate staff to "fix" the child, followed by their disillusionment and frustration that therapeutic "magic" could not provide a quick fix. I had good intentions, but it was difficult to hold the child in mind. I asked: Who is my client?

The child in the system

When reviewing "promising programme models and innovative practices" in TRC, Whittaker (Whittaker, del Valle, & Holmes, 2015, p. 332) describes that when the components are taken together, they intensify the search for "active ingredients" that are necessary, sufficient, and the "glue" that holds these components together to achieve desirable outcomes for children in TRC.

The "therapeutic" consensus includes a "purposely constructed multi-dimensional environment" in which to structure, "provide treatment, socialisation, support, and protection", and improve children's mental health in collaboration with their families and community (Whittaker, del Valle, & Holmes, 2015, p. 24).

My main findings demonstrated that "organisational readiness" is the glue binding all therapeutic work that leads to improved outcomes for the child, and hence an ethical requirement of TRC. Eclectic-TRCs can learn from TCs to understand the essential qualities and foundations embedded in the psychoanalytically informed milieu. The evidence-based models or active ingredients in (re)designed TRC act as an enabler for trauma-informed therapeutic relationships (the glue).

Eclectic-TRC is supported by an integrative therapeutic approach with a psychoanalytic foundation. The macro-level glue (i.e. political/social/cultural aspects) requires urgent attention; TRC's professional status should be raised, children's voices need amplifying, and unconscious bias needs to be explored.

The organisation ("Org") and organisational readiness

When considering Org as my client, I ask myself the following questions: What kind of caregiver and provider is Org? How might I support Org as my client? What feelings arise in me? What relational patterns emerge? Can Org look inward and outward, stay with difficult feelings, and develop an emotional language that expresses the reality of the trauma Org contains? Will my client and I remain "task focused" (Bion, 1961)? And perhaps most importantly, what are Org's blocks to seeing the child?

Organisational readiness is an ethical thread through six key areas of Org's personality that require reflection and attention, in which Org may come to a place of readiness for achieving outcomes for the children in Org's care. The six key areas are:

1. The child
2. Staff/carers
3. Models of care
4. Therapeutic interventions and psychoeducation
5. Culture/climate
6. Leadership

What follows are perspectives of these six key areas, taken as though Org were an individual or a one-to-one client.

The child: what the child may need, imagined in the child's voice

Be responsible for me. I ask the sector and Org to communicate more effectively. Share your good practice, and develop systematic ways of seeking, recording, and analysing my views and experiences, including how they change over time (The Children's Commissioner, 2017). I need high-quality assurance to help improve my life in TRC (Lyman & Wilson, 1992, in Brady & Caraway, 2002; The Children's Commissioner, 2017).

Everyone involved with my care and decisions for my life, please understand the impact of trauma and be my cortex when I experience limbic hijacking. Sequentially Regulate, Relate, and Reason with me (Perry, 2020). See my relational challenge and symptoms of PTSD (i.e. numbing). Depression and fear increase when I lose agency with my future plans (Brady & Caraway, 2002).

I need a person, not a staff member. Please better understand the importance of my need for relationship. Carers are an essential therapeutic resource for my well-being and improved interrelational skills. I want to feel wanted by forgiving carers who want to be there; a sense of belonging; and a freedom to be myself. Train and emotionally support my carers; this predetermines my continued sense of belonging during and beyond TRC (Carter, 2011). I need empathy, availability, sensitive listening, reliability, honesty, and resilience (Harder, Knorth, & Kalverboer, 2017), and for my carers to survive my trauma and forceful and destructive emotions because I blame myself as I "fail up" (Stuck, Small, & Ainsworth, 2000) to TRC (Brady & Caraway, 2002).

Do you *really* understand loss? When I change placements, I feel sadness, anger, disappointment, stress, weariness, loneliness, and loss of connection (family, siblings, friends). Professional counselling supports me through changes, and more one-to-one time with adults would support my feeling of loneliness. Changing schools is emotionally challenging and distressing, and the changeover of social workers decreases trust and causes apathy. I get feelings of rejection and destabilisation; it is traumatic to repeat my past. I want transparency and a chance to say goodbye, a safe space for a meeting (home), a crossover of old/new social workers to ease the process, and the new social worker to be well-informed. Having a constant professional makes it easier to adapt (a teacher, an Independent Reviewing Officer, or a counsellor) (The Children's Commissioner, 2019). Without understanding loss and how your systemic responses and policies interrupt my relational permanence, you paradoxically perpetuate trauma in your attempt to treat it! My voice needs to be heard and prioritised.

I am less interested in (or unaware of) techniques/models you use, and more interested in relationship-based practice. I am dependent upon Org's readiness and devotion to teach my carers and emotionally contain them because they are my **key objects** of growth (Harder, Knorth, & Kalverboer, 2017; Carter, 2011). Your (re)designed models enable trauma-informed relationships. Even better is when you provide a therapeutic community for me that understands my relationship with the whole system, and here I live and learn in open communication with my carers (Bloom & Sreedhar, 2008; Haigh, 2013; McLoughlin & Gonzalez, 2014; Price et al., 2018; Rose, 2002; Whitwell, 2002), as these provide what I missed in my early development ("secondary emotional development", Haigh, 2013, p. 6).

Staff/carers: perspectives on therapeutic residential care, imagined in the carer's voice

We share/parallel the child's feelings (mentioned above). Eclectic-TRC, please take better care of our mental and emotional needs because the children depend on us, and we depend on our leaders, managers, and Org. We need to be the village to raise the children.

We often feel ill-equipped. Children's needs are understandably complex and challenging. We need more training than a Level 3 Diploma in Residential Childcare; we need there to be a minimum training standard agreed across the UK (Narey, 2016). You, Org, are responsible for selecting staff with emotional sophistication, training, support, and managerial fidelity (including in models/approaches). We experience trauma, burnout, resilience, and loss of self-agency, and rely on coping and/or survival strategies. We feel alone, a loss of control, emotional detachment, and blame culture. We require regular supervision and reflective practice, team consultation, training (including managers), shared risk-planning, and to understand how to care for ourselves and each other (Carter, 2011; Brown, Chadwick, Caygill, & Powell, 2019; Steckley, 2012; Graham & Killick, 2019; Harder, Knorth, & Kalverboer, 2017). Training alone is not enough; we benefit from a reflective space to think about the children and explore how we cope because a high staff turnover means further loss for the child.

As trauma-informed carers, we create a sense of safety for children. Children feel emotionally contained, known, and held in mind by us through their ongoing challenges and the distress caused by transitions, loss, and trauma, and their outcomes are better (Izzo, Smith, Sellers, Holden, & Nunno, 2020). Containing and psychologically holding relationships (glue), before the model or treatment (active ingredient), enable us to create the right environment (Andersson & Johansson, 2008).

Models of care: the identity of Org, and the ontology of TRC that Org has emerged from

There are differences geographically and culturally. Nordic countries such as Denmark, Norway, Finland, and Sweden, the UK, and the United States share similarities and differences, yet cross-national collaboration is closing the gap. The variation of evidence-based (re)designed TRC models was created to respond to children's complex needs in the socially constructed living environment (Cameron & Das, 2019; Izzo et al., 2020; Nordoff & Madoc-Jones, 2014).

Understanding the model is essential. The model is Org's heartbeat, which enables the trauma-informed relationships that facilitate the reparation of trauma. Principally, models grounded in a relational and/or organisational approach, such as CARE (Izzo, Smith, Sellers, Holden, & Nunno, 2020) or Sanctuary (Bloom & Sreedhar, 2008; Rivard et al., 2004) held weight in my findings. However, like many models, they lack attachment and trauma psychoeducation and clinical assessment.

TCs: the embedded milieu *is* the model. Originally rooted in psychoanalysis, the milieu and therapy are joined up. TC provides a primary developmental experience that children have lacked in their early lives, and this is the heart of the milieu. Winnicott's "potential space" (Winnicott, 1960a, p. 43) is the metaphorical space between the infant and mother, creating learning for them both; therefore, this psychic space is at the heart of the milieu (Whiteley, 2004). Children are supported to attach to the community. Staff selection is crucial for awareness and understanding of transference and countertransference because children with trauma are experts at pressing carers' buttons (Whitwell, 2002). Sensitive leadership and management (including awareness of the danger of misinterpreting one's own countertransference), and staff encouragement and involvement, are fundamental and a multilayered feature of the ethos of a therapeutic community and milieu. TCs can be perceived as inward-looking and mysterious and are difficult to measure because the psychoanalytic foundations are embedded into the fabric.

Social pedagogy (SP): macro, micro, and culture. There are stark differences between Nordic and UK social pedagogy in how society views and treats looked-after children. In the UK, the system is the place for the problem child, and neither the child nor the sector is embraced by the heart of society. Unconscious bias in society leads to petitions being signed to keep TRC homes off local streets by the same people who donate to charities afar. Here the ego splits off (Klein, 1946) from the painful reality of trauma up close, and instead guilt may be consoled through an act of charitable kindness.

We can learn from Nordic countries if we know their ontology. Adopting a model by removing a complex adaptive system and placing it into another does not work. SP stems from complex philosophical origins that lead to a "child-friendly" (Timonen-Kallio & Hämäläinen, 2019) culture and climate. In the UK, silo behaviour enables the enigmatic Org to avoid networking, and therein lies an undertone of possession of the child; therefore, shared responsibility no longer lives in a social network ("our child" becomes "Org's child").

Unlike the UK, a Nordic social pedagogue holds a higher level of qualification and works systemically around the child's community and in direct relationship with the child (personal and professional role). The UK lacks trained professionals to think and behave in networked patterns, to bring the child, TRC, and the sector towards social identity and socially competent members of society.

(Re)designed models. From the further (re)designed models, my findings reiterated Macdonald and Millen's (2012, pp. 34–46)—that (re)designed models offer TRC and all staff a framework and **shared**

language that is crucial to think about their work, self-awareness/reflection, improved practice and responses to their own and children's behaviour, improved job satisfaction, insight and skill, and consistency within the team. The limitations and concerns suggest that at best, models provide a theory of change; complex systems vs complex interventions, possible misuse of power within Org, and the hurdle of waiting for organisational readiness all present complexities around the model that mean the model itself is not the glue, it is an active ingredient.

Therapeutic interventions and psychoeducation: key considerations

Therapeutic interventions are more effective when the therapist works **not solely with the child, but also the system**, the milieu, and the supporting relationships. Therapeutic evidence-based interventions (i.e. TF-CBT, EMDR) appear effective in clinical settings, but less promising with children in TRC (Cohen et al., 2016: Greenwald et al., 2012) unless the system and supportive relationships are incorporated. Otherwise, there is little difference in the varied therapies (i.e. CBT, psychodynamic) (Carr, 2008; Weisz, McCarty, & Valeri, 2006; Kelley, Bickman, & Norwood, 2010) unless organisational readiness is thoroughly addressed, often with costly training (Cohen & Mannerino, 2008) and high investment in train-the-trainer approaches (Hambrick et al., 2018).

Complications can also arise, including culture and climate, fidelity, buy-in, and risk aversity blocking access to therapy. Success is dependent upon a therapist's ability to work systemically around the child in a stable, validating, trauma-informed system that can explore underlying reasons for behaviour rather than simply managing it. This reduces restraints and critical incidents, and empowers staff to be proactive rather than reactive, encompassing the other twenty-three hours of the day when the child isn't in therapy as an assimilative, embedded model of care.

Complimenting the (re)designed model is the background work of **integrative psychotherapy**, the intensive intervention. It is most effective and most sustainable if the system around the child does not become vicariously traumatised.

Psychoeducation. The train-the-trainer approach supports embedding a theoretically grounded (re)designed model, which avoids clinical terminology, with relationship-focused reflective practice. Key themes are complex trauma (seven domains) and ACEs, a neurosequential model, behaviour as a function of communication, polyvagal theory, dissociation, attachment, psychoanalytical defences, transference and countertransference, PACE, blocked care, vicarious trauma, self-care, therapeutic parenting, shame, food and nurture, loss, and neurodiversity.

The evidence base. TRC has an ethical responsibility to the children it serves to support **growing research** (i.e. university partnerships), otherwise business-as-usual focuses on profit and staffing (ratio rather than training and support). However, this warrants mindful attention to the nuanced relational, theoretical, and systemic influences; better creative, innovative measuring is required. The glue remains in the power of trauma-informed relationships and their healing quality. Understanding the therapeutic milieu vs manualised treatments can be complex when there are many systemic influences. Pressure to demonstrate evidence for funding dominates. There are cross-national concerns that an empirical "medical model" aims to treat but does not "contextualise" the human experience (Wampold & Imel, 2015), that arrogance can be displayed over one model for another, impacting the "spirit of science", leading to "power politics", and that research methodologies become "self-fulfilling prophecies" and "marketing"-focused (Wachtel, 2016: 24:28–27:38). Fonagy (2010, p. 84), however, encourages the psychodynamic field to use more rigorous specified therapeutic methods.

The evidence base race pervades the mental health space and TRC. While there are excelling examples of Eclectic-TRC, the lack of inward reflection (organisational readiness) limits its ability to recognise itself, losing a psychic space for essential psychotherapeutic reverie. Research, therefore, provides an active ingredient.

Climate/culture: systems and group dynamics

Bloom and Farragher (2011) highlight risks of **trauma re-enactment** in the uninformed and uncontained Org. TCs and (re)designed models that include group dynamics understand the necessity of clinical consultation or coaching to strengthen these foundations.

The alexithymic Org (Bloom & Farragher, 2011, pp. 259–261) is unable to talk about the issues that remain unsolvable. Org's chronic stress and destructive processes mirror or parallel the children's processes. Managerial failure to recognise the importance of these qualities can cause unhealthy, toxic environments (Haigh, 2013, p. 6) and abuse enquiries where "charismatic leaders are somewhat suspect for demanding collusive loyalty" (Whitwell, 2002, p. 8).

Finally, **grief and traumatic loss become commonplace.** Staff can feel increasingly angry, demoralised, helpless, and hopeless about the children they are working to serve, and they become burned out, hence the need for sophisticated and organisationally structured clinical supervision (consultancy, coaching, staff support, specialist training, team processes) (Rose, 2002; Collie, 2008; Whitwell, 2002). Bion's (1961) group dynamic theory supports the understanding of "dependency, fight or flight, and pairing" as survival mechanisms in action. Menzies-Lyth (1960) introduced staff "defences against anxiety".

Trauma lies in the fabric of Org's life and is to be expected. Support alone is not the answer, but containment is the focus, and Org's design is responsible for providing effective containment for staff anxieties. Organisational readiness ethically holds culture and climate in its structural design, a foundation for the "purposely constructed multi-dimensional environment" to structure and "provide treatment, socialisation, support, and protection" (Whittaker, del Valle, & Holmes, 2015, p. 24).

Leadership

Here lies the void.

Systems within systems: combining the sociopolitical factors

Certain questions arise when reflecting upon Org (TRC). Has Org (TRC) lost the meaningful roots from which the therapeutic shoots and growth emerge, limiting the rich embodiment and narrative of TRC? Is Org acting out in the wider transference, the instant gratification race for the gold medal of randomised controlled trials (RCT) over a longer-term care model with high efficacy for looked-after children? Does Org struggle to look inwards where internal (unconscious) conflicts lie dormant and hidden? Is it possible to "link" (Bion, 1962, pp. 58–60) feeling and thinking, in which to know oneself, develop some resilience and tolerance for discomfort (being the human condition Org holds), and develop ego-strength and reflective qualities (organisational readiness) to reduce reactivity? Can Org and the private sector look at the internalised authority parent of the political economy? Where are the institutional power dynamics in the commodified wider family system?

Conway indicates that well-intentioned policy will always be at risk of breaking down at vulnerable "fault lines" (2009, p. 18) in the system, with children's needs falling into the gaps if we fail to extend psychoanalytical awareness to systemic behaviour. On reflection of governmental policies, and analysing gaps in communication, Conway finds splits, divisions, rivalries, and a failure to communicate within and between services for vulnerable children. Conway refers to a pervasive blame culture and abundant complaints.

Org and its private sector family risk becoming a dysfunctional family laced with insidious systemic trauma and messy communication.

Post research: has profit become a dirty word?

The learning is painfully slow, and repetitious cycles continue. Josh MacAlister's (2022) Review magnifies TRC's "fault lines" (Conway, 2009) and the state of the sector and the political and social landscape. Stanley (2022) highlighted MacAlister's (2021) "case for change" as the need to address relational permanence for children, better access to education, and a societal shared responsibility for the looked-after child. MacAlister recognised these problems and recommendations for change have been longstanding. Achieving change has proved "stubbornly difficult", the conversation will cause "tensions", and "debates" may be "uncomfortable for many working in the system", such as changing the "profit path" (MacAlister, 2021).

My concern is that of blind repetition, albeit with good intention: focusing on the right areas (profit and leadership) but in the wrong way.

An integrative, assimilative, and systemic lens is crucial, and possibly not enough!

Feinstein et al. (2022), as members of the Review group, share their reflections on the risks of "reforming in haste and repenting at leisure", echoing the call for change with caution. They offer some constructive perspectives on the evidence base underpinning the Review's recommendations:

- This is not a systematic review of all research evidence but a framework for policy and practice reform. They refer to wider "evidence" of interdependencies, crucial to avoid unintended consequences. There is limited evidence in the new leadership proposed (Regional Care Cooperatives) that may hinder current mechanisms, while pressures build to "reform" to manage "marketing". Caution lies in this becoming an expensive distraction (as seen in the NHS reform).
- There are power imbalances in the system. A focus towards family support in line with the Children's Act is required. Evidence lies in the socio-economic drivers associated with family involvement in child protection services.
- Control, support, and care are not separate. Early years support is fundamental.
- Skilled, knowledgeable practitioners are essential to a functioning system. The proposed Early Career Framework (care workers, social workers) is welcome, but with warning that this does not have the research backing. Training has limited impact on practice without understanding the organisational context and climate. Power and influence lie in supervision, leadership, and culture.
- There is concern around the political longevity and sustainability required for whole-systems change. Attention to the wider interdependencies avoids risking fragmenting the system further. Government must act as a whole system itself if it desires system change for children and families; this requires government departments to share ownership of complex and intersecting social issues and ensure the wider infrastructure which supports family life does not decline further.
- Equality and attention to rights is essential. Those who experience social care services are marginalised and scrutinised in society, their

voices go underheard, and they experience an overuse of surveillance with not enough support. Ethical data control is required.
- Before the Review's recommendations are executed, it is essential to understand research on the implementation of policies and practices within health systems. Trusting relationships that are empathic, authentic, and collaborative are key to effective implementation.
- Government must position itself as an enabler to the sector in humility and collaboration. Policy reform needs more than passion; critical thinking, skill, and judicious use of evidence are also required. It should be "done with" and not "done to" those it is seeking to influence.

The media took the ethical and moral debate around the system outside of the sector and into society, homes, and hearts. The emotive narrative sparked an emotive response, such as in Michael Sheen's BBC Wales documentary *Lifting the Lid on the Care System* (2022), which "[I]nvestigates ... a shocking insight into the lives of young people in care who say they were put at serious risk by the very system meant to protect them".

Attention to the huge profits made from young people's inadequate care thankfully led to tighter regulations. This implicitly suggested that all TRC follows an immoral path. The Welsh government (2022) leaped into "Proposed changes to primary legislation in relation to social care and continuing NHS Healthcare" (p. 1), a reactive policy to "eliminate profit" in an attempt to eliminate the problem. The Children's Homes Association (CHA) provided a collective response from its members and providers in the sector. Sandiford (2022) explained the policy:

> [F]ocuses on delivery models and their governance, not child focused outcomes to support and protect vulnerable children and develop social value and increased prosperity ... [and has] flaws incapable of remedy. (p. 4)

Sandiford's concerns include diminishing the availability of TRC for vulnerable children who need it, challenge to recruitment and staffing, and loss of expertise and knowledge in a vulnerable sector. Another reactive policy hindering outcomes. Is this the "Re-thinking" that Org, Org's family, and the village will benefit from?

Reactivity as a defence blocks thinking, reflection, and the unbearable feeling (Freud, 1923b). The feeling is split off (Klein, 1946) and projected into the bad-Other with black and white thinking. The emotional neurological limbic response lacks the thoughtful cortex reflection required for problem-solving. Failing to feel the discomfort required to live in the contradiction of caring fails to place the child at the centre and "model the model" (Treisman, 2021, p. 62). Where is the effective leadership? Western's (2015) strategic frame explores emotions to thinking and thinking to action. Bypassing thinking leads to reactive solutions.

The CHA (2022, p. 12) suggests an "outcomes focused approach" to eliminate excessive profit that seeks to advance the sector and represent social value, work with local authorities, and achieve a resilient marketplace. If profit ethics are present, what led to excess?

Children deserve more than pragmatism and reactivity. Repetitious thought patterns create the same well-intended efforts, funding, projects, and idealistic "visionary" characters on a familiar road of old knowledge. Different epistemologies and ontologies are required to avoid the "noise" of "knowledge" to "penetrate through to the wisdom" (Bion, 1978, 24:14).

How has Org come to look away, and why the lure towards "excessive" profit? How emotionally containing has the market been while Org holds trauma, "survives", and "competes"?

New leadership: ways forward

Change is only possible when essential questions are identified. Through Western's five frames (depth analysis, relational analysis, leadership analysis, network analysis, and strategic analysis), I offer a road map of thought-signposts to Org. If Org is ready and willing to bear discomfort, some deeply meaningful work may be achieved. In a contained space, curiosity is the antidote of blame to really think. These frames are fluid and adaptive, they would cross over in natural conversation, and they are not linear or prescriptive.

Depth analysis

Org, what is your "symptom"? Why have profit and money become the issue? What does it signify through unconscious desire (Lacan, 1994)? Why might this be attractive? Like the carers' painful feelings paralleled the children's, is this a symptom of the family village? Is there a shared felt sense of worthlessness, lack of "value", and emptiness (trauma in the system) that not only contributes to these splits, divides, and rivalries, but also attempts to self-soothe, to fill up our cavities with smoke, food, and consumerism (money)? Winnicott (1971, pp. 216–218) reminds us that feelings of deprivation may lead to feeling owed and entitled to "take" something from the environment.

Have you internalised an affectless parent (Alvarez, 2012, pp. 11–25), feeling empty and worthless, and what might this say about the wider village (society)? In *The Selfish Society*, Gerhardt (2010) says "We All Forgot to Love One Another and Made Money Instead". Can you see beyond the money you make to the money wasted? The current cost of children's social care is £10 billion per year (Maskell, 2022). Org, can you bear the discomfort, stretch your "window of tolerance", regulate your nervous system, and avoid reactive instant gratification; the "solution"? Are you entrapped in the pleasure of the pain (Lacan, 1992)? How might we put your symptom to work (Freud, 1930a) for the sake of staying with the task ahead? Can you imagine reconnecting with meaning and purpose in your work, feeling reward in relational connections with the children and carers (all staff), rather than the external object—the "big-Other" (Lacan, 1994)?

Signpost: What is being "filled"? Identify your symptom.

Relational analysis

Org, what is the picture of your relational dynamics (inside and out, teams, family, friends, authority figures, social groups, and distinct roles)? What might you be carrying on behalf of these? What presents for us? Do these patterns feel familiar to you?

Cybernetics is concerned with the way things work, symbiosis, interdependence and interconnectedness (not just technology)

(M. Bateson, 2014). We need to bring disciplines together to meet the complexity of the systems. The sector and society assume competition, and here lies the problem: how do we reverse the patriarchal conversation (transference) from "go get" and "achieve" to "gather together in support and shared responsibility"? This is where we are, entrapped in familiar scripts. Genuine generosity is required, not altruism, starting by showing up and paying attention.

How might you unravel from the unhealthy relationships and patterns and move closer to those who will strengthen you? What are your desires? Where might change be possible?

How might you creatively celebrate the remarkable children in your care and support them to tell their stories, to be witnessed? Can you enlighten society to the richness of these incredible children (confidentially) and the power of the relationships of TRC? How might you bring success stories to support children to imagine their future selves (Cherry, 2022)?

Signpost: Identify unhealthy patterns. Where is the richness? How can you celebrate and educate?

Leadership analysis

Org, what is your leadership style (and those dominant inside and outside of you)? Where do you lead and follow? How do personality and context (over competency) help you take up authority and power?

Controller leadership

Org, are you transactional? Do you lean on science and rationality? Numbers, audits, and measuring culture (algorithms), management control systems, and performance outcomes are helpful and necessary. Can your assessments inform you while you remain in the spirit of the nuanced, contextual, complex, less measurable contributing factors to human life? Are you a complex self-regulating system or cogs of a machine?

Signpost: How might your "Quantifiable Self" (Western, 2019, p. 180) (graphs/charts/percentages) talk to your "creative self" (celebrating/

expressing diversity) with reverie and human concern? Are the children visible or "heads on beds" and a means to an end: profit?

Therapist leadership

Org, how do you embrace relationships, humanise, democratise, create participation? Can you describe your philosophy, vision, values, ethics, and culture? Can you assimilate therapeutic practice, hold reflective practice spaces, support staff teams, and manage defences and team dynamics? Are you leaning too heavily on "motivational management" through measuring (happiness surveys) as quick-fix emotional tools (solution focus) to avoid the messy feelings?

Signpost: Pathologise cautiously and notice dependencies.

Messiah leadership

Org, can you explore your charismatic "transformational" and visionary self and strong culture? Can you see the "idealized transference" (Coopey, 1995, p. 207) in your loyal followers, who may become dependent? Is your monoculture open or silencing to challenging questions? What is your unconscious desire? (To fill a lack?)

Signpost: Can you think about corporate culture, corporate parenting, power, and reinvestment and redistribution? Can you guide and be guided by your followers?

Eco-leadership

Org, do you identify with your ethical mind? Who and what are you connected to and dependent upon as "eco-systems within eco-systems" (Western, 2019, p. 259)? Can you shift from hierarchy towards emergence, organic growth, and strategic planning and influence change through devolved power?

Where is your human spirit beyond material gain, and meaningful/kinship connections (partnerships, consortiums, communities, creativity, and imagination)? Can you reclaim collective wisdom from unusual places?

Signpost: To be a part of a principle-based society, how can you put people before profit (then profit will return)?

Network analysis

Org, where does power lie in your connections, nodal points, and clusters? How would you describe your internal family or external village? Can we empower and reveal opportunities for influence and change? Whose voices are heard and silenced? Can we look differently at the "network"?

Clearly, a shared language and cross-disciplinary knowledge is crucial for a thread of connection to hold the child in mind, to create a "net-that-might-work".

The antidote to projection is to look closely at ourselves with self-compassion, humility, and curiosity, to learn how we play a key role in perpetuating the existence of what we hope to change. "Moral capitalism" is to look beyond shareholder value (Krantz, 2021, 27:11).

Signpost: Org, can you identify and locate your discomfort and where you take psychic flight? Is there real worth and value there, and where else might it be? Do you "full-fill" or want to be fulfilled? Where do you experience connection, love (oxytocin), reward (serotonin), and joy (dopamine)? How do you handle money (hoarding, redistribution)? How do you value values? Where is true richness celebrated?

Strategic analysis

What is needed in creating an intentional and emergent strategy, following on from the Review? You have an ethical responsibility to understand the leadership that is required to "know yourself", Org, and the characters you grow within you. Alongside this, you also grow your identity, purpose, and meaning. But this is only achievable if you and your conscious leaders reciprocate commitment and responsibility to each other in relatedness. The following are some suggestions to consider.

What follows are strategy perspectives on the wider system.

What: Government to model the model—review the Review:

- Governmental departments to align and connect with essential voices within the network *before* implementing the Review's recommendations and review the "re-think".
- Review these against evidenced-based research and representatives for the child (and care-experienced adults), carers, TRC organisations, psycho/education, mental health (all disciplines), early years, LA (Child in Need and Child Protection) and "actors" (Latour, 2005) (technology, media platforms, social movements, creative arts, etc.).
- Enable trauma-informed relationships to improve outcomes for children (and future generations). Model the regulation of reactive impulses, relating through a shared language, and reason and reflect on the evidence base and systemic interdependencies with experts from all departments.

How: Steering committee to hurry slowly:

- A round table in which power is distributed and where a *shared responsibility* for the child can emerge.

What: Sector to model the model:

- Address splits, silos, defences, competition, and ethics and explore how these impact our ability to recognise our interdependence and interrelatedness and hence, responsibility to each other on behalf of the child in our care.

How: Connecting spaces:

- A regulated commitment to social and professional spaces or a community of communities, essential for strengthening good relations and connectivity. Modelling a psychologically held and contained system that embraces all TRC organisations to influence a healthy culture.

What: Raise the generic standard of TRC:

- Allow room for variation and specificity of TRC to meet children's varying needs. Identify a core ethical, evidence-based standard to be met across all TRC to instil confidence and restore (epistemic) trust in a (parental) system of "care" ethics, allowing for complexities, contradiction, and control where required.

How: Rigorous review of organisational readiness, a policy of system guidelines:

- Evidence Org's responsibility to: child, staff/carers, models, therapeutic interventions (trauma-informed) and psychoeducation, culture/climate, and leadership. Identify gaps and seek support.

What: University and TRC partnerships:

- Explore gaps in research that bridge mental health, leadership, systems, and transdisciplinary thought to embrace complexity and systems.

How: Guided by the evidence, or lack thereof:

- Establish where to pitch training courses from identified gaps.
- Include contextualised research methods.

What: Eco-leadership to embrace social movements via networks:

- To inspire, educate, and embrace the heart of communities/society via all mediums to better understand the child in care, the complexity of trauma, induce relational value, worth, enjoyment, connectivity, community and hence, pride and a shared responsibility.

How: Connecting clusters and nodes and creative spaces and projects that combine:

- Care-experienced voices.
- Artists, poets, the spoken word, drama, music.
- The media's influence of social movements.
- The personal/professional career.
- Inspiration for communities, businesses, and enterprises to support TRC.

What: Profit:

- Moral capitalism.

How: TRC to report on:

- How it reinvests profit to develop social value and increased prosperity for the child.
- How it reinvests a percentage of excess profit to benefit the child's local community to support connectivity in society.
- Joining local organisations in caring for the planet.

Final reflections

Fault lines in the system cannot be ignored. To stop children falling through the gaps, we must first identify the gaps. Change is desired by society, but the complexity of living in caring is contradictory. Human defences take hold, driving a paradoxical, emotionally reactive, unconscious "gaze" of the child in care and care homes themselves. Defences in the sector may cling to an imperfect system, favouring its entrapments above fear of the unknown.

It is time for change. Children call to us. Let us unite in allyship, kinship, and warriorship.

References

Alvarez, A. (2012). *The Thinking Heart: Three Levels of Psychoanalytic Therapy with Disturbed Children*. Hove, UK: Routledge.

Andersson, B., & Johansson, J. (2008). Personal approaches to treatment among staff in residential care: A case study. *Journal of Social Work, 8*(2): 117–134.

Arendt, H. (1978). *The Life of the Mind: The Groundbreaking Investigation on How We Think* (McCarthy, M. Ed.). New York: Harcourt Brace Jovanovich.

Bateson, G. (n.d. 2019). *How We Know What We Know—Part 1—Gregory Bateson*. 13 August 2019. https://youtu.be/D0fR1RGRQsM (last accessed 12 January 2023).

Bateson, M. (2014). *Cybernetics in the Future* (Introduction by Mary Catherine). George Washington University. https://youtu.be/nXQraugWbjQ (last accessed 12 January 2023).

BBC Wales (2022, 11 July). *Michael Sheen: Lifting the Lid on the Care System.* https://www.bbc.co.uk/programmes/m0018vld (last accessed 12 November 2022).

Bion, W. R. (1961). *Experiences in Groups.* London: Tavistock.

Bion, W. R. (1962). *Learning from Experience.* London: Heinemann.

Bion, W. R. (1978). *Tavistock Clinic Seminars*—4/8 1978. https://www.youtube.com/watch?v=kuE_JepuqDwnterpretation (24:14) (last accessed 12 January 2023).

Bloom, S. L., & Farragher, B. (2011). *Destroying Sanctuary: The Crisis in Human Service Delivery Systems.* Oxford: Oxford University Press.

Bloom, S. L., & Sreedhar, S. Y. (2008). The sanctuary model of trauma-informed organizational change. *Reclaiming Children and Youth, 17*(3): 48–53.

Bowlby, J. (1988). *A Secure Base: Parent–Child Attachment and Healthy Human Development.* London: Routledge.

Brackett, K. (2020). What are the "active ingredients" and "glue" (Whittaker et al., 2015: 323) that bind and underpin Therapeutic Residential Care, and how does it serve Looked After Children and Young People? [Unpublished master's. See: https://www.grammarly.com/blog/masters-degree/dissertation]. Terapia, Middlesex University: London.

Brady, K. L. S., & Caraway, J. (2002). Home away from home: Factors associated with current functioning in children living in a residential treatment setting. *Child Abuse & Neglect, 26*(11): 1149–1163. DOI: 10.1016/s0145-2134(02)00389-7

Brown, A. M., Chadwick, R., Caygill, L., & Powell, J. (2019). One moment you're covered in blood and next it's what's for tea? An interpretative phenomenological analysis of residential care staff's experiences of managing self-harm with looked after children. *Scottish Journal of Residential Child Care, 18*(3).

Cameron, R. J. S., & Das, R. K. (2019). Empowering residential carers of looked after young people: The impact of the emotional warmth model of professional childcare. *The British Journal of Social Work, 49*(7): 1893–1912. https://doi.org/10.1093/bjsw/bcy125

Carr, A. (2008). Depression in young people: Description, assessment and evidence-based treatment. *Developmental Neurorehabilitation, 11*(1): 3–15

Carter, J. (2011). Analysing the impact of living in a large-group therapeutic community as a young person—Views of current and ex-residents. A pilot study. *Journal of Social Work Practice*, 25(2): 149–163. https://doi.org/10.1080/02650533.2010.541231 (last accessed 12 November 2022).

CHA (2022). CHA response to Welsh government policy to eliminate profit from the care of looked after children. 01 September. The Children's Homes Association (the-cha.org.uk) (last accessed 13 November 2022).

Cherry, L. (2022). *The Brightness of Stars: Stories from Care Experienced Adults to Inspire Change*. Oxfordshire: Wilson King.

Child Exploitation and Online Protection Centre (2011). Out of mind, out of sight: breaking down the barriers to understanding child sexual exploitation. London: Child Exploitation and Online Protection Centre.

The Children's Commissioner (2017). A rapid review of sources of evidence on the views, experiences and perceptions of children in care and care leavers. https://www.childrenscommissioner.gov.uk/wp-content/uploads/2019/07/cco-childrens-voices-childrens-experiences-of-instability-in-the-care-system-july-2019.pdf (last accessed 18 December 2022).

The Children's Commissioner (2019). Children's voices. Children's experiences of instability in the care system. https://www.childrenscommissioner.gov.uk/wp-content/uploads/2019/07/cco-childrens-voices-childrens-experiences-of-instability-in-the-care-system-july-2019.pdf (last accessed 27 November 2022).

Cohen, J., & Mannarino, A. P. (2008). Disseminating and implementing trauma-focused CBT in community settings. *Trauma, Violence, & Abuse*, 9(4): 214–226. https://doi.org/10.1177/1524838008324336

Cohen, J. A., Mannarino, A. P., Jankowski, K., Rosenberg, S., Kodya, S., & Wolford, G. L. (2016). A randomized implementation study of trauma-focused cognitive behavioral therapy for adjudicated teens in residential treatment facilities. *Child Maltreatment*, 21(2): 156–167. https://doi.org/10.1177/1077559515624775

Collie, A. (2008). Consciously working at the unconscious level: Psychodynamic theory in action in a training environment. *Journal of Social Work Practice*, 22(3): 345–358. https://doi.org/10.1080/02650530802396676

Conway, P. (2009). Falling between minds: The effects of unbearable experiences on multi-agency communication in the care system. *Adoption & Fostering*, 33(1): 18–29. https://doi.org/10.1177/030857590903300103

Coopey, J. (1995). The learning organization, power, politics and ideology introduction. management learning. In: S. Western, *Leadership: A Critical Text* (pp. 193–213). London: Sage, 2008.

Csibra, G., & Gergely, G. (2009). Natural pedagogy. *Trends in Cognitive Sciences*, *13*, 148–153.

Daw, E., & Gill, A. (2017). From care to where? Care leavers' access to accommodation. Centrepoint Policy report. https://centrepoint.org.uk/media/2035/from-care-to-where-centrepoint-report.pdf (last accessed 27 November 2022).

DeJong, M., (2010). Some reflections on the use of psychiatric diagnosis in the looked after or "in care" child population, *Clinical Child Psychology and Psychiatry*, *15*(4): 589–599. https://doi.org/10.1177/1359104510377705

Department for Education. (2015). Care leavers' transition to adulthood. HC 269 SESSION 2015–16 17 JULY 2015. https://dera.ioe.ac.uk/23504/1/Care-leavers-transition-to-adulthood.pdfDfE (2019). Department for Education. Children looked after in England (including adoption), year ending 31 March. https://assets.publishing.service.gov.uk/government/uploads/system/uploads/attachment_data/file/850306/Children_looked_after_in_England_2019_Text.pdf (last accessed 27 November 2022).

Department for Education. (2019). Children looked after in England (including adoption), year ending 31 March 2019. National Statistics Publication Template (publishing.service.gov.uk) (last accessed 7 January 2022).

Department for Education. (2022) Reporting Year 2022: Children looked after in England including adoptions. https://explore-education-statistics.service.gov.uk/find-statistics/children-looked-after-in-england-including-adoptions/2022 (last accessed 27 November 2022).

Eluvathingal, T. J., Chugani, H. T., Behen, M. E., Juhász, C., Muzik, O., Maqbool, M., Chugani, D. C., & Makki, M. (2006). Abnormal brain connectivity in children after early severe socioemotional deprivation: A diffusion tensor imaging study. *American Academy of Pediatrics*, *117* (6): 2093–2100. DOI: 10.1542/peds.2005-1727.

Engler, A. D., Sarpong, K. O., Van Horne, B. S., Greeley, C. S., & Keefe, R. J. (2022). A systematic review of mental health disorders of children in foster care. *Trauma, Violence, & Abuse*, *23*(1): 255–264. https://doi.org/10.1177/1524838020941197

Fallon, D., & Broadhurst, K. (2015). Preventing unplanned pregnancy and improving preparation for parenthood for care-experienced young people: A comprehensive review of the literature and critical appraisal of intervention studies. University of Manchester and Lancaster University on behalf of Coram.

Feinstein, l., MacDonald, G., Bywaters, P., Simmonds, J., Broadhurst, K., Forrester, D., & Holmes, D. Some members of the Care Review Evidence Group reflect on the risks of reforming in haste and repenting at leisure. University of Oxford Department of Education (2022). Category: Blog. https://www.education.ox.ac.uk/some-members-of-the-care-review-evidence-group-reflect-on-the-risks-of-reforming-in-haste-and-repenting-at-leisure/#_ftn8 (last accessed 17 December 2022).

Fonagy, P. (2010). Psychotherapy research: Do we know what works for whom? *British Journal of Psychiatry*, *197*(2): 83–85. doi:10.1192/bjp.bp.110.079657

Freud, S. (1923b). *The Ego and the Id. S. E. 19*. London: Hogarth.

Freud, S. (1930a). *Civilization and its Discontents. S. E., 21*. London: Hogarth.

Gerhardt, S. (2010). *The Selfish Society: How We All Forgot to Love One Another and Made Money Instead*. London: Simon & Schuster.

Gov.uk (20 July 2012). Radical scheme to rescue NEETs, [Government press release]. https://www.gov.uk/government/news/radical-scheme-to-rescue-neets (last accessed 12 January 2023.)

Graham, A., & Killick, C. (2019). Developing team resilience to prevent burnout in statutory residential care. *Scottish Journal of Residential Child Care*, *18*(3): 1–28.

Greenwald, R., Siradas, L., Schmitt, T., Reslan, S., Fierle, J., & Sande, B. (2012). Implementing trauma-informed treatment for youth in a residential facility: First-year outcomes. *Residential Treatment for Children & Youth*, *29*(2): 141–153. https://doi.org/10.1080/0886571X.2012.676525

Haigh, R. (2013). The quintessence of a therapeutic environment. *Therapeutic Communities: The International Journal of Therapeutic Communities*, *34*(1): 6–15. https://doi.org/10.1108/09641861311330464

Hambrick, E. P., Brawner, T. W., Perry, B. D., Wang, E. Y., Griffin, G., DeMarco, T., Capparelli, C., Grove, T., Maikoetter, M., O'Malley, D., Paxton, D., Freedle, L., Friedman, J., Mackenzie, J., Perry, K. M., Cudney, P., Hartman, J., Kuh, E., Morris, J., & Strother, M. (2018). Restraint and critical incident reduction following introduction of the neurosequential model of therapeutics (NMT). *Residential Treatment for Children & Youth*, *35*(1): 2–23. https://doi.org/10.1080/0886571X.2018.1425651

Haraway, D., & Latour, B. (2020). Donna Haraway & Bruno Latour | Discussion of the Film *Storytelling for Earthly Survival*. 25 June 2020. https://www.youtube.com/watch?v=j-2r_vI2alg 44:38 (last accessed 11 January 2023).

Harder, A. T., Knorth, E. J., & Kalverboer, M. E. (2017). The inside out? Views of young people, parents, and professionals regarding successful secure residential care. *Child & Adolescent Social Work Journal, 34*(5): 431–441. https://doi.org/10.1007/s10560-016-0473-1 (last accessed 11 January 2023).

Havel, V. (1991). *Disturbing the Peace.* New York: Vintage Books.

Izzo, C. V., Smith, E. G., Sellers, D. E., Holden, M. J., & Nunno, M. A. (2020). Improving relationship quality in group care settings: The impact of implementing the CARE model. *Children and Youth Services Review, 109.* https://doi.org/10.1016/j.childyouth.2019.104623

Kelley, S. D., Bickman, L., & Norwood, E. (2010). Evidence-based treatments and common factors in youth psychotherapy. In: B. L. Duncan, S. D. Miller, B. E. Wampold, & M. A. Hubble (Eds.), *The Heart and Soul of Change: Delivering What Works in Therapy* (pp. 325–355). New York: American Psychological Association. https://doi.org/10.1037/12075-011

Klein, M. (1946). Notes on some schizoid mechanisms. *The International Journal of Psychoanalysis, 27*: 99–110.

Krantz, J. (2021). The century of the system with James Krantz. *Edgy Ideas: Apple Podcasts* [Podcast]. September 2023. Available at https://podcasts.apple.com/gb/podcast/the-century-of-the-system-with-james-krantz/id1507167521?i=1000536336183 (last accessed 11 January 2023).

Lacan, J. (1992). *The Ethics of Psychoanalysis.* London: Routledge.

Lacan, J. (1994). *Le séminaire. Livre VIII: Le transfert,* 1960–1961. (Jacques-Alain Miller, Ed.). Paris: Seuil.

Lammy, D. (2016). Review of racial bias and BAME representation in criminal justice system announced. Published 31 January 2016. https://assets.publishing.service.gov.uk/government/uploads/system/uploads/attachment_data/file/643001/lammy-review-final-report.pdf (last accessed 11 January 2023).

Latour, B. (2005). *Reassembling the Social: An Introduction to Actor-Network-Theory.* Oxford: Oxford University Press.

Lee-Izu, M., & Perry, L. (2022). Improving health for all rests on getting it right for children. *The Impact of the Health and Care Bill: A Special Report by the Leaders Council of Great Britain and Northern Ireland* (pp. 46–48). https://www.leaderscouncil.co.uk/special-reports/The-Impact-of-the-Health-and-Care-Bill-A-special-report-by-The-Leaders-Council (last accessed 12 January 2023).

Lyman, R. D., & Wilson, D. R. (1992). Residential and inpatient treatment of emotionally disturbed children and adolescents. In: K. L. S. Brady & J. Caraway (2002). Home away from home: factors associated with current functioning in children living in a residential treatment setting. *Child Abuse & Neglect*, 26: 1149–1163.

MacAlister, J. (2021). The case for change. The independent review of children's social care. https://childrenssocialcare.independent-review.uk/wp-content/uploads/2022/06/IRCSC_The_Case_for_Change_27.05.22.pdf (last accessed 12 January 2023.)

MacAlister, J. (2022). Final report. The independent review of children's social care. https://childrenssocialcare.independent-review.uk/wp-content/uploads/2022/05/The-independent-review-of-childrens-social-care-Final-report.pdf (last accessed 12 January 2023.)

Macdonald, G., & Millen, S. (2012). Therapeutic approaches to social work in residential childcare settings: Literature review. Social Care Institute for Excellence. Retrieved from www.scie.org.uk

Maskell, R. (2022). House of Commons. Parliamentlive.TV. Thursday 24 November 2022 https://parliamentlive.tv/event/index/c88e95f7-a639-4222-9dc3-acd1a216ca69?in=13:51 (last accessed 11 January 2023).

McLoughlin, P. J., & Gonzalez, R. (2014). Healing complex trauma through therapeutic residential care: The Lighthouse Foundation therapeutic family model of care. *Children Australia*, 39(3): 169–176. https://doi.org/10.1017/cha.2014.22

Menzies-Lyth, I. (1960). A case-study in the functioning of social systems as a defence against anxiety. A report on a study of the nursing service of a general hospital. *Human Relations*, 13(2): 95–121.

Missing People & ECPAT UK. (March 2022). Away and at risk: The scale of exploited children going missing from care in the UK, 2018–2020. https://www.missingpeople.org.uk/wp-content/uploads/2022/03/Exploitation-report-FINAL.pdf (last accessed 12 January 2023.)

Narey, N. (2016). Residential care in England. Report of Sir Martin Narey's independent review of children's residential care. Last accessed 12 January 2023. https://assets.publishing.service.gov.uk/government/uploads/system/uploads/attachment_data/file/534560/Residential-Care-in-England-Sir-Martin-Narey-July-2016.pdf (last accessed 12 January 2023.)

The National Network for the Education of Care Leavers (29 June 2022). A summary of some of the latest data on care experienced students. https://www.nnecl.org/resources/32-data (last accessed 12 January 2023).

Nordoff, J., & Madoc-Jones, I. (2014). Aiming higher: More than "on the job" training for residential child care workers. *Journal of Children's Services*, 9(1): 42–57. http://dx.doi.org/10.1108/JCS-12-2013-0037

Perry, D, B. (2020). 4. Regulate, Relate, Reason (Sequence of Engagement): Neurosequential Network Stress & Trauma Series. 2 April 2020 https://youtu.be/LNuxy7FxEVk (last accessed 18 December 2022).

Porges, S. W. (2007). The polyvagal perspective. *Biological Psychology*, 74(2): 116–143. https://doi.org/10.1016/j.biopsycho.2006.06.009

Price, H., Jones, D., Herd, J., & Sampson, A. (2018). Between love and behaviour management: The psychodynamic reflective milieu at the Mulberry Bush School. *Journal of Social Work Practice*, 32(4): 391–407. https://doi.org/10.1080/02650533.2018.1503167

Public Health England (2021, June 10). Young people's substance misuse treatment statistics 2019 to 2020: report. https://www.gov.uk/government/statistics/substance-misuse-treatment-for-young-people-statistics-2019-to-2020/young-peoples-substance-misuse-treatment-statistics-2019-to-2020-report (last accessed 30 December 2022).

Ribeiro-Addy, B. (25 November 2021). The care-to-prison pipeline shows our failure of looked-after children. *Independent*. https://www.independent.co.uk/voices/children-in-care-prison-social-care-b1964142.html?amp (last accessed 12 January 2023).

Rivard, J. C., McCorkle, D., Duncan, M. E., Pasquale, L. E., Bloom, S. L., & Abramovitz, R. (2004). Implementing a trauma recovery framework for youths in residential treatment. *Child and Adolescent Social Work Journal*, 21(5): 529–550. https://doi.org/10.1023/B:CASW.0000043363.14978.e6

Rose, M. (2002). Therapeutic communities for children and adolescents: A renaissance of heart and mind. *Residential Treatment for Children & Youth*, 19(3): 1–15. https://doi.org/10.1300/J007v19n03_01

Sandiford, P. (2022). Response of the Children's Homes Association (CHA) to the policy to "Eliminate profit" from the care of looked after children. Children's Homes Association. https://members.the-cha.org.uk/documents/e38678aa-3348-4723-a37f-fd705fcc7598.pdf (last accessed 12 January 2023).

Sissay, L. (2012). Lemn Sissay: A child of the state. TEDx Houses of Parliament. 24 October 2012. https://www.youtube.com/watch?v=sLiM2-izFl4&t=658s (last accessed 12 January 2023).

Sissay, L. (2017). On care. Hay Festival. YouTube: https://www.youtube.com/watch?v=QNicvw_iUFM (last accessed 12 January 2023).

Stanley, J. (2022). A political economy of Residential Child Care: National Centre for Excellence in Residential Child Care (NCERCC). https://ncercc.co.uk/wp-content/uploads/2022/07/NCERCC-A-political-economic-history-of-RCC-0722-revised.pdf (last accessed 12 January 2023).

Steckley, L. (2012). Touch, physical restraint and therapeutic containment in residential child care. *British Journal of Social Work*, *42*(3): 537–555. https://doi.org/10.1093/bjsw/bcr069

Stuck, E. N., Jr., Small, R. W., & Ainsworth, F. (2000). Questioning the continuum of care: Toward a reconceptualization of child welfare services. *Residential Treatment for Children & Youth*, *17*(3): 79–92. https://doi.org/10.1300/J007v17n03_12

Taylor, E., Di Folco, S., & Lou, Y. (2018). Resilience and resilience factors in children in residential care: A systematic review. *Children and youth services review*, (89): 83–92. https://doi.org/10.1016/j.childyouth.2018.04.010

Timonen-Kallio, E., & Hämäläinen, J. (2019). Social pedagogy-informed residential child care. *International Journal of Social Pedagogy*, (7): 1. DOI: 10.14324/111.444.ijsp.2019.v7.1.010; https://www.patricktomlinson.com/therapeutic-model-development-a-long-history-and-international-research-patrick-tomlinson-2021/77

Treisman, K. (2021). *A Treasure Box for Creating Trauma-Informed Organizations: Volumes 1 & 2*. London: Jessica Kingsley.

Van der Kolk, B. A. (2014). *The Body Keeps the Score: Brain, Mind, and Body in the Healing of Trauma*. New York: Viking.

Wachtel, P. L. (2016). On psychotherapy integration: From psychoanalysis and behavior therapy to the future. Psychotherapy expert talks. https://youtu.be/igEqlf68_5s 38:33–39:13 (last accessed 12 January 2023).

Wampold, B. E., & Imel, Z. E. (2015). *The Great Psychotherapy Debate: The Evidence for What Makes Psychotherapy Work* (2nd ed.). New York: Routledge.

Weisz, J. R., McCarty, C. A., & Valeri, S. M. (2006). Effects of psychotherapy for depression in children and adolescents: A meta-analysis. *Psychological bulletin*, *132*(1): 132–149. https://doi.org/10.1037/0033-2909.132.1.132

Welsh Government (2022). Proposed changes to primary legislation in relation to social care and continuing NHS Healthcare. https://gov.wales/sites/default/files/consultations/2022-08/consultation-document-summary_0.pdf (last accessed 12 January 2023).

Western, S. (2008). *Leadership: A Critical Text,* London: Sage. (Third edition reprinted London: Sage, 2019.)

Western, S. (2012). *Coaching and Mentoring. A Critical Text*. London: Sage.

Western, S. (2015). A-N Coaching System™ http://www.simonwestern.com/a-n-coaching-system.html (last accessed 12 January 2023).

Whiteley, S. (2004). The evolution of the therapeutic community. *Psychiatric Quarterly*, 75(3): 233–248. https://doi.org/10.1023/B:PSAQ.0000031794.82674.e8

Whittaker, J., del Valle, J., & Holmes, L. (2015). *Therapeutic Residential Care for Children and Youth: Developing Evidence-based International Practice*. London: Jessica Kingsley.

Whitwell, J. A. (2002). Re-framing Children's Services. *NCVCCO Annual Review Journal No.3*. Edited by Keith J White. London: National Council of Voluntary Child Care Organisations.

Winnicott, D. W. (1949). Hate in the counter-transference. *International Journal of Psychoanalysis*, (30): 69–74.

Winnicott, D. W. (1960a). The theory of the parent–infant relationship. In: *The Maturational Processes and the Facilitating Environment: Studies in the Theory of Emotional Development*. London: Karnac.

Winnicott, D. W. (1960b). Ego distortion in terms of the true and false self. In: *The Maturational Processes and the Facilitating Environment: Studies in the Theory of Emotional Development*. London: Karnac.

Winnicott, D. W. (1971). *Therapeutic Consultations in Child Psychiatry*. New York: Basic Books.

CHAPTER 12

Working through play on the mentalizing capacity of controlling-caregiving children who suffered early relational trauma

Nadja Rolli

In this chapter, I introduce Sophie, Simon, and the Family Smith. These vignettes involve children who are controlling-caregiving after having experienced significant attachment disruptions and emotional neglect. I have worked with them over two years and have been able to witness several hopeful developments in their search for their sense of self and a stronger mentalization capacity. With the help of the vignettes, I hope to bring the theoretical background of my work as an integrative child psychotherapist to life by interlinking conceptual and clinical reflections on the relationship between the controlling-caregiving child and the development of the mentalizing capacity.

Mentalization

Mentalizing is a form of imaginative mental activity that involves the ability to differentiate between what is in one's mind and what is in another's mind (Fonagy & Target, 1997). It describes the individual's capacity to reflect and respond to the mental state of another and make people's behaviour meaningful and predictable. The operationalisation of this psychological process is called "reflective function"

(Fonagy, Gergely, Jurist, & Target, 2002). The ability to mentalize helps children to develop a sense of identity and enhances their understanding of their own feelings and motivations, as well as those of others. This understanding results in better psychosocial functioning, such as emotional intelligence, social-emotional maturity, the ability to self-regulate, and developing empathy. There is a crucial distinction between mentalizing explicitly and mentalizing implicitly. Mentalizing explicitly is when one names a feeling or a thought, or consciously interprets behaviour. Mentalizing implicitly is the automatic natural emotional resonance to another that takes place without thinking about it. The person's capacity to mentalize and the accuracy of that mentalization are linked to their own story and emotional state. Implicit mentalization is impaired when the person is frightened, angry, or ashamed, and when defensive mechanisms are active (Allen, 2013, p. 136). In this sense, secure mentalizing is the ability to distinguish the internal state from external reality; pretend from real modes of functioning; and intrapersonal mental and emotional processes from interpersonal communications (Fonagy, Gergely, Jurist, & Target, 2002, pp. 24–25).

Everyone is born with the capacity to mentalize, but its development is modulated through the quality of early relationships (Allison & Fonagy, 2012; Bateman & Fonagy, 2019). Numerous studies (Allison & Fonagy, 2012; Bateman & Fonagy, 2019; Steele & Steele, 2005, among others) focus on the importance of a secure attachment within the parent–child relationship, specifically the parent's ability to reflect on children's state of mind, to support the development of the mentalizing capacity of young children. There is a strong association between insecure-avoidant or disorganised attachment behaviour and impairment of the reflective function (Fonagy, Gergely, Jurist, & Target, 2002). If the caregivers are not able to demonstrate an insightful and accurate understanding of the child's emotional state, the child does not learn how to understand their own thoughts, feelings, and motivation or the thoughts, feelings, and motivations of others. A child with impaired mentalization will tend to struggle to integrate and differentiate mental states, especially under conditions of high emotional arousal. Impaired mentalization is defined as either undermentalization or hypermentalization. Undermentalizing refers to a diminution in the ability to understand and attribute mental states, whereas hypermentalizing involves making assumptions about other people's mental states that go far beyond observable data (Sharp et al., 2011).

Case study: Sophie

I first met six-year-old Sophie during a home visit at her adoptive parents' home. The white middle-class couple adopted her and her younger brother when Sophie was five years old. Both children had been removed from their birth parents three years earlier, after several domestic incidents had been reported to the authorities. Investigations brought to light that the birth parents had a history of drug and alcohol abuse and often neglected the physical and emotional needs of their children. Furthermore, the children occasionally were given into the care of a family friend, whom the authorities suspected might have physically and sexually abused the children, especially the brother. Before the children met their adoptive parents, they were looked after by a foster family. Leaving the foster family and settling into the forever family was difficult for both children, as the foster parents had established a loving bond with the children. I was made aware that especially Sophie had created the coping strategy of telling people about her life story without any filter in an attempt to maintain a sense of control over her life.

My work with Sophie initially involved meetings with her, her brother, and the adoptive parents, to help them form a positive and nurturing attachment with each other. In these sessions, Sophie defined her role as being the caregiver of the emotional needs of the family and struggled to experience a space of intimacy where her emotional needs were taken into consideration by adults.

Attachment theory provides a developmental model for understanding the affectionate bonds created by close relationships, initially with primary carers (Bowlby, 1980). The bond aims to protect the child from fear and harm and provides love, nurturance, security, and encouragement for exploration. As a result of interactions with their primary caregivers, the infant creates an internal working model (IWM). IWM describes the development of mental representations of oneself, specifically the worth of the self and expectations of others' behaviour in relation to oneself (Verschueren, Marcoen, & Schoefs, 1996). This psychological construct allows the infant to imagine interactions with others based on previous experiences, which are then generalised to other relationships. Although some life events may modify IWM, it tends to be change-resistant (Fraley, 2002) unless the individual undergoes specific treatment. Depending on the early experiences of the infant with the primary caregiver, the infant develops attachment strategies, known as: a) secure, as with a positive relational pattern; b) anxious–ambivalent, as with an anxious or angry relational pattern; c) anxious–avoidant, as with an untrusting and self-sufficient relational pattern; or d) disorganised, as with no predictable relational pattern (Ainsworth, Blehar, Waters, & Wall, 1978; Bowlby, 1980). Disorganised attachment behaviour is often linked to abuse, emotional neglect, and unavailability of the primary carer (Alexander, 2013). The trauma that unfolds out of the interactions with emotionally neglectful caregivers has an impact on the child's emotional and psychosocial development.

> Individual child psychotherapy for Sophie and her brother started once the family felt that they had established a strong relationship with each other and had established a family dynamic that allowed the children to feel held in mind. After discussions with my supervisor, I made the decision that it was important for both children to have their separate time to ensure that their different therapeutic needs had a safe space to be expressed and processed.
>
> Once Sophie attended individual sessions, it felt that I finally had the chance to meet her true person. Around her family, Sophie loved being in charge and giving orders to all members. However, when she was alone with me in the room, she did not know what to play. She often lined up toy figurines or art materials without having the capacity to hold an idea long enough in her mind to be able to play. When she tried to create a craft activity, she easily gave up on things and felt frustrated with her own skills. Hence, in early sessions, Sophie often preferred to engage with me through talking, not playing. She also expressed the wish that I should lead our sessions, rather than her being in charge. On the level of the countertransference, I could feel her emotional overwhelm, as she was not able to predict our interactions in the sessions, and this provoked fear and anxiety. Her usual coping strategy of catering to the wishes of others did not work in the therapeutic setting.

As research (Hesse & Main, 1999; Green & Goldwyn, 2002; Lyons-Ruth, Yellin, Melnick, & Atwood, 2005) suggests, it is the display of frightening parental behaviour, or behaviour that is frightened, that results in a high likelihood of infant disorganisation. The child paradoxically needs to turn for comfort to the attachment figure who is causing the child's fear (Hesse & Main, 1999). Green hypothesises that the child perceives the emotionally unavailable mother as alive but psychically dead. The mother's inability to show interest in the emotional world of her child brings loss of love, followed by loss of meaning for the child; nothing makes sense anymore. "She [the mother] is lost to the subject, but at least, however afflicted she may be, she is there. Dead and present, but present nonetheless. The subject can take care of her, attempt to awaken her, to cure her" (Green, 1986, p. 164). By the age of six, the disorganised child tends to evolve their attachment pattern into controlling conduct towards the primary carer, either into controlling-punitive behaviour or controlling-caregiving behaviour (Main & Cassidy, 1988). Controlling-caregiving children are often perceived as adaptable, less hyperactive, and less demanding (Moss, Cyr, & Dubois-Comtois, 2004), hence there is a risk that these children will not be identified as being emotionally vulnerable.

> I was aware that I needed to not be seduced into Sophie's established behavioural pattern of unconsciously nurturing my needs, but to gently support her to find her own expression. By mindfully giving the leading of the session back to her, I created a space that invited her to connect with her own desires rather the desires of others. Sophie found this incredibly challenging, as her desire was to please me. At that time, the play in the session often felt confusing and emotionally empty. She had the tendency to move from one activity to the next without the ability to create meaning. I tried to be as transparent in my emotions as possible by communicating how difficult it can be to make choices or playing what she liked. I aimed to make my internal processes available to allow her to go on the journey to find her own sense of self. At times, I noticed that this emptiness started to lull my awareness into sleep and disassociation; and, together with my supervisor, I worked on containing the heaviness and exhaustion from the sessions.
>
> For a long time, there was no change in the therapeutic process, and I, like Sophie, felt at a loss. A shift finally occurred when, in one session, Sophie found the box with the fidget, wiggle, and squeezy toys. With

newfound interest, she started to explore the wide range of materials and soon entered a flow state (Csikszentmihalyi, 2002), which Winnicott (1971) describes as the first relational interaction when the baby plays in the presence of the mother and enters a potential space of being. Through the sensory play, Sophie's body and facial expressions came to life with wonder, curiosity, and the excitement of discovering new things. Through the physical exploration of touch, sound, and movement, Sophie started to develop a body-self, which is essential for the development of identity (Jennings, 1999, p. 51.) Soon, Sophie added water, syringes, and shaving foam to enhance her sensory experiences, and we had many enjoyable sessions moving water from one container to another. Later, she discovered the ready-made poster paint and started to mix colours, making handprints and all kinds of water-paint potions. By exploring the varied materials in the here and now and without any risk of failure, Sophie started to connect with her inner world. She created moments where she repudiated and reaccepted the play object, in the same way as a "baby has the capacity to find and being herself waiting to be found" (Winnicott, 1971, p. 63).

Childhood trauma

According to van der Kolk (2005), traumatic childhood experiences are highly common and may be the most important public health challenge of our time. Being exposed to multiple and prolonged experiences of abuse and neglect has an excessive impact on the individual's mental health. The Adverse Childhood Experiences (ACE) study (Felitti et al., 1998) found a highly significant relationship between ACE and depression, suicide attempts, alcoholism, drug abuse, sexual promiscuity, domestic violence, cigarette smoking, obesity, physical inactivity, and sexually transmitted diseases later in life. Furthermore, the study also found a significant relationship between ACE and a person developing heart disease, cancer, stroke, diabetes, skeletal fractures, and liver disease.

Despite the common belief that babies are too young to remember traumatic events and are therefore less impacted, research (Brazelton, 1982; van den Bergh, Dahnke, & Mennes, 2018; van der Kolk, 2014; Yahuda & Lehrner, 2018) has shown that a) a history of severe trauma in the parent's life can change the baby's genetic makeup; b) prenatal stress leaves the baby at high risk of alterations in brain structure, brain function, and intrinsic brain networks, and increases the baby's risk of born less resilient to life's stresses; and c) early trauma—especially trauma at the hands of a caregiver—can alter a child's perception of self and the world, undermine their trust in others, and hinder the establishing of secure attachment (Terr, 1990; Ogden, Minton, & Pain, 2006). Alexander (2013, p. 40) pointed out that "even though mothers and fathers do not differ in their rates of behaviours that are frightening to children, infant disorganisation is more likely to result from maternal than paternal disruptive behaviour".

Impact of trauma on the nervous system

Studies (Schore, 2001; Perry, 2001) have found that the brain develops hierarchically from the bottom up and the inside out, mirroring the progression in which the upper-brain centres regulate the primitive reactivity of the lower- and central-brain centres. It is known (De Bellis & Zisk, 2014) that early-life trauma leaves its imprint on the anatomy and physiology of the brain and is associated with the development of dysfunctional neural circuits. Chronic trauma interferes with neurobiological development and the capacity to integrate sensory, emotional, and cognitive information into a cohesive whole (van der Kolk, 2005). Grabbe and Miller-Karas (2018) summarised that trauma causes alterations in neuroendocrine and neurotransmitter systems and in brain areas associated with mood regulation. It leaves "scars" on emotional control, learning (problem-solving skills and concentration), executive functioning, and memory.

A person's ability to manage states of emotional arousal is dependent on staying regulated. A child cannot regulate emotions or access learning if they are hypo- or hyper-aroused. If the child is in a state of fear, they miss the necessary sensory information to allow adaptive reactions to a perceived threat, and everyday situations may be misinterpreted. This can potentially result in fight, flight, or freeze stress responses to situations that seem insignificant to others (van der Kolk, 2003; Siegel, 2020). Any experience that disturbs the development of a sense of safety and secure attachment at a time of heightened dependence will lead to impaired development of the neural pathways that subserve emotional behaviours. Without the necessary support, the resulting impaired emotional regulation is likely to persist throughout the individual's lifetime (Sarkar & Adshead, 2006).

Neuroimaging research on stress and trauma responses (Haase et al., 2016; Herringa, Phillips, Almeida, Insana, & Germain, 2012; van der Kolk, 2014, among others) indicates that the insula oversees positive adaptation in the context of adversity. The insula, which is surrounded by the limbic system and the cortical executive control centres, is thought to be responsible for empathy, social interactions, and sense of self. It has a sharply reduced activity in people who have experienced developmental trauma. Survival becomes the focus of the child's interactions, and adapting to the demands of their environment takes priority. They cannot afford to explore their ideas or interests and may lose themselves in the process of coping with ongoing threats to their survival. Often, they come to internalise the idea that there is something inherently wrong with them, and believe that they are at fault, unlovable, hateful, helpless, and unworthy of protection and love (Fonagy, Gergely, Jurist, & Target, 2002). As such, distress is intolerable and overwhelming, and these experiences cannot be integrated on a symbolic level. Hence, there is an elevated risk that the child may split them off in the form of dissociation. Dissociation is a disconnection in the integration of memory, consciousness, emotion, perception, and identity; therefore, it affects all areas of the personality functioning of the self (Heim & Nemeroff, 2001). Childhood abuse or neglect is regarded as an event so intense that it fosters a pathological active formation of impaired personality functioning. Thus, it is reasonable to predict that ACE hinders the development of good mentalizing abilities (Wagner-Skacel, Riedl, Kampling, & Lampe, 2022) and interferes with the ability to gain an understanding that another person's emotional state is responsible for what is happening to them.

Case study: Simon

Simon was referred to child psychotherapy after having had several unprovoked anger outbursts. He was ten years old and living with his adoptive parents, a male couple, as well as his three-years-younger brother in a house in a suburban area. When I spoke with his adoptive fathers, they described

Simon as very caring and helpful but also displaying strong separation anxiety and the desire to please them at all costs. Furthermore, they spoke about how guilty and anxious Simon would feel after each anger outburst and that after such an outburst, he would tell them that it is all his fault and that he will try to do better. They also revealed that sometimes it felt like Simon would not trust them, even in moments of loving intentions and emotional warmth. His eyes would vigilantly keep scanning the environment to ensure that there was no threat. Graham Music (2019, p. 39) talks about how other adopting parents report similar experiences in his group work.

As mentioned earlier, 66–75 per cent of children who display a disorganised attachment as toddlers reorganise their attachment behaviour into a controlling, role-reversed pattern (Main & Cassidy, 1988; Moss, Cyr, Bureau, Tarabulsy, & Dubois-Comtois, 2005; Wartner, Grossman, Fremmer-Bombik, & Suess, 1994), such as controlling-punitive behaviour or controlling-caregiving behaviour. Children who are classified as controlling-punitive use hostile, confrontational, and combative behaviour with the caregiver, whereas controlling-caregiving children direct the parent's activities by structuring interactions in a helpful and emotionally positive manner (Moss, Cyr, & Dubois-Comtois, 2004). Main and Cassidy (1988) explain this shift as the child's attempt to resolve the paradox of the frightening/frightened parent by assuming the role of the caregiver. Moss, Cyr, and Dubois-Comtois (2004), as well as Solomon and George (2008), found that the controlling-caregiving pattern is associated with a history of loss in the family, which was highly significant in Simon's case. He and his brother were removed from their birth parents when the authorities became alarmed for the children's well-being, caused by the birth father falling seriously ill and the birth mother facing a long prison sentence after being arrested for theft.

> In our first meeting, Simon presented himself as a confident child who was happy to engage with me. Only his eyes and his hands displayed the level of distress Simon was feeling: his hands were forming fists and his eyes restlessly never settled. Maté (1999, p. 133) speaks about this automatic scanning as the brain circuitry created when the child learned to constantly scan the mother's withdrawn or depressed features to seek her contact and presence. When Simon and I spoke about the reasons why he would come to

see me, he shared many loving memories of his birth parents and expressed how much he was missing them, but they would have sent him away, as he was so badly behaved. It seemed to me that, even though he felt very settled and happy with his adoptive parents, he mourned the loss of his mother and blamed himself for the loss, not understanding that it was the inability of his birth parents that had caused the separation. His recent anger outbursts were confusing and scary to him and he expressed his wish for them "just to go away".

Main and Cassidy (1988) highlight that controlling-caregiving children have the tendency to internalise their emotions and are not typically aggressive towards others but have an IWM that is marked by inhibition and anxiety. As controlling-caregiving children tend to have positive interactions with peers and teachers, there is a significant risk that their underlying emotional needs and experiences around developmental trauma will not be identified and therefore will not receive child therapeutic support. However, it is known that, without early intervention and support, mental health problems among teens and adults result in significant personal, relational, societal, and economic costs (Knapp & Wong, 2020; Early Intervention Foundation, 2021).

Simon's initial sessions, similar to Sophie's, often felt emotionally disconnected. He engaged with me through football or other ball activities; however, I struggled to attune to his mind. At this time, Simon expressed emotions of not feeling anything and not knowing what he wanted. I decided to adopt a "not-knowing stance" and to have an inquisitive, curious mindset about what was happening in the room and what he may have been thinking or feeling at that moment. This active questioning about Simon's mental state helped to make my mind available to him, demonstrated my interest in understanding him, and reinforced his sense of "being seen". We also started to integrate body awareness exercises such as breathing techniques, mindful meditation, and mirror games into the football games. These types of activities helped Simon to strengthen his self-awareness, embodying a sense of self, and helped him to become more aware and trustful of the space surrounding him. It was important for him to have the experience that his body existed in a safe space. Jennings (1999, p. 29) describes this kind of activity as the proto-play that enhances the development of a sense of safety through satisfactory physical experiences of being stimulated with sufficient nurture.

After enacting proto-play for several months, Simon moved on to initiate sword fights. During our first fight of many, I was taken by surprise by the strength of his presence. Until then, I always encountered Simon as a shy boy; however, with the sword fight play, a new side of him entered the room. It felt like an outburst of emotions that finally was allowed to be acknowledged. He instructed me about how he wanted me to fight, how much strength I should have as his enemy, and how he would kill me in the game. Each kill was followed by a resurrection of the next enemy, which he would again strike down. Simon made it clear that I always represented a female figure as the enemy. On the level of the countertransference, it felt that Simon was finally able to express his hurt and anger towards his birth mother, without needing to worry about any consequences.

Losing the mother makes the development of one of the first milestones in the healthy development of a human being more difficult: the achievement of basic trust. Children who are separated from their birth mothers need to go through stages of grief to process the loss (Verrier, 1993). Even after the child has become attached to a new parent, which Simon has with his fathers, there is always fear of further loss, the loss of another parent abandoning him. Simon not only needed to grieve for his mother, he also needed to process his anger about her inability to keep him emotionally safe before the separation happened.

It is established that parental sensitivity and attunement are key to children's acquisition of self-regulation and understanding their own minds. This means that a parent with a disorganised attachment style and impaired mentalizing capacity cannot regulate an infant's emotional arousal (Fonagy, Steele, & Steele, 1991; Sroufe, 1996). They will not be able to hold the emotional state of the child in mind and may fail to decode the emotional component of a situation. Therefore, children who grow up with dysregulated, unpredictable, frightening, and distanced caregivers may not learn healthy emotional responses by making sense of the situation and reading the mind of the parent correctly to predict a possible emotional reaction from them. As a result, the child does not have the opportunity to acquire appropriate emotion regulation strategies (Sroufe, 1996; Brumariu, 2015).

In play, Simon was able to control his environment and felt regulated by my capacity to hold his emotional state in mind. Hence, he created something that was not there before—a space where he was able to manipulate external reality to create a bodily experience that was satisfying (Winnicott, 1971, pp. 69–70). As the interaction was full of fun and reciprocal enjoyment, Simon's nervous system was not at risk of feeling overwhelmed or dysregulated, even though he was processing highly triggering emotions. Over time, the sword fights became more sophisticated, with each of us building forts and having different weapons, as well as creating banners to mark our territory. What initially started as expression of his hurt became an opportunity for creativity and enhancement of his skills. A new world started to appear in front of him, with new possibilities and new adventures ahead.

The controlling-caregiving child and the ability to self-regulate and mentalize

Fonagy, Gergely, Jurist, & Target (2002, p. 56) point out that the inability of the parent to respond contingent to the infant's self-state evokes intense anxiety, either through frightening behaviour or behaviour suggesting fear. Infants growing up in a high-stress environment often respond by developing hypermentalization—being a precocious and anxious mind-reader of the mother's mental state in an attempt to reconnect with her—or by appearing to disengage from the mental state of the mother as a defence mechanism. In both scenarios, the child's interest in their own mental state decreases consequently (Allison & Fonagy, 2012, p. 25), compromising the development of a mentalizing self. The disorganised child anticipates that their emotional needs will be rebuffed and learns to disengage their attachment needs by not being an inconvenience to their mother and diminishing their painful emotions when offered comfort. Paradoxically, not bothering their mother too much serves to maintain the attachment—at a distance.

Furthermore, a study (Mansueto, Schruers, Cosci, & Van Os, 2019) indicated that early childhood experiences of being frightened and emotionally neglected had an observable negative impact on the development of neurocognitive functions and mentalizing abilities. Interestingly, the study pointed out that this relation was more prominent in male children than in female children.

Emotional regulation strategies become more sophisticated in middle childhood, when they start to include the awareness of multiple complex emotions and the employment of emotion "scripts" in social situations (Skinner & Zimmer-Gembeck, 2007).

Brumariu, Kerns, Guiseppone, and Lyons-Ruth (2021) conducted a study to evaluate the link between disorganised/controlling attachment behaviours and children's emotional regulation in later middle childhood. The study is based on the theory that when controlling-caregiving children attempt to regulate their parents' emotions and behaviour, they become precociously attuned to understanding others' emotions, whilst showing a poor awareness of their own emotions. The mature role in their relationship may force them to learn to "suppress" negative emotions and to project positive affect to cheer up and engage the parent. After assessing the interactions of eighty-seven mother–child dyads in a family problem-solving task, the results indicated that, in late middle childhood, controlling-caregiving children do not have a specific pattern of difficulties with emotion regulation. On the contrary, they demonstrated a greater level of emotional awareness than the control group. This can be explained by the fact that controlling-caregiving children might gain emotions skills, such as unusual vigilance to the parent's needs (hypermentalization). Brumariu, Kerns, Guiseppone, and Lyons-Ruth (2021) pointed out that the results may indicate that a controlling-caregiving child is internalising their emotional distress and therefore the apparent lack of difficulty in emotional regulation needs to be understood with caution. The resemblance of children's controlling behaviour to adulthood relationships characterised by violence or vulnerability to violence is remarkable (Alexander, 2013).

This statement is supported by the results of another study (Lyons-Ruth, Bureau, Holmes, Easterbrooks, & Brooks, 2013), which highlighted that nineteen-year-old adolescents with controlling-caregiving attachment behaviour have an increased risk of suicidality or self-injury and a high association with abuse towards romantic partners, dysfunction in peer relationships, and greater depressive and dissociative symptoms. Thus, the negative effects of the controlling-caregiving attachment may become increasingly evident with the increased demands and responsibilities of adolescence (Brumariu, Kerns, Guiseppone, and Lyons-Ruth, 2021).

The healing parameters

Part of the therapeutic work with controlling-caregiving children aims to repair the shortcomings of their environment in the early years, which may have been characterised by a lack of the contingent, responsive, and sensitive care that is essential for the development of brain functions to support the child's capacity to calm distress (Schore, 1994). When a child grows up in a family where abuse and fear are ongoing, self-reflection is discouraged, which in turn impedes the development of self-agency. For older children, the impact of ongoing threat-based arousal is likely to trigger implicit automatic reflexive mentalizing (Redfern, 2019).

As a therapist, it is crucial to spend time understanding the acute and chronic impact the maltreatment had on the child's functioning. As stated before, the controlling-caregiving child has learned to suppress their painful emotions to maintain the attachment to the parent, hence difficult feelings such as anger, distress, and neediness may never have been experienced as safe enough to be expressed towards the other. The therapist's capacity to reflect on the child's autonomous needs, feelings, and thoughts is crucial to understand why the child may display some of the behaviours witnessed. Equally important is the therapist's own capacity to mentalize, as working with a child with a disorganised attachment style frequently requires the therapist to effectively separate out the self from the other. "This often becomes particularly difficult in the face of high arousal, where, again, the influence of implicit mentalizing dominates and guides quick and automatic interpretation of behaviour" (Redfern, 2019, p. 271). It is important that a controlling-caregiving child experiences the therapist's direct expressions of commitment to their emotional state, as such expressions reinforce the sense of self-worth and provide more emotional exchanges and interactions between the child and therapist.

It is known that for psychotherapy to succeed when working with trauma, "the child must be sufficiently regulated, organised, grounded and present, such that language, imagination, and symbolic expressive function can emerge" (Warner, Koomar, Lary, & Cook, 2013, p. 730). Thus, it will be important that the therapeutic alliance initially creates a sense of safety, stability, control, and competence to manage distressing symptoms (Herman, 1997) before the child is able to start working on the underlying trauma. Once an awareness of containment and safety has been established, the psychotherapeutic interaction functions as a reparative attachment relationship (Schore, 2001, p. 213) for clients who experienced attachment pathologies and resulting developmental disorders of self-regulation. Still, the child's history and age will have a significant impact on how long it takes before a real change is seen in the child's capacity to build trust in the therapeutic relationship.

Numerous authors, such as Winnicott (1971), Jennings (1999), and Sunderland (2016), highlight the importance of integrating play therapy skills and techniques as well as sensory-based interventions into the work with children to support a sense of safety and strengthen the ability to self-regulate. By naming and describing what can take place between two people, the therapist incorporates herself or himself into the child's play without taking the lead in the play activity itself. This is especially important when working with children who hypermentalize, as these children will be so attuned to the needs of the adult that it has become their second nature to create whatever they believe the adult desires. It can be challenging to increase enjoyment and playful positive interactions when the child has withdrawn from their own source of creativity and struggles to be aware of their own needs.

In these cases, the play often has the quality of being monotonous, repetitive, and featuring compulsive/obsessive components; there is a substantial risk that the child will disassociate from the bleakness of not having a sense of self, as such wounding is intolerable and impossible to integrate into the expression of play. Moreover, many children cannot describe with words that they feel empty or without any ties (Zevalkink, Verbeugt-Pleiter, & Fonagy, 2012). It is the therapist's responsibility to help the client to make sense of what kind of feelings they experience and to gain an understanding of how miscommunication or misunderstanding of these feelings may lead to challenging social interactions. The therapist's capacity to mirror back the child's emotional experience in a marked way labels the emotions and communicates that those emotions are governable (Fonagy & Campbell, 2015). "Marked mirroring" describes how a person represents with a soothing voice an exaggerated display of the child's affect to mitigate the potentionally arousing effect of direct imitation (Gergely & Unoka, 2008). This forms a secondary representation of the child's experience in its mind and gradually forms a sense of self.

Case study: Family Smith

When working with hypermentalizing children, it is important to keep the parent–child relationship in mind as well. This may involve also working with the parent, often the mother, to enhance her reflective function ability. Helping the mother to understand her child and recognise her feelings can hopefully decrease the probability of an intergenerational cycle of disorganised attachment behaviours and low mentalizing capacity.

The mother of the Family Smith was suffering from borderline personality disorder, and both children displayed behavioural difficulties at school. The oldest child, the daughter (seven years old), often acted within the family setting as the carer, whereas the younger brother (five years old) displayed severe anger outbursts towards peers and teachers. Furthermore, the family had suffered the loss of the father, who he had died from an illness several years before. At the stage of the referral, social services were involved with the family, and there was a risk that the children might be taken into care if the mother would not engage with mental health support.

After the initial assessment of the family circumstances and resources, I decided to start the therapy by offering the mother individual meetings to help her to build a trusting and supportive relationship with me. When working with a frightened parent, the bond between therapist and parent is not easily established and often remains fragile. It is important that the parent experiences a sense of being represented in the mind of the therapist (Debbané & Bateman, 2019). Through integrating the parent into the psychotherapeutic process, the therapist can gain awareness of the parent's perception of the child. By inviting the parent to reflect and understand these perceptions—and, if necessary, challenge the experience—the therapist can help the parent to explore her own underlying emotions and how these representations may interfere with the ongoing relationship with her child (Redfern, 2019).

Once our therapeutic relationship was established, the mother soon started to compare her own childhood experiences with the way she was parenting her children. This was very painful for her, and she recognised her need to attend individual psychotherapy alongside our sessions to contain her own wounding and painful past experiences. In our sessions together, we were focusing on her ability to stay in the present moment. As I would work with children, we started to use play as a medium, and we integrated a wide range of sensory experiences, such as exploring different tactile sensations, such as gardening and creating art, to help the mother to become aware of her felt sense.

My focus during these sessions was to share with my client her excitement when she achieved a drawing the way she wanted, or her disappointment when things did not work out. I was marked mirroring her emotions and often expressed how joyful, satisfying, frustrating, or annoying the activities felt. When hearing these statements, the mother regularly made eye contact and studied my face carefully. I simply held her gaze and allowed her to take her time to look at me. It became a ritual in our sessions that we gazed into each other's eyes and that I was transparent about my own thoughts and perceptions. After a few of these sessions, the mother said to me: "I always know what you are thinking. It is very helpful." This observation led us to further explore who else's mind she could read and if she could read the minds of her children. This helped her to become more aware about her own facial expressions.

As a next step, we invited her children into the sessions, and so the family attended the psychotherapy as a unit. Several models, such as the mentalization-based treatment for families (Keaveny et al., 2012), promote the benefit of working simultaneously with the parent and child or adolescent through therapeutic interventions. Within this scenario, the key component of the therapist's work is holding the balance for each family member between thinking and feeling, between action and reflection, and between implicit mentalizing and explicit mentalizing (Asen & Midgley, 2019). The therapist needs to focus on three relationships at once: those between therapist and parent, parent and child, and therapist and child. The balance between the three relationships is extremely sensitive:

> If the clinician gives too much attention to the mother, the infant may remain invisible in the treatment. If the clinician gives too much attention to the infant, this may elicit jealousy in the mother, in two diverse ways: the mother may feel intimidated in her own motherhood, thinking that the clinician is a better parent than she is; or she may feel jealous about the fact that the child gets the attention that she needs for herself. (Suchman, Pajulo, Kalland, DeCoste, & Mayes, 2012, p. 319)

In the sessions, I introduced a wide range of relational play activities, such as interacting with each other with hand puppets, or "mirror–mirror games", where a person needs to copy the other person's facial expression and movements. The aim was that the children were able to strengthen their bond with their mother by experiencing her as attentive and caring but also emotionally available in a child-led activity. During play, I supported the mother's reflecting thinking by using circular questioning (i.e., "When you look at your daughter's face, what do you think that she may feel just now? How do you know? What facial clues has she given you?") to reflect on the emotional well-being of each family member, as well as their relationship to each other. This work helped the mother to learn to keep the minds of her children in her own mind and not to project her own representation onto her children. Over time, the bond between the mother and the children became more playful, and the school reported improvements in the boy's behaviour towards peers and staff members.

Conclusion

This chapter focuses on the relationship between the controlling-caregiving child and the development of the mentalization capacity. The current theoretical concepts classify the controlling-caregiving attachment behaviour as a pattern that emerges from the disorganised attachment style. Preschool-aged children often reorganise their attachment behaviour into a role-reversed, controlling pattern to cope with the frightening parental behaviour. The shift is explained as an attempt to resolve the paradox of the frightening/frightened parent by assuming the role of the caregiver. Research has been presented that highlights the current understanding that a child who grows up with a frightening/frightened parent will not learn healthy emotional responses to arousing situations and therefore is at risk of not having the opportunity to acquire emotional regulation strategies. It is likely that children will respond to the high-stress situation by developing hypermentalizing skills in an attempt to reconnect with the parent by being a highly attentive and anxious mind-reader. Becoming precociously attuned to understanding the parent's emotions compromises the development of a healthy mentalizing self. Further studies also highlight the high association between controlling-caregiving children learning to suppress negative emotions to protect their fragile relationship with the parent and having an increased risk of suicidality and self-harm with the augmented demands and responsibilities of adolescence.

These findings have an important impact on the work as an integrative child and adolescent psychotherapist. The chapter presents three case studies to demonstrate the significance of the relational aspects in a clinical setting when working with controlling-caregiving children. The therapist uses the capacity to mentalize as a model for the client and interacts within the therapeutic stance of "not knowing". This mindset as to what is happening at the moment supports a person's awareness of their state of mind. Marked mirroring and transparency about the therapist's mental state allow the client to feel seen and to discover their own inner experiences in relation to external reality. Even though in this chapter these principles are used in integrative child psychotherapy, the same concept can be adapted to adult psychotherapy, as building up the capacity to mentalize is not age specific.

Therapeutic play enables the child to integrate the inner experiences and create moments where he or she can repudiate and reaccept the object, and creates a potential space where the child can manipulate the external reality in a satisfying way without the nervous system being at risk of feeling overwhelmed and dysregulated.

References

Ainsworth, M. D. S., Blehar, M. C., Waters, E., & Wall, S. (1978). *Patterns of Attachment: A Psychological Study of the Strange Situation*. Hillsdale, NJ: Erlbaum.

Alexander, P. C. (2013). Relational trauma and disorganized attachment. In: J. D. Ford, & C. A. Courtois (Eds.), *Treating Complex Traumatic Stress Disorders in Children and Adolescents* (pp. 39–61). New York: Guilford Press.

Allen, J. G. (2013). *Mentalizing in the Development and Treatment of Attachment Trauma*. London: Karnac.

Allison, E., & Fonagy, P. (2012). What is mentalization? In: N. Midgley, & I. Vrouva (Eds.), *Minding the Child* (pp. 11–34). Hove, UK: Routledge.

Asen, E., & Midgley, N. (2019). Working with families. In: A. Bateman, & P. Fonagy (Eds.), *Handbook of Mentalizing in Mental Health Practice*

(2nd ed.) (pp. 135–149). Washington, DC: American Psychiatric Association Publishing.

Bateman, A. W., & Fonagy, P. (2019). *Handbook of Mentalizing in Mental Health Practice* (2nd ed.). Washington, DC: American Psychiatric Association Publishing.

Bowlby, J. (1980). *Attachment and Loss, Vol. 3: Loss, Sadness and Depression*. London: Basic Books.

Brazelton, T. B. (1982). Pre-birth memories appear to have lasting effect. *Brain/Mind Bulletin, 7*(5): 2.

Brumariu, L. E. (2015). Parent–child attachment and emotion regulation. In: G. Bosman, & K. A. Kerns (Eds.), Attachment in middle childhood: Theoretical advances and new directions in an emerging field, special issue. *New Directions for Child and Adolescent Development, 2015*(148): 31–46.

Brumariu, L. E., Kerns, K. A., Guiseppone, K. R., & Lyons-Ruth, K. (2021). Disorganized/controlling attachments, emotion regulation, and emotion communication in later middle childhood. *Journal of Applied Developmental Psychology, 76*: 101324. https://doi.org/10.1016/j.appdev.2021.101324 (last accessed 22 October 2022).

Csikszentmihalyi, M. (2002). *Flow: The Classic Work on How to Achieve Happiness*. London: Rider.

Debbané, M., & Bateman, A. (2019). Psychosis. In: A. Bateman, & P. Fonagy (Eds.), *Handbook of Mentalizing in Mental Health Practice* (2nd ed.) (pp. 417–429). Washington, DC: American Psychiatric Association Publishing.

De Bellis, M. D., & Zisk, A. (2014). The biological effects of childhood trauma. *Child and Adolescent Psychiatric Clinics of North America, 23*: 185–222.

Early Intervention Foundation (2021). Why it is good for children and families? www.eif.org.uk/why-it-matters/why-is-it-good-for-children-and-families (last accessed 27 August 2021).

Felitti, V. J., Anda, R. F., Nordenberg, D., Williamson, D. F., Spitz, A. M., Edwards, V., Koss, M. P., & Marks, J. S. (1998). Relationship of childhood abuse and household dysfunction to many of the leading causes of death in adults: The Adverse Childhood Experiences (ACE) Study. *American Journal of Preventive Medicine, 14*(4): 245–258.

Fonagy, P., & Campbell, C. (2015). Bad blood revisited: Attachment and psychoanalysis. *British Journal of Psychotherapy, 31*: 229–250.

Fonagy, P., & Target, M. (1997). Attachment and reflective function: Their role in self-organization. *Development and Psychopathology, 9*: 679–700.

Fonagy, P., Gergely, G., Jurist, E. L., & Target, M. (2002). *Affect Regulation, Mentalization, and the Development of the Self.* New York: Other Press.

Fonagy, P., Steele, H., & Steele, M. (1991). Maternal representations of attachment during pregnancy predict the organization of infant–mother attachment at one year of age. *Child Development, 62*(5): 891–905.

Fraley, C. R. (2002). Attachment stability from infancy to adulthood: Meta-analysis and dynamic modelling of developmental mechanisms. *Personality and Social Psychology Review, 6*: 123–151.

Gergely, G., & Unoka, Z. (2008). Attachment and mentalization in humans: The development of the affective self. In: E. L. Jurist, A. Slade, & S. Bergener (Eds.), *Mind to Mind: Infant Research, Neuroscience and Psychoanalysis* (pp. 50–87). New York: Other Press.

Grabbe, L., & Miller-Karas, E. (2018). The trauma resiliency model: A "bottom-up" intervention for trauma psychotherapy. *Journal of the American Psychiatric Nurses Association, 24*(1): 76–84.

Green, A. (1986). *On Private Madness.* Abingdon, UK: Routledge, 2018.

Green, J., & Goldwyn, R. (2002). Annotation: Attachment disorganisation and psychopathology: New findings in attachment research and their potential implications for developmental psychopathology in childhood. *The Journal of Child Psychology and Psychiatry, 43*(7): 835–846.

Haase, L., Stewart, J. L., Youssef, B., May, A. C., Isakovic, S., Simmons, A. N., Johnson, D. C., Potterat, E. G., & Paulus, M. P. (2016). When the brain does not adequately feel the body: Links between low resilience and interoception. *Biological Psychology, 113*: 37–45.

Heim, C., & Nemeroff, C. B. (2001). The role of childhood trauma in the neurobiology of mood and anxiety disorders: Preclinical and clinical studies. *Biological Psychiatry, 49*(12): 1023–1039.

Herman, J. (1997). *Trauma and Recovery: The Aftermath of Violence from Domestic Abuse to Political Terror.* New York: Basic Books.

Herringa, R., Phillips, M., Almeida, J., Insana, S., & Germain, A. (2012). Posttraumatic stress symptoms correlate with smaller subgenual cingulate, caudate, and insula volumes in unmedicated combat veterans. *Psychiatry Research, 203*: 139–145.

Hesse, E., & Main, M. (1999). Second-generation effects of unresolved trauma in non-maltreating parents: Dissociated, frightening, and threatening parental behaviour. *Psychoanalytic Inquiry, 19*: 481–540.

Jennings, S. (1999). *Introduction to Developmental Playtherapy: Playing and Health.* London: Jessica Kingsley.

Keaveny, E., Midgley, N., Asen, E., Bevington, D., Fearon, P., Fonagy, P., Jennings-Hobbs, R., & Wood, S. (2012). Minding the family mind: The development and initial evaluation of mentalization-based treatment for families. In: N. Midgley, and I. Vrouva (Eds.), *Minding the Child* (pp. 98–112). Hove, UK: Routledge.

Knapp, M., & Wong, G. (2020). Economics and mental health: The current scenario. *World Psychiatry*, *19*(1): 3–14. doi.org/10.1002/wps.20692. (last accessed 22 October 2022).

Lyons-Ruth, K., Bureau, J. F., Holmes, B., Easterbrooks, A., & Brooks, N. (2013). Borderline symptoms and suicidality/self-injury in late adolescence: Prospectively observed relationship correlates in infancy and childhood. *Psychiatry Research*, *206*: 273–281.

Lyons-Ruth, K., Yellin, C., Melnick, S., & Atwood, G. (2005). Expanding the concept of unresolved mental states: Hostile/helpless states of mind on the Adult Attachment Interview are associated with disrupted mother-infant communication and infant disorganisation. *Development and Psychopathology*, *17*: 1–23.

Main, M., & Cassidy, J. (1988). Categories of response to reunion with the parents at age 6: Predictable from infant attachment classifications and stable over a 1-month period. *Developmental Psychology*, *24*: 415–426.

Mansueto, G., Schruers, K., Cosci, F., & Van Os, J. (2019). Childhood adversities and psychotic symptoms: The potential mediating or moderating of neurocognition and social cognition. *Schizophrenia Research*, *206*: 183–193.

Maté, G. (1999). *Scattered Minds: The Origins and Healing of Attention Deficit Disorder*. London: Vermilion.

Moss, E., Cyr, C., & Dubois-Comtois, K. (2004). Attachment at early school age and developmental risk: Examining family contexts and behaviour problems of controlling-caregiving, controlling-punitive, and behaviourally disorganised children. *Developmental Psychology*, *40*(4): 519–532.

Moss, E., Cyr, C., Bureau, J. F., Tarabulsy, G., & Dubois-Comtois, K. (2005). Stability of attachment between preschool and early school-age and factors contributing to continuity/discontinuity. *Developmental Psychology*, *41*: 773–783.

Music, G. (2019). *Nurturing Children from Trauma to Growth Using Attachment Theory, Psychoanalysis and Neurobiology*. Abingdon, UK: Routledge.

Ogden, P., Minton, K., & Pain, C. (2006). *Trauma and the Body: A Sensorimotor Approach to Psychotherapy*. New York: Norton.

Perry, D. B. (2001). The neurodevelopmental impact of violence in childhood. In: D. Schetky, and E. P. Benedek (Eds.), *The Textbook of Child and Adolescent Forensic Psychiatry*, (Chapter 18, pp. 221–238). Washington, DC: American Psychiatric Press.

Redfern, S. (2019). Parenting and foster care. In: A. Bateman, & P. Fonagy (Eds.), *Handbook of Mentalizing in Mental Health Practice* (2nd ed.) (pp. 265–279). Washington, DC: American Psychiatric Association Publishing.

Sarkar, J., & Adshead, G. (2006). Personality disorders of attachment and affect regulation. *Advances in Psychiatric Treatment*, *12*(4): 297–305.

Schore, A. N. (1994). *Affect Regulation and the Origin of the Self: The Neurobiology of Emotional Development*. New York: Psychology Press.

Schore, A. N. (2001). The effects of early relational trauma on right brain development, affect regulation, and infant mental health. *Infant Mental Health Journal*, *22*: 201–269.

Sharp, C., Pane, H., Ha, C., Venta, A., Patel, A. B., Sturek, J., & Fonagy, P. (2011). Theory of mind and emotion regulation difficulties in adolescents with borderline traits. *Journal of the American Academy of Child and Adolescent Psychiatry*, *50*(6): 563–573.

Siegel, D. J. (2020). *The Developing Mind: How Relationships and the Brain Interact to Shape Who We Are* (3rd ed.). New York: Guilford Press.

Skinner, E. A., & Zimmer-Gembeck, M. J. (2007). The development of coping. *Annual Review of Psychology*, *58*: 119–144.

Solomon, J., & George, C. (2008). The measurement of attachment security and related constructs in infancy and early childhood. In: J. Cassidy, & P. R. Shaver (Eds.), *Handbook of Attachment: Theory, Research and Clinical Applications* (2nd ed.) (pp. 383–416). New York: Guilford Press.

Sroufe, L. A. (1996). *Emotional Development: The Organization of Emotional Life in the Early Years*. New York: Cambridge University Press.

Steele, H., & Steele, M. (2005). Understanding and resolving emotional conflict: The London Parent–Child Project. In: K. E. Grossmann, K. Grossmann, & E. Waters (Eds.), *Attachment from Infancy to Adulthood: The Major Longitudinal Studies* (pp. 137–164). New York: Guilford Press.

Suchman, A., Pajulo, M., Kalland, M., DeCoste, C., & Mayes, L. (2012). At-risk mothers of infants and toddlers. In: A. Bateman, & P. Fonagy (Eds.), *Handbook of Mentalizing in Mental Health Practice* (pp. 309–346). Arlington, TX: American Psychiatric Association Publishing.

Sunderland, M. (2016). *What Every Parent Needs to Know* (2nd ed.). London: DK UK.
Terr, L. (1990). *Too Scared to Cry: Psychic Trauma in Childhood*. New York: Basic Books.
Van den Bergh, B. R. H., Dahnke, R., & Mennes, M. (2018). Prenatal stress and the developing brain: Risks for neurodevelopmental disorders. *Development and Psychopathology*, 30: 743–762.
Van der Kolk, B. A. (2003). The neurobiology of childhood trauma and abuse. *Child and Adolescent Psychiatric Clinics of North America*, 12: 293–317.
Van der Kolk, B. A. (2005). Developmental trauma disorder: Toward a rational diagnosis for children with complex trauma histories. *Psychiatric Annals*, 35(5): 401–408.
Van der Kolk, B. A. (2014). *The Body Keeps the Score: Mind, Brain and Body in the Transformation of Trauma*. New York: Penguin Books.
Verrier, N. N. (1993). *The Primal Wound: Understanding the Adopted Child*. London: CoramBAAF.
Verschueren, K., Marcoen, A., & Schoefs, V. (1996). The internal working model of the self, attachment, and competence in five-year-olds. *Child Development*, 67(5): 2493–2511.
Wagner-Skacel, J., Riedl, D., Kampling, H., & Lampe, A. (2022). Mentalization and dissociation after adverse childhood experiences. *Scientific Reports*, 12: 6809.
Warner, E., Koomar, J., Lary, B., & Cook, A. (2013). Can the body change the score? Application of sensory modulation principles in the treatment of traumatized adolescents in residential settings. *Journal of Family Violence*, 28: 729–738.
Wartner, U. G., Grossman, K., Fremmer-Bombik, E., & Suess, G. (1994). Attachment patterns at age six in south Germany: Predictability from infancy and implication for preschool behaviour. *Child Development*, 65: 1014–1027.
Winnicott, D. W. (1971). *Playing and Reality*. London: Routledge.
Yahuda, R., & Lehrner, A. (2018). International transmission of trauma effects: Putative role of epigenetic mechanisms. *World Psychiatry*, 17(3): 243–257.
Zevalkink, J., Verbeugt-Pleiter, A., & Fonagy, P. (2012). Mentalization-informed psychoanalytic psychotherapy. In: A. Bateman, & P. Fonagy (Eds.), *Handbook of Mentalizing in Mental Health Practice* (pp. 129–158). Arlington, TX: American Psychiatric Association Publishing.

Index

Indexer: Dr Laurence Errington

abandonment fears, 175
Abram, David, 9
abuse, 46, 48, 249, 281, 286
    FGM as, 119
    sexual, 48, 281
acceptance (therapist's stance), 186, 188, 207
acculturation, 95–97, 109, 110, 111
    strategies, 95–97, 110
    stress of, 95, 96, 97, 101, 104, 109, 110
activism, internal and external, 17
Adaku (Nigerian refugee), 79–87
ADHD *see* attention deficit hyperactivity disorder
Adiche, Chimamanda Ngozi, 52
adolescence, biological changes and psychic struggles, 102–103
adoption, 95, 281, 286–287, 289
    prenatal alcohol exposure and, 217–238
adventure therapy, 5

adverse childhood experiences (ACE), 284, 286
    fetal alcohol spectrum disorder and, 214–215
advocates (therapists as)
    prenatal alcohol exposure and, 237
    refugees, 78, 79
Afghani refugee (Ali), 67–79
Africa
    FGM, 120, 121, 136
    West, culture, 99–100
African Americans, 170
Alayarian, Aida, 66–67, 68, 76–77, 77, 80
alcohol, prenatal exposure (PAE), 213–238, 213–241
alexithymic Org, 258
Ali (Afghani refugee), 67–79
Alice and Freddie (cases with prenatal alcohol exposure), 217–238
Alvarez, Anne, 34, 35, 263
Amna Refugee Trauma Initiative, 93
Amnesty International, 94

INDEX

anger, 148
   in case studies, 100, 128, 176–177, 286–287, 288
Anna Freud Centre, 93
antenatal period *see* prenatal period
anti-Semitism, xxx, 147, 149–151, 151
anxiety, climate change, 16
anxious–ambivalent attachment, 282
anxious–avoidant attachment, 280, 282
arousal
   hyper-arousal, 7, 30, 72, 285, 292
   hypo-arousal, 30, 31, 285
Aspheleia, 93
assimilation acculturation strategy, 96, 110, 111
Association of Visitors to Immigration Detainees, 94
asylum seekers, 65
   legal help sources, 94
attachment
   anxious–ambivalent, 282
   anxious–avoidant, 280, 282
   autism and, 206, 208
   disorganised, xxxi, 280, 282, 283, 285, 287, 289, 290, 291, 292, 296
   insecure (and obstacles to attachment), 38, 280
   to place/nature/landscape, 3–19
   prenatal alcohol exposure and, 215, 221, 233–234, 238
   relational trauma and, 280, 281–282, 283, 285, 287, 289, 290, 291, 292, 296
   secure, 280, 282, 285
   theory, 281–282
attention deficit hyperactivity disorder (ADHD), 10
   cases, 104, 105, 107, 189, 218, 219
   fetal alcohol spectrum disorder and, 218, 219, 220, 225
   medication, 218, 219, 220, 223
attunement, 289
   in autism, 193

authoritarian parenting style, 85
autism (autistic spectrum disorder; ASD), 185–211, 189
   fetal alcohol spectrum disorder, 218, 225
   somatic countertransference and, 21–43
autonomic nervous system/states, 72, 196, 198, 203
awareness (of body)
   nature and, 6, 7
   in somatic countertransference, 27, 28, 29, 33, 35

babies and infants
   attachment *see* attachment
   FGM, 136
   Gina Ford method with, 25
   guilt-stricken, 173–174
   Lenny (case) regressing to, 54
   observing *see* observation
   traumatic events, 284–285
   see also prenatal period
BACP (British Association for Counselling and Psychotherapy), 46, 127
BAME (black, Asian, and minority ethnic) communities, 96, 102, 110, 111, 246
Barnardos, 93
Baobab Centre for Young Survivors in Exile, 75, 93
Barrows, Anita, 11, 16
beliefs (client's), Orthodox Jews and respect for, 155–157
belonging (feeling/sense of)
   ethnicity/race and, 97, 100, 103, 104, 106, 108, 110
   female genital mutilation and, 120
   looked-after children, 246, 252
   refugee, 83–84
Berger, Ronen (ecotherapist), 8
biology incl. physiology
   adolescence, 102–103
   brain and trauma, 285

birth mother
  fetal alcohol exposure, 228
  separation from, 289
  see also adoption
black, Asian, and minority ethnic (BAME) communities, 96, 102, 110, 111, 246
Black Lives Matter protests, 111
black people/children
  African American, 170
  Caribbean heritage, 96, 99, 165, 169
  social injustice and collective grief, 169, 170, 172
Blackwell, Dick, 67, 73, 76, 77, 83, 84, 86, 87, 88
blame, prenatal alcohol exposure, 228
body
  awareness of *see* awareness
  grounding, 29–31
  mind and, connection, 9
  therapist's, and somatic countertransference, 21, 22, 23, 30
  see also embodiment *and entries under* somatic
body scan, 197
Bowlby, John, 102, 166, 198, 249, 281, 282
Brady (case study) and ecotherapy, 9–11
brain
  brain-based needs and psychoeducation with prenatal alcohol exposure, 221, 227, 233–234, 237
  interpersonal brain-to-brain communication, 22
  limbic system, 252, 262, 286
  trauma and, 285, 292
  uniquely wired, xxx–xxxi, 185–211
  see also nervous system *and entries under* neuro-
break-it-down boards, 234
British Association for Counselling and Psychotherapy (BACP), 46, 127

Brothers Grimm, 50
brown skin, 101, 102, 103, 106, 108, 170

campaigners for refugees, 94
care
  systems *see* systems
  therapeutic residential *see* residential care
CARE model, 254
carers *see* controlling-caregiving children; father; mother; parents; staff
Caribbean heritage (black), 96, 99, 165, 169
Carroll, Roz, 29
Chalquist, Craig (ecotherapist), 6, 9
Child Psychotherapy Council (CPC), xxi
Childline, 93
Children and Families Across Borders, 93
Children's Homes Association, 261, 262
Children's Society, 93
chronic trauma, 285
Cinderella, 49
circumcision (female genital mutilation), xxx, 117–144
Clare, Anthony, 52
climate (organisational), 255, 256, 257, 258
climate change anxiety, 16
clitoris in FGM, 120
cognitive capacities, male–female differences, 52
collective grief, 169–172
colour of skin *see* skin
communication
  brain-to-brain (interpersonal), 22
  embodied, 27, 28, 35
  by impact, 22, 32
  social, 187, 204, 217
  see also language; speech
community
  Orthodox Jews, xxx, 145–162
  refugees and, 73, 74, 75, 78, 85
  therapeutic (TC), 249, 250, 254–255, 255, 257

compassion, therapist's feelings of, 55, 70, 74, 85, 174, 177, 179
complex trauma, 88, 257
confidentiality
   FGM and, 124
   Orthodox Jews and, 152
   outdoors and, 8
containing/containment/container, 58, 76, 77, 130, 267, 293
   Orthodox Jews' beliefs and, 155
   somatic countertransference and, 27, 28, 30, 32, 33, 34, 35
   therapeutic residential care and, 250, 254, 258, 262, 267
controller leadership, 264–265
controlling-caregiving children, 279–302
controlling-punitive children, 283, 287
Coram Children's Legal Centre Advocacy Service, 94
Coram Legal Centre Migrant Children's Project, 94
co-regulation, 193, 198, 200, 204, 207, 209
cost (financial) of prenatal alcohol exposure, 227–228
co-therapist, 233
   nature as, 5, 8, 9–11
countertransference, 247
   culturally-specific, 153
   reactive, 193
   somatic, 21–43
COVID-19 pandemic, xxii
criminal justice system, 170, 236, 246
cultural homelessness, 102
cultural identity, 83–84, 99–100, 103, 110, 175
   see also belonging
cultural idioms of distress, 71–73
culture
   countertransference and, 153
   idioms of illness and distress (Ali - refugee), 71–73
   therapeutic residential care and, 254, 255, 257–258
cybernetics, 263–264

dads *see* fathers
Daughters of Eve, 139
dead mother (psychically), 283
death, 164
   parent (bereavement), 14, 33, 57, 165, 166, 167, 175
   as taboo, 164
decision-making (client) in therapeutic residential care, 252
defences (unconscious/psychic)
   controlling-caregiving child, 290
   refugee, 69, 73, 76, 87
depression, postnatal, 25
developmental, individual-difference, relationship-based (DIR) Floortime, 186, 198–206
developmental age
   autism and, 186
   grief and, 164, 178
   prenatal alcohol exposure and, 227
   see also neurodevelopmental disorders
diagnosis (and its impact)
   fetal alcohol spectrum disorder/prenatal alcohol exposure, 215
   grief of autism diagnosis, 203
   stigma or shame, 189
Diagnostic and Statistical Manual of Mental Disorders (DSM), 66
   DSM-5, 66, 80, 249
Dicken's Fagin in *Oliver Twist*, 150
Dimension of Personal Identity Model (PIM), 154
DIR Floortime, 186, 198–206
disabilities in prenatal alcohol exposure, 235, 237
   primary, 222–223, 230, 231, 232, 233, 234, 237
   secondary, 221, 224–225, 226, 228, 231–232, 233, 235, 236, 237
   tertiary, 235, 236, 237
disassociation *see* dissociation
disorganised attachment, xxxi, 280, 282, 283, 285, 287, 289, 290, 291, 292, 296

dissociation/disassociation, 7, 286, 293
   momentary, 76
distress (emotional)
   autism (preschool child) and, 201, 207–208
   controlling-caregiving children, 291, 292
   cultural idioms of, 71–73
diversity
   LGBTQ+, 157
   training, 156
Doctors of the World, 94
domestic violence, 9, 46
   child to parent, 219, 227
drawing, 31, 82, 98–99, 100–101, 176, 194, 197
DSM *see* Diagnostic and Statistical Manual of Mental Disorders
Duncan, Roger (systemic psychotherapist), 6
Dylan (case study), 169–172, 179
dynamic leadership, 248
dysregulation, 193, 194

Early Career Framework, 260
eating disorders (incl. minimal eating), 86, 191, 192
   neurodiversity and, 196
Eclectic-therapeutic residential care, 249, 251, 253, 257
eco-leadership, 265–266
economic realities for refugees, 77–79
   see also cost
ecopsychotherapy, xxviii–xix, 3–19
eco-systems within eco-systems, 265
education *see* psychoeducation; school
embodiment
   of communication, 27, 28, 35
   of countertransference, 31, 34
emotional arousal *see* arousal
emotional capacities, male–female differences, 52
emotional distress *see* distress
emotional neglect *see* neglect
emotional regulation *see* regulation
emotional revolution (Schore's), 25–26

End-FGM-European-Network, 121
ending of therapy
   bearing witness to, 172–178
   female genital mutilation and, 135, 136–137
environment
   adverse, prenatal alcohol exposure and, 232–233
   natural, attachment to, 3–19
envy (therapist), 153
equality, 260–261
erotic transference, 48, 54
ethical issues, 154, 157
   therapeutic residential care, 247, 250, 251, 257, 258, 261, 266, 267–268
ethnic/racial identity, 95, 96, 97, 102, 109, 110, 170
ethnocultural groups, 95–96, 109–110
evidence-based research, therapeutic residential care, 256, 257, 260, 267, 268
experiencing and experiences, 28
   sensory, 9, 75, 195, 284
   see also adverse childhood experiences
eye contact (looking into other's face), 99, 105, 106, 123, 132
   autism and, 193, 195, 206–207
   mother–therapist, 295

Fagin in *Oliver Twist*, 150
fairy tales, 49–50
faith *see* religion and faith
family
   autism and, 189, 191, 192, 198
   controlling-caregiving children and, case study, 294–296
   fetal alcohol spectrum disorder and, 217–238
   FGM and, 118–119, 121, 122–123, 125
   neurodivergence in, 189
   Orthodox Jews, 145, 147, 155, 157
   racial trauma and, 98–99
   refugee's, 84–87
   see also fathers; mothers; parents

fathers/dads, 33, 49–58
  absent, 47, 56, 57
  Flora's (case study), 23–24, 25
  Jessica's (case study), 57–58
  Lenny's (case study), 54–55
  Nuru's (case study), 122–123, 123–125, 134, 137
  Sara's (= Phillip; case study), 200, 208, 209
  training and the position of, 53–54, 55
  see also parents
fear brought into therapy, 193
feelings (of child) in therapeutic residential care, 251, 253
female genital mutilation (FGM), xxx, 117–144
females (and women), men and, cognitive and emotional differences, 52
femininity and womanhood, 51, 52, 53, 56, 59
fetal alcohol spectrum disorders (FASD), xxxi
FGM (female genital mutilation), xxx, 117–144
financial issues *see* cost; economic realities; profit
Floortime, 186, 198–206
Flora (case study), 23–25, 30–31, 36–37, 38
Floyd, George, killing, 170, 172
focusing (by Missy in a session), 103
Ford (Gina) method with babies, 25
Fostering Network, 94
Franklin, Michael (art therapist), 56
Freddie and Alice (cases with prenatal alcohol exposure), 217–238
freedom, refugee, 82
Freedom from Torture, 93
Freud, Sigmund, xx, 71, 262, 263
  as secular Jew, 150

games *see* play
gender, 59
  disparity (in profession), 7, 45, 55, 59
  social construction of, 51, 56, 58
  spectrum of, 59
  stereotypes, male therapists and, 47, 48–49, 50, 53, 56, 57, 58, 59
genital mutilation, female, xxx, 117–144
geographic differences in therapeutic residential care, 254
Gerhardt, Sue, 190, 198, 263
Ghana and Ghanaian culture, 106, 107
Girl from Mogadishu, 138
Gomez, Lavinia, 58
government and therapeutic residential care, 261, 266–267
grandmother
  Lenny's, 46
  Lucia's, 175, 176, 178, 179
Grenadian heritage, 99, 100
grief, xxx, 163–181
  of autism diagnosis, 203
  bearing witness, 165
  collective, 169–172
  ecotherapy, 14–17
  prenatal alcohol exposure and, 227
  therapeutic residential care and, 258
Grimm Brothers, 50
grounding the body, 29–31
group dynamics in therapeutic residential care, 257–258
guilt-stricken infant, 173–174
gut, trusting one's, 37–38

Hassidic Orthodox Jewish community, 156
Helen Bamber Foundation, 93
Hickman, Caroline (climate psychologist), 16
historical background, xx–xxi
historical interests of client, 166
holding, 14, 17, 35, 52, 58, 130, 254
Holocaust, 151
homelessness, 245
  cultural, 102
Hrdy, Sarah Blaffer, 52
Human Rights Watch, 94
  see also rights
hunter, fairy tales, 50
hunter-gatherer societies, 52

hyperactivity *see* attention deficit hyperactivity disorder
hyper-arousal, 7, 30, 72, 285, 292
hypermentalization, 280–281, 290, 291, 293, 296
hypo-arousal, 30, 31, 285
hypomentalization (undermentalization), 280

identity (personal)
    autism and, 189, 193
    cultural, 83–84, 99–100, 103, 110, 175
    racial/ethnic, 95, 96, 97, 102, 109, 110, 170
    therapist's, 154
    see also belonging
Ifrah and *Girl from Mogadishu*, 138
Ike (case study), 95, 104–109, 109, 110–111
illness, cultural idioms of, 71–73
immigration and sources of support, 94
impact, communication by, 22, 32
infants *see* babies and infants
infibulation (narrowing of vaginal opening), 119
influencing leadership, 247–248
insecure attachment (and obstacles to attachment), 38, 280
insula, 286
insularity, Orthodox Jews, 147, 150, 155
integration assimilation strategy, 96, 97, 110, 111
interdisciplinary support *see* multidisciplinary support
internal working model (IWM), 46, 249, 281–282, 288
interoception, 197
interventions in therapeutic residential care, 256–257
introjection, 197
    toxic masculinity, 58

Jasmine (case study), 165–169
Jessica (case study), 57–58
Jews, Orthodox, xxx, 145–162
Jordan, Martin, 8
Jung, Carl Gustav, 56
Just for Kids Law, 94
justice system (criminal), 170, 236, 246

Kenya, FGM, 117, 120
kinship, 18, 265
kirigu, 118, 120
Klein, Melanie, 101, 153, 173–174, 176, 262
    guilt-stricken infant, 173–174
    phantasies, 100, 108, 174
kukeketa (tohara; tahara; Swahili for FGM), 117, 120, 140

landscape, attachment to, 3–19
language, 207, 233, 236–237
    autism and, 207
    delays, 217
    Orthodox Jews, 148
    prenatal alcohol exposure and, 217, 223, 233, 234, 236–237
    shared, in therapeutic residential care, 255–256, 266, 267
    see also communication; speech
law *see* legal dimensions
Lawrence, Stephan, murder, 170, 172
Le Vay, David (play therapist), 47–48, 53
leadership, 247–248, 268
    new, 260, 262–266
legal dimensions/issues
    FGM, 136
    refugees, 69, 94
Lenny (case study), 45–46, 54–55
LGBTQ+
    Orthodox Jews and, 157
    Rainbow Migration, 94
life story work, fetal alcohol spectrum disorder, 225
Lifting the Lid on the Care System, 261
limbic system, 252, 262, 286
Little Red Riding Hood, 49, 50
lived experience, 83, 102
    Blackwell's six dimensions of, 67, 88
Lizzie (case study), 14–15
looked-after children *see* residential care
loss (of relationship)
    anger at unfairness of, 177
    therapeutic residential care and, 252–253, 258
    see also death; grief; mourning
Lucia (case study), 175–178, 179

MacAlister's Social Care Review, 246–247, 259, 260, 266
Macy, Joanna, 3
males (and men), 45–61
    patriarchal system affecting, 52
    psychotherapists, xxix, 45–61
    women and, cognitive and emotional differences, 52
    see also fathers; masculinity; patriarchal system
manhood and masculinity, 47, 49, 50, 51, 52, 53, 56–57, 58, 59
marked mirroring, xxxi, 293, 295, 297
Marshall, Hayley (outdoor therapist), 7
masculinity and manhood, 47, 49, 50, 51, 52, 53, 56–57, 58, 59
meaning (and needing or finding it)
    clients, 70, 86
    male practitioners and, 50
medication (for ADHD), 218, 219, 220, 223
melting pot (ethnocultural), 96, 111
Melzak, Sheila, 67
men see males
mental health workers and services, refugee children, 69, 78
mental representations see representations
mentalization, 279–302
Merchant of Venice, Shylock, 149–150
Messiah leadership, 265
metaphor, nature as, 11–14
Migrant Help, 93
Migrant Rights Network, 94
Mila na Desturi, 137–1389, 140
milieu and therapy, 254–255
mind (psyche)
    body connection with, 9
    dead mother concept, 283
minority group(s), 137
    male psychotherapist as, 55
    Orthodox Jews and other groups, 155, 157
mirror, nature as, 11–14
mirroring, 103
    marked, xxxi, 293, 295, 297

Missy (case study), 95, 97, 97–104, 109, 110–111
mixed race heritage, 97, 100, 101
mothers/mums, 33
    Adaku's (case), 79, 84, 85, 86, 87
    dead (psychically), 283
    death, 14, 57, 165–166, 167
    emotionally unavailable/psychically dead, 283
    fetal alcohol spectrum disorder and, 228
    Flora's (case), 23, 25
    grief and, 165, 166, 167, 176, 179
    Ike's (case), 104
    Jasmine's (case), 165, 166, 167
    Lenny's (case), 46
    Lucia's (case), 176
    Missie's (case), 98, 100, 103
    Nuru's (case), 122–125, 131, 132, 134, 135, 137
    Sara's (= Penny in case study), 199, 200, 201, 202–203, 204, 205, 206
    Simon's (case), 286–287
    training and, 53, 55
    see also birth mother; grandmother; parents; pregnancy
mourning, 163, 164, 166, 168, 173, 176, 178
multiculturalism, 96, 111, 146, 154
multidisciplinary (interdisciplinary) support
    prenatal alcohol exposure, 222, 223
    refugee, 4, 78, 85, 87, 93
    "team around the child", 4, 78, 85, 87
mummy-daddy, child describing male therapist as, 50–51
    see also mothers
Music, Graham, 34, 287

Nafsiyat Intercultural Therapy Centre, 93
National Education Union, 94
National FGM Centre, 132, 135, 139

INDEX

National Health Service (NHS) and FGM, 132, 139
National Society for the Prevention of Cruelty to Children (NSPCC) and FGM, 132, 139
nature, attachment to, 3–19
NEET (Not being in Education, Employment, or Training), 245
neglect, xxxi, 34, 48–50, 249, 282, 286, 290
    postnatal, 214
Nell (case study), 12–13
nervous system
    autonomic, and autonomic states, 72, 196, 198, 203
    trauma and, 285–290
    see also brain *and entries under* neuro-
network analysis, 266
neurodevelopmental disorders/conditions (NDD), 187
    prenatal alcohol exposure and, 214, 215, 218, 227, 229, 231, 232
neurodivergent and uniquely wired children, xxx–xxxi, 185–211
neuroimaging, stress and trauma, 286
NHS (National Health Service) and FGM, 132, 139
Nigerian refugee (Adaku), 79–87
Nordic countries, therapeutic residential care, 254, 255
Not being in Education, Employment, or Training (NEET), 245
NSPCC and FGM, 132, 139
nursery observation *see* observation
Nuru (case study), 121–138

object
    primary, 33, 176
    transitional, 30, 190–191
observation (nursery/infants)
    autistic child, 201–202
    in training, 55
Oliver Twist, Fagin, 150
Orbach, Susie, 29, 30, 34

organisation (Org), 251–259, 262, 263, 264, 265, 266
    readiness, 247, 250, 251, 253, 256, 257, 258, 259, 268
Orthodox Jews, xxx, 145–162
othering, 75, 107
outdoors, attachment to, 3–19
overmentalization (hypermentalization), 280–281, 290, 291, 293, 296

parents (and other primary carers)
    attachment to *see* attachment
    authoritarian parenting style, 85
    autism
        adolescent (case), 187–188, 189, 191, 192
        in Floortime therapy, 198
        preschool child (case), 199–204, 208
    controlling-caregiving behaviour, 279–302
    controlling-punitive behaviour towards, 283, 287
    death (bereaved child), 14, 33, 57, 165–166, 167, 175
    Orthodox Jews, 153, 155, 156
    racial trauma and, 98, 100, 106–107, 108, 109, 111
    reflective work *see* reflective work
    refugees and, 84–87
    unavailability, xxxi, 282
    violence towards, 219, 227
    see also adoption; controlling-caregiving children; family; father; grandmother; mother
pathological demand avoidance (PDA), 189
patriarchal system, 47, 52, 118, 119
    oppression, 47, 52
pedagogy, social, 255
Perrault's fairy tales, 49–50
personal identity *see* identity
phantasies (Kleinian), 100, 108, 174
physiology *see* biology

play and games, 126
   autism and, 197, 205, 206–207
   controlling-caregiving children, 282, 283, 289, 290, 293, 294, 295, 296, 297
   grief and, 165, 167, 168, 169, 170, 171
   prenatal alcohol exposure and, 233
   projective play, 56, 82, 125
   role play *see* role play
   sand play/tray, 81, 125–126, 196, 201
Play-Doh, 103, 205, 207
Plotkin, Bill, 12, 13–14
political issues *see* asylum seekers; sociopolitical issues
postnatal period
   depression, 25
   neglect, 214
post-traumatic stress disorder (PTSD)
   Holocaust survivors, 151
   refugees, 66, 80
poverty, refugee, 70
power (in therapeutic residential care), 264, 265, 266, 267
   imbalances, 260
pregnancy, 55
   teenage, 246
   see also postnatal period; prenatal period
prenatal (antenatal) period
   alcohol exposure (PAE), 213–238, 213–241
   stress, 284–285
preschool child
   attachment *see* attachment
   autism (case), 199–209
   death as seen by, 171
   prenatal alcohol exposure (case - Freddie), 217–238
primary carers *see* parents
primary object, 33, 176
prison, from care to, 247
private sector, xxvi
   therapeutic residential care, 249, 259
profit, therapeutic residential care, 259–262, 266, 269
projective play, 56, 82, 125

proprioception and autism, 202, 205, 209
psyche *see* mind
psychodynamic psychotherapy, 103
psychodynamic theory, 103
   leadership and interrelational dynamics, 247
psychoeducation, 257
   FGM, 133–134
   prenatal alcohol exposure, 221
   therapeutic residential care and, 257
"psychosocial influencing dynamic model" of leadership, 247
PTSD *see* post-traumatic stress disorder
puberty, 102

Rabbis, Orthodox Jewish, 145–146, 147–149, 155
racial (ethnic) identity, 95, 96, 97, 102, 109, 110, 170
racial socialisation, 108, 110, 111
racism (and traumatic effects), xxix–xxx, 95–118, 189
   refugee, 74
Rainbow Migration (LGBTQ+), 94
Rakesh (case study) and ecotherapy, 3–4
reactive countertransference, 193
Red Cross, 93
(re)designed therapeutic residential care models, 250, 253, 254, 255–256, 257
reflective work (parents/carers)
   prenatal alcohol exposure, 220, 221, 224, 227, 229–230, 237
   refugees, 84, 87
refugee(s), xxix, 65–94
   trafficking, 69, 73, 138
Refugee Action, 94
Refugee Council, 93
Refugee Effective Partnership, 93
Refugee Therapy Centre, 93
regression, 30
   Lenny (case), 54
   therapist's, 32
regulation/self-regulation
   autism, 202, 206, 209
      dysregulation, 193, 194

controlling-caregiving child, 289, 290–291
prenatal alcohol exposure, 222
see also co-regulation; dysregulation
relational dynamics/analysis, 263–264
relational traumas, 279–302
early, xxxi, 279–302
prenatal alcohol exposure, 225, 235
relationships
autism and, 198, 199, 200, 202, 208
loss *see* loss
therapeutic *see* therapeutic alliance
religion and faith
countertransference and, 153
Orthodox Jews, xxx, 145–162
refugees, 86–87
representations, mental, 281–282
of parent, 174
research, therapeutic residential care, 257, 261, 267, 268
evidence-based, 256, 257, 260, 267, 268
residential care, therapeutic, xxxi, 245–278
fault lines, 246, 259, 269
leavers, 245, 246
models, 255–256
social work, xix–xx, 252
resources, xxvii
refugee support, 93–94
respect, responsibility, integrity, competence, concern (RRICC) model, 154
responsibility (therapeutic residential care), 251–252, 257, 266, 268
shared, 255, 259, 267
rights (human)
FGM and, 117, 119
therapeutic residential care and, 260–261
risk assessment, outdoor therapy, 17
Roberts, Vega Zagier, 47
rocking behaviours in autism, 201–202
Rogers, Carl, 165, 195, 196
role play, 56, 105, 106, 233
grief, 167, 171–172, 176, 178–179

Safe Passage, 94
safeguarding, school, 67, 70, 85, 127, 133, 135
safety
prenatal alcohol exposure and, 234
refugee's internalised sense of, 70–71
therapeutic residential care and, 250
Samuels, Andrew, 27, 31
Sanctuary model, 254
sand play/tray, 81, 125–126, 196, 201
Sarah (case), 199–209
Save the Children, 94
Scandinavian (Nordic) countries, therapeutic residential care, 254, 255
school (incl. teachers and education), 190
autism and, 191, 196, 197, 201–202
case studies, 10, 23, 37, 67, 68, 70, 74, 79, 80, 82, 85, 87, 88, 97, 98, 100, 104–105, 106, 107, 108, 109, 133, 134, 135, 152, 165, 169, 170, 172, 175, 191, 196, 217, 218, 219, 220, 294, 296
ecopsychotherapy, 10
neurodiversity and, 186, 190
prenatal alcohol exposure and, 217, 218, 219, 220, 222
racial trauma and, 97, 98, 100, 104–105, 106, 107, 108, 109
refugee children, 67, 68, 70, 74, 79, 80, 82, 85, 87, 88
safeguarding, 67, 70, 85, 127, 133, 135
therapeutic residential care, 245
Schore, Allan N., 25–26, 285, 292, 293
Schowalter, John E., 31, 32, 33, 37
secondary (vicarious) trauma, 77, 138, 256
secularism, Jewish, 150, 151, 152, 156
secure attachment, 280, 282, 285
self (the), autism and, 202
self-disclosure, 195
self-esteem and autism, 190, 198, 200, 209
self-exploration (therapist), 154
self-harm/injury, 57–58, 177, 196, 246, 291, 297

self-regulation *see* regulation/
    self-regulation
The Selfish Society, 263
sensory experiences, 9, 75, 195, 284
sensory system and autism, 197–198,
    204, 205, 206
separation, 173, 174, 175, 176, 289
    in early childhood, 173
    at end of therapy, 173, 174, 175, 176
    see also adoption
sexual abuse, 48, 281
sexualised transference, 48, 54
sexuality
    FGM and, 123
    refugee and, 83
    see also LGBTQ+
Shakespeare, William, 149
shame, 108
    of diagnosis, 189
    fetal alcohol spectrum disorder and,
        220, 228, 232, 233
    Orthodox Jewish community,
        151–152
    therapist's, 48
shared language in therapeutic
    residential care, 255–256,
    266, 267
shared responsibility (in therapeutic
    residential care), 255, 259, 267
Sheen's (Michael) BBC documentary
    *Lifting the Lid on the Care
    System*, 261
Shtisel, 156
Shylock in *Merchant of Venice*, 149–150
Siegel, Daniel, 7, 30
silo behaviour, 255
Simon (case study), 286–290
Sissay, Lemn, xx, 245, 248
skin colour, 101, 102
    brown, 101, 102, 103, 106, 108, 170
Smith family (case study), 294–296
Social Care Review (MacAlister's),
    246–247, 259, 260, 266
social communication, 187, 204, 217
social construction of gender, 51, 56, 58
social cues of reciprocity, 203–204
social dynamics of leadership, 247

social injustice, bearing witness,
    169–172
social pedagogy, 255
social work, residential, xix–xx
socialisation, racial, 108, 110, 111
sociocultural dimensions
    male therapists, 47
    refugee (case study), 73–77
sociopolitical issues
    refugees, 75
    therapeutic residential care, 258–259
Solace (Yorkshire), 93
Somalia, FGM, 120
somatic countertransference, 21–43
somatic presentations, Ali (refugee),
    71–73
Sophie (case study), 281–284
soulwork/soulcraft, 11–14
speech
    Orthodox Jews, 148
    prenatal alcohol exposure, 223,
        237–238
    see also communication; language
splitting, 32, 34, 97, 255, 286
staff (carers in therapeutic residential
    care), 252, 253–254, 255, 258
stereotypes
    gender, male therapists and, 47,
        48–49, 50, 53, 56, 57, 58, 59
    Orthodox Jews and, 154
    racial trauma and, 109, 110
    refugees and, 84
Stern, Daniel, 6, 14, 15, 31, 32
stigma
    of diagnosis, 189
    Orthodox Jewish community,
        151–152
Stoller, Robert, 52–53
stories and tales, 248
    fairy tales, 49–50
strategic analysis, 266–267
stress
    acculturative, 95, 96, 97, 101, 104,
        109, 110
    family life and fetal alcohol
        spectrum disorder and,
        229

neuroimaging, 286
see also post-traumatic stress disorder
substance use, 165, 214, 246
suicidality, 70, 76, 250, 291
Swahili words for FGM, 117, 120, 140
system/systems (of care), 250–251, 255, 256, 257, 260, 261, 268
    fault lines, 269
    systems within, 258–259
systemic work, refugees, 84

taboo, death as, 164
tahara/tohara (Swahili for FGM), 117, 120, 140
Tavistock Institute, xx
teachers *see* school
"team around the child", 4, 78, 85, 87
teenage pregnancy, 246
Terapia, xxii, xxiii, xxv, xxvi, xxvii–xxviii
therapeutic alliance/relationship/bond
    controlling-caregiving children, 292–293
    culturally specific countertransference and, 153
    grief and, 169, 173, 174, 175
    mother's eye contact with, 295
    Orthodox Jews and, 148, 153, 156
    refugees and, 70, 71, 75, 79
therapeutic community (TC) model, 249, 250, 254–255, 255, 257
therapeutic residential care *see* residential care
therapist(s)
    advocacy *see* advocates
    autism and triad of parent and child and, 204
    body, somatic countertransference and, 21, 22, 23, 30
    envy, 153
    leadership by, 265
    male, xxix, 45–61
    regression, 32
    self-exploration, 154
    see also co-therapist

therapist(s) shame, 48
tohara/tahara (Swahili for FGM), 117, 120, 140
tolerance, 6, 30, 31, 259
    window of, 7, 30, 263
Totton, Nick, 17
trafficking (refugees), 69, 73, 138
training, 45–46, 53–58
    diversity, 156, 156
    male trainees, 45–46, 53–58
    Orthodox Jews, 146, 156, 158
    in residential care, 253, 256, 257, 260
    Terapia, xxv, xxvi, xxvii–xxviii
transference, eroticised or sexualised, 48, 54
transgenerational trauma, 80, 87, 151, 157
transitional object, 30, 190–191
trauma, 279–302
    chronic, 285
    complex, 88, 257
    relational *see* relational traumas
    therapeutic residential care and, 249, 252, 253, 254, 255, 256, 257, 258, 267
    transgenerational, 80, 87, 151, 157
    vicarious/secondary, 77, 138, 256
    see also female genital mutilation; post-traumatic stress disorder; racism; triple trauma paradigm
trauma-informed carers in therapeutic residential care, 254
trauma-informed relationships in therapeutic residential care, 253, 254, 257, 267
triple trauma paradigm, 66
28-Too-Many, 121

UK *see* United Kingdom
ultra-Orthodox Jews, xxx, 145–162
UN *see* United Nations
unaccompanied asylum-seeking children (UASCs), 65
unaccompanied refugee minors (URMs), 65
uncertain future, refugee, 70, 77–78

unconscious level/processes
    defences *see* defences
    racial bias, 109
undermentalization, 280
uniquely wired and neurodivergent children, xxx–xxxi, 185–211
United Kingdom (UK)
    acculturative shift, 111
    ethnocultural groups and acculturation in, 110
    fetal alcohol spectrum disorder prevalence, 216
    FGM and, 133, 135, 136, 139
    legal issues *see* legal dimensions
    refugees, 66
        case study, 67–87
        sources of support, 93–94
    therapeutic residential care, 249, 253, 254, 255
United Kingdom Council (UK Council) for International Student Affairs, 94
United Kingdom Council for Psychotherapists (UKCP), xxi, 47
United Kingdom Trauma Council (UK Trauma Council), 93
United Nations (UN)
    UNHCR (High Commission for Refugees), 94
    UNICEF, 94
United States (US)
    alcohol in pregnancy, 216, 227
    racial trauma, 110
university–therapeutic residential care partnerships, 268

vagal system, 202
vaginal opening, narrowing (infibulation), 119
Verhaeghe, Paul, 51
vicarious trauma, 77, 138, 256
Virgin Mary, 51

walk and talk therapy, 5
Waterloo Community Counselling https, 93
weather system (how one is feeling today), 8
Weinrach, Stephen G., 146, 149, 150, 151
West African culture, 99–100
Western, Simon, 247–248, 262
Western culture, 48–49, 51
WHO (World Health Organization)
    female genital mutilation, 117–118, 119, 120
    refugees, 78
window of tolerance, 7, 30, 263
Winnicott, Donald W., xxvi, 4, 9, 30, 58, 78, 88, 146, 171, 174, 190–191, 198, 207, 247, 248, 254, 263, 284, 293
wisdom, 31–33, 109, 262
witness (bearing)
    to end of therapy, 172–178
    to grief, 165–172
    to social injustice, 169–172
wolf in fairy tales, 49, 50
women *see* females; femininity; mother; pregnancy
World Health Organization *see* WHO
worthlessness, 108, 263

young children *see* babies and infants; preschool child
YoungMinds, 93
Young Roots, 93

Zoom meetings with parents (in autism), 187, 188, 191, 205, 208